Lexi's clean kitchen

150 delicious paleo-friendly recipes to nourish your life

Alexis Kornblum Davidson

VICTORY BELT PUBLISHING INC.

LAS VEGAS

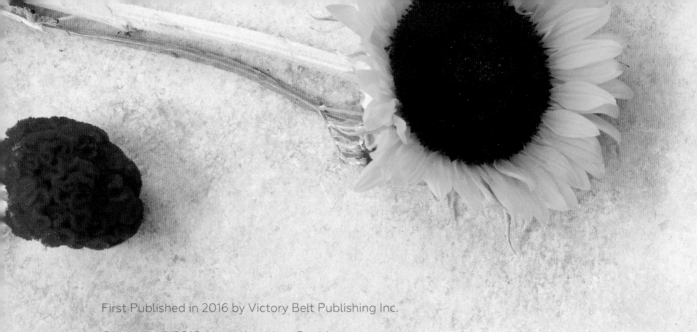

First Published in 2016 by Victory Belt Publishing Inc.

Copyright © 2016 Alexis Kornblum Davidson

ISBN-13: 978-1-628601-08-4

This book is for entertainment purposes. The publisher and author of this cookbook are not responsible in any manner whatsoever for any adverse effects arising directly or indirectly as a result of the information provided in this book.

Book design by Yordan Terziev and Boryana Yordanova

Cover photography by Sarah Fennel

Photos on pages 4, 8, 12, 20, 24, 29, 39, 71, 183, 255, 273, and 361 by Kristin Chalmers Photography

Printed in Canada

TC 0116

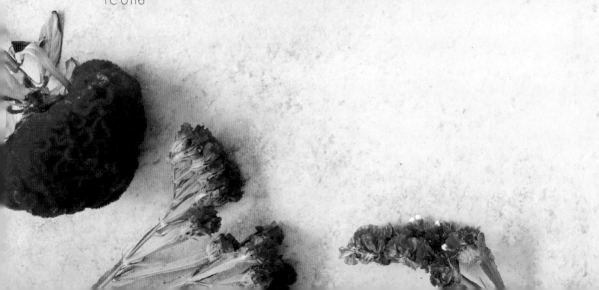

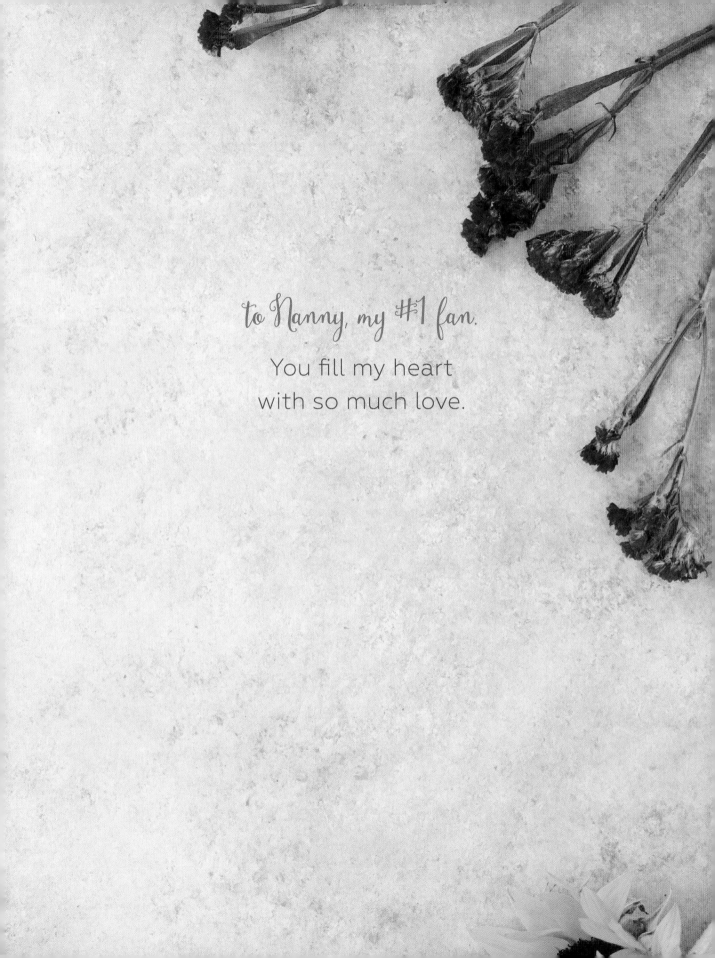

to Nanny, my #1 fan.

You fill my heart
with so much love.

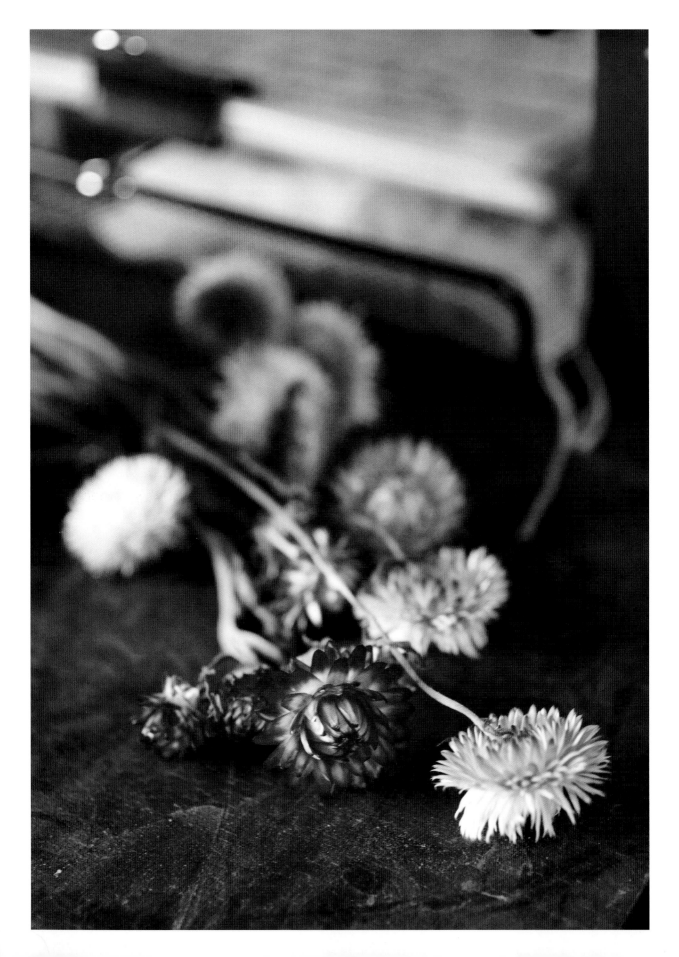

CONTENTS

ACKNOWLEDGMENTS

To my readers, thank you forever, because there wouldn't be a Lexi's Clean Kitchen, and now a *Lexi's Clean Kitchen Cookbook*, without you. Thank you from the bottom of my heart for following me, growing with me, making my recipes, sharing them on social media, and trusting me when creating nourishing meals for yourself and your loved ones.

Mike, thank you from the bottom of my heart for encouraging me to pursue Lexi's Clean Kitchen in the first place and for persuading me to leave my teaching job and take a leap to make my dream a reality. Thank you for being by my side through this crazy journey that is our life—for supporting me, loving me unconditionally, and being the greatest, most honest taste-tester there is. I love you, and I am lucky to go through life with you by my side.

Mom, my best friend and my joy in this world, thank you for being you! You believe in me and support me through every life endeavor, lift me up when I'm down, laugh with me, cry with me, and love me through it all. You are the strongest person I know, and I am lucky every single day that you are my mom. *I love you more and bigger, bigger and more.*

Adam, my rock, words can't begin to describe how blessed I am that you are my brother. Thank you for shaping me into the person I am today. Every day I hope that I am for you half the loving, supportive, and encouraging person that you are for me. I love you, Addy!

Dad, I am so lucky to have inherited your artistic eye, your love, and your compassion. You are the most creative and talented person I know, and I'm fortunate to have received even a fraction of that!

Marcy, Marvin & Daniel, growing up I could only have dreamed of having people who so lovingly welcomed me into their family as you have. Moving to a new state almost five years ago wasn't always easy, but you instantly made it feel like home. Thank you for your endless love and support.

to the village it took
TO BRING THIS BOOK TO LIFE

A huge thank you to those who helped make this book as magnificent as it is. I am forever grateful to each and every one of you.

To the entire hardworking team at Victory Belt Publishing, for bringing this vision to life and for being so excited to be in my corner. A special thanks to Erich Krauss, Holly Jennings, Lance Freimuth, Susan Lloyd (my soul sister), and Pam Mourouzis for every precious minute that you put into this book. Thank you for guiding me and encouraging me, for the endless phone calls and pep talks, and ultimately for making this book possible. I am grateful every day.

To Sabrina, for all your help on the day-to-day details of Lexi's Clean Kitchen. You are wonderful, and I am so grateful to have you on the team.

To Jim, for taking a chance on my blog, and me, way back when—and sticking with me for the ride. There's truly no Lexi's Clean Kitchen without you!

To my agent, Andrea, who believed in me and in this book way before this book was even a thought! Thank you, thank you, thank you.

To Kristin Chalmers and Sarah Fennel, for your amazing photography contributions to this book; **to Dominique Pasquarosa,** for the countless glam days and making me look beautiful throughout the book; and **to Miriam Hope Rieder** of *TASTE by Spellbound,* for coming and playing decorator with my cakes and cupcakes. This book is beautiful because of all of you.

To all my virtual blogging friends who are near and dear to my heart, your passion motivates me, your words of encouragement guide me, and your support pushes me every day to achieve. I am grateful for our community and for each and every one of you.

To my friends who are like my family, who have listened endlessly about the writing of this book and have kept me sane throughout this process, I am truly grateful for your friendship. Thank you always.

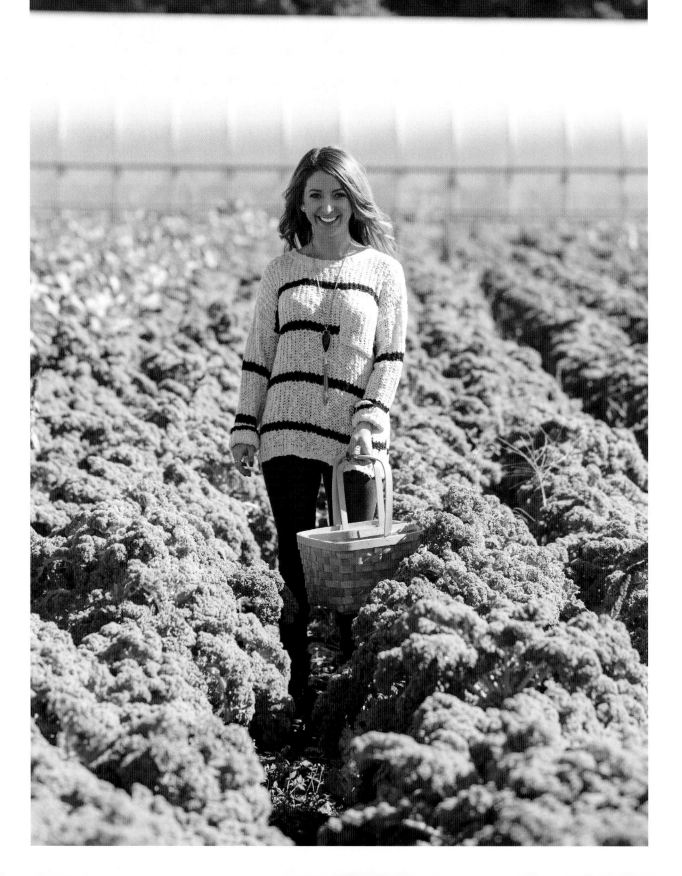

introduction

Welcome! Welcome! Welcome! I am thrilled that you are here reading away, and I simply cannot wait for you to dive into the recipes! But first, I'd love to share a little of my story and how I have arrived at where I am today.

I have always had a passion for food. My childhood photos are full of me holding a bag of pretzels or beaming from ear to ear over my (or anyone else's) birthday cake. As a kid, I coveted my hidden stash of junk food and candy. Later, during my art career (in college), my work subconsciously revolved around food (seriously, I only painted candy for a long time). And from the time I was tall enough to reach the counter, I loved being in the kitchen and helping my mom prepare dinner. Simply put, food, in one way or another, was always *my thing*. And it still is.

I wasn't raised a healthy eater. I mean, we never had soda or *really* terrible junk food in the house, but my mom was a hardworking lady, and after-school snacks typically were prepared by me or my brother. Like any kid would do, we opted for things like pretzels and tortilla chips, frozen pizza bites, packaged cookies, and grilled cheese, or we ordered pizza or Chinese food—you get the idea. At the time this was fun and delicious, of course, but I really do believe that the food I was eating all those years had a direct impact on my health over time.

In college, while still eating poorly and with my weight slowly creeping up, I started thinking more about how we indulge as a society, how food is portrayed in the media, and what the food we eat is eating. This ended up being what I wrote my thesis on! I became interested in these topics in part because I constantly had horrible stomachaches, hormone and skin issues, and other ailments. Though I wasn't ready to change my lifestyle at the time (wish I could give my twenty-year-old self a kick in the butt!), I did start educating myself about the food we consume and its effect on our bodies and our society. I cut out meat for over a year. I couldn't afford good-quality meat at the time, and I thought that going without meat was a good alternative. Makes sense, right? Wrong! Because I felt hungry a lot of the time, I ended up eating a ton of non-meat junk food to compensate. This experience taught me an invaluable lesson: realizing that my initial reasoning was faulty ended up being a huge step in the right direction.

It wasn't until after graduate school that I started thinking more intentionally about diet and exercise and paying closer attention to how I was feeling physically, mentally, and emotionally. I began to exercise more regularly, but my gastrointestinal issues were worse than ever and started to affect my daily life. I didn't want to go out and do things because I was so bloated and felt sick all the time. I'll spare you the details, but when you can't go to the bathroom for days and days, it's not a fun feeling.

Something needed to change. It was pretty clear to me that all of the ailments I was experiencing were gut related, so I researched foods that can cause inflammation and prevent proper digestion. I decided to cut out gluten and dairy, and I was pretty strict about it. Just ask my now-husband, Mike, who was shocked when I declined the bread basket at dinner during the first few weeks of my new regimen. Guess what? Almost instantly, I started feeling pretty good. Not amazing, but I definitely began seeing improvements across the board.

I *slowly* began to eliminate other trigger foods, such as grains, soy, and refined sugars (I put emphasis on *slowly* because I don't love an all-or-nothing approach to diet). That was the turning point. I really started to see a dramatic change in my health. I was going to the bathroom regularly, I wasn't bloated all the time, I was feeling confident in my body, and I started to have more energy. On top of all that, I was excited to make delicious meals with the clean ingredients that were fueling my recovery. Since I still wanted to be able to eat the meals and certain comfort foods that I loved, I became more creative in the kitchen.

Soon I began to realize that there were likely many people out there, like me, struggling to heal various ailments *or* just wanting to eat healthier. This motivated me to reach out and share my clean-eating experiences, hoping that they could help others. Simply for fun, I started an Instagram account.

My Instagram account didn't start as Lexi's Clean Kitchen. It was Alexisk916, and it was pretty bad iPhone pictures with recipes written out below. Looking back, it was pretty comical. Still, my following was growing, and people kept asking for a place to find all of my recipes. So I started the Lexi's Clean Kitchen website, and in three short years it has evolved into a robust and vibrant resource for recipes, cooking guides, travel tips, and so much more. It is a place where I can be creative, have fun with photography, create and test delicious recipes, and interact with readers on a daily basis. I couldn't be happier and more grateful for this little corner of the Internet that I have built.

let's move forward **TO THE PRESENT DAY**

Later on I started seeing a naturopathic doctor and furthered the healing (through food, experimentation, and supplementation) of what I now know was/is a combination of *Candida* overgrowth and leaky gut, along with a few other things. I do believe that the healing of our bodies is a process, and as a result I am always learning and doing more to improve my health and feel my best. I work daily on managing stress, creating a less toxic home, and so on.

Today I can tell you that I don't struggle with the gut issues I used to suffer from daily, I have more energy, my weight fluctuates less, and overall I feel pretty great—healthy and happy. I have also found a path of comfort and healing in mindfulness, meditation, and yoga practices. Now, do I ever go out and indulge in cocktails and junkier food? YES, I do, and I am completely comfortable sharing that! It is important to remember to have balance and to know and listen to your body.

When I was sick all the time, I couldn't go out and indulge and enjoy because I would feel terrible afterward. Now, I have gotten my body to the point where I can and I do! If and when *you* decide that your body has healed enough to indulge in the occasional treat that falls outside the clean-eating protocol, my best advice is to make sure (as best as you can) that it's made with high-quality ingredients, without preservatives, chemicals, additives, or fake flavorings. Don't drive yourself crazy, though. You need to live your life, too!

Think of it as an 80/20 or 90/10 approach, where you let yourself enjoy and have what you want some of the time, but for the larger percentage of the time you are eating clean (and that doesn't mean boring!).

why i wrote this book

I truly believe in the power of food.

I believe that food brings us together. It creates a sense of tradition and culture, and it can be a catalyst for healing. Can you tell how much I *love* food?!

Simply put, I love sharing my experiences and recipes with you, and I encourage you to join me on this path to living a fruitful, energized life. Whether you're taking baby steps, you already eat healthy, or you've decided to try something new, it's no secret that real, clean food is the answer. I just know you will feel wonderful!

I wrote this cookbook to give you a robust resource for making your hectic life a little bit healthier. I wrote this cookbook to show you that eating clean does not have to be tasteless and boring, and that it can in fact be fun and exciting. I wrote this cookbook to encourage you to get creative and find enjoyment in the kitchen. But most of all, I wrote this cookbook so that you can nourish your body with real food—so that you can feel healthier and more confident and live life to the absolute fullest, because you deserve that!

Lexi

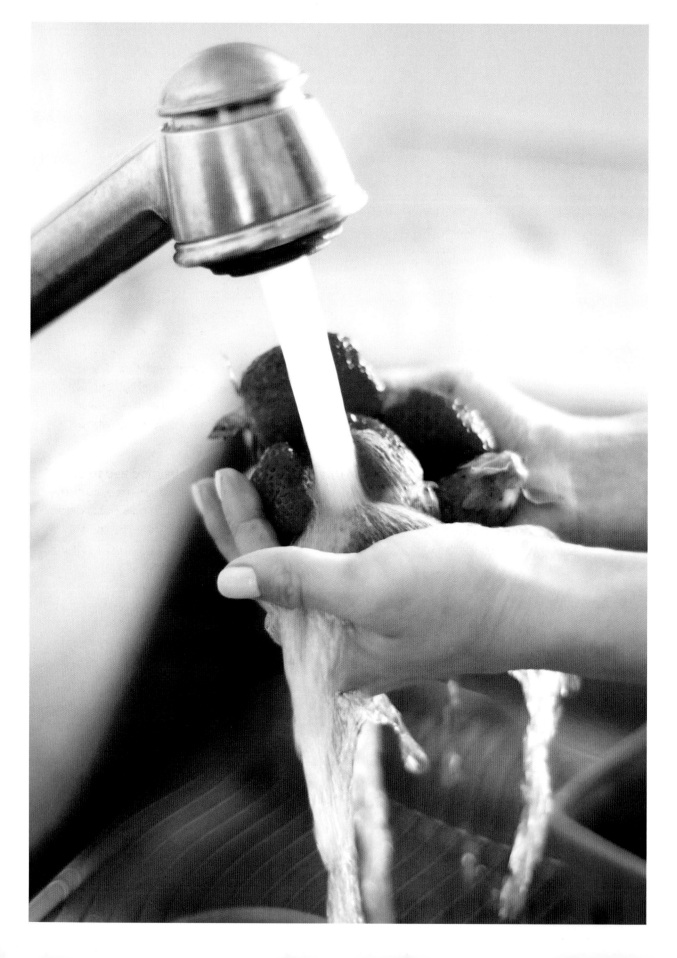

clean EATING 101

Clean eating is a practical and customizable framework for your daily food choices. At its core, clean eating is about eating whole foods and replacing processed and refined foods with healthier options to ultimately improve your health and well-being. But perhaps above all, eating clean is not a fad diet. It's an intuitive lifestyle approach to eating that transcends dietary labels and becomes part of who you are and how you live. It has staying power.

HOW DOES A PALEO LIFESTYLE FIT INTO *clean eating?*

Seamlessly! Paleo, just like clean eating, is a framework for improving how you feel by eating real food. I think Paleo gets a bad rap: too often people assume that it is a strict, complicated diet and means "eating like a caveman," but in truth it's much more straightforward than that. At its heart, just like clean eating, Paleo is really about eating *real, nutrient-dense food*. Often people hear that a Paleo diet is about eating tons of bacon and other meat, regardless of the quality. That's one of my least favorite misconceptions. Similar to clean eating, Paleo is *so much* about the quality of the ingredients.

Almost all of the recipes in this book are, or can easily be modified to be, gluten-free, grain-free, dairy-free, soy-free, and refined sugar–free, so they work for anyone following a Paleo protocol. Recipes that fit this description are marked as Paleo-Friendly. When slight modifications must be made to make the recipe dairy-free and/or Paleo-friendly, such as swapping out butter for coconut oil, these adjustments are clearly indicated.

how is clean eating DIFFERENT FROM PALEO?

Clean eating is a less strict, more flexible way of eating. Even more than Paleo, it's based on doing what works for you rather than following rules and regs. Too often people think Paleo is an all-or-nothing, super-strict approach. I often hear people ask, "How can you eat that? It's not Paleo!" I believe that if your body is fine with something, even if it's not considered Paleo-friendly, then you should go for it! (Though I wouldn't suggest having something like legumes or grains make up the majority of your meals.) In short, I view clean eating as a customizable approach that can, after a process of elimination and healing and the ongoing process of listening to your body, result in a larger umbrella of allowed foods.

so, WHAT SHOULD I EAT?

You might think that clean eating is all about taking things away from your diet, but I totally disagree! There is a huge variety of healthy foods for you to choose from:

- Meat
- Poultry
- Eggs
- Fish

- Nuts and seeds
- Veggies
- Fruit
- Healthy fats

When a recipe in this book calls for dairy, meat, chicken, or eggs, try to buy organic, grass-fed, and pasture-raised options whenever possible! (*Note:* If you can't find pasture-raised eggs, the next best bet is "free-range.")

and WHAT SHOULD I AVOID?

If you do a quick Internet search about which foods to avoid when cleaning up your diet, you'll see that you should probably steer clear of soda and other sugary drinks, fast food, candy, cereal, and foods with added preservatives. But I'm going to make a leap and assume that you probably already know that those things aren't awesome for you.

When I decided that I needed to change my diet and lifestyle—after experiencing GI issues, hormonal issues, and more for way too long—I cut out negative health instigators like gluten, grains, most dairy, and refined sugars in addition to the obvious things listed above. I healed, and continue to heal, my body through food, but ultimately I just *feel awesome* eating this way.

Now, I don't like telling you what you should and shouldn't eat. Ultimately, you need to listen to your own body when creating your list of "No" foods. Here is my personal list of foods that I do *not* consider to be part of a clean-eating lifestyle:

- Artificial sweeteners
- Most dairy
- Processed foods
- Soy and other legumes

- Gluten
- Most grains
- Refined sugars

Why ditch these foods? Often, they are instigators of inflammation and other ailments, and most people find that they feel and function better without them. Once you learn to cook tasty meals without these ingredients, I promise you won't miss them!

Like I said above, though, if your body breaks down some of these foods (for example, legumes) just fine, then adding them to some dishes is okay. Remember, it's not all-or-nothing!

the importance OF BALANCE

My personal approach to clean eating has a strong emphasis on *balance*. I find that when I keep balance front and center as an essential principle in my life and in the way I eat, I don't need to worry about counting calories, comparing myself to others, or subscribing to dietary labels, and if I want to indulge in something, I can do so without guilt. The recipes in this book are a reflection of the way I eat—a balanced, practical approach. We all want a slice of pizza every now and again, or a bowl of pasta, or a brownie after dinner, or a slice of cake on a special occasion. I've included cocktails in this book because, hey, sometimes we want a cocktail! Not depriving yourself is important. I created this book so that you can have all of the things you want to eat and feel good about eating them. By making cleaner choices and using better-quality ingredients, you can feel better about including those occasional indulgences!

IT'S NOT *an all-or-nothing* APPROACH

Don't feel like you need to cut a million things out of your diet at once. Start slowly and jot down foods that don't make you feel awesome. Then simply see how you feel and go from there. It's a process, and it shouldn't stress you out!

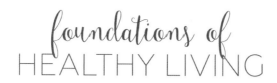

foundations of HEALTHY LIVING

The foundations of a healthy lifestyle go beyond what you eat (yes, even though this is a cookbook!). I have found so much healing and so many wonderful health benefits when, in addition to eating clean, I make the effort to exercise regularly and work on developing practices to manage stress and ensure sound sleep. The following four categories are the foundations of healthy living that I find are truly essential.

STRESS *management*

It's no secret that stress can cause an unbelievable number of issues. I believe wholeheartedly that managing stress and living a less stressful life will benefit everyone. Now, stress *is* going to affect you. Life is not always easy, and stress will come and go, often related to events and situations that are out of your control. What you *can* control is how you manage stress, and the best way to do that is to develop coping mechanisms that work for you as an individual. Often it's a matter of finding a balance in life, making sure to fit in time for restorative activities.

THINGS I DO: I practice mindfulness and meditation. I take breaks. I get outside in nature. I make lists and prioritize tasks. I focus on positive energy. I surround myself with people who have positive attitudes. I prioritize time for family, fun, and shutting off.

SLEEP

A good night's sleep is critical. Too often we sit looking at computer screens or watching TV or do all sorts of other stimulating activities before bed (like drinking coffee late in the day). These activities tell our brains that it's not bedtime, and many of us don't get adequate sleep as a result. It's time to make sleep a priority. When your sleep improves, you will see major benefits in your energy and outlook, not to mention increase your odds for good long-term health.

THINGS I DO: I put the phone away an hour before bed. I wear blue light–blocking glasses when I'm on the computer or phone or watching TV in the evening. Before bed, I do some light reading, breathing, or meditating; I take a soothing Epsom salt bath; drink some caffeine-free hot tea; and I supplement with magnesium, which aids in good sleep (as well as healthy digestion).

DIET

I've already talked about how food choices have improved my life in amazing ways. Good food choices have helped heal my ailments, regulate my digestion, provide me with energy, and so much more. A healthy diet, among these other pillars, is essential to a healthy lifestyle. It is so important to listen to your body and analyze what's going on, then see how you can improve naturally. For example, if you feel like you need a nap every day at 4 p.m., the types of foods you're eating throughout the day may be spiking your blood sugar. After making some minor dietary changes, you may find that you have more energy and don't need that nap! A good start is to take note of how you feel throughout the day, especially after meals, and how your digestion is. From there, you can experiment with the types of foods you eat and when you eat them—with the ultimate goal of eating to fuel your body and mind, have adequate energy, and just *feel great!*

THINGS I DO: I eliminate foods for at least one month and then reintroduce them, keeping a food journal or notes in my cell phone to document changes in my energy, mood, and digestion. (If you're feeling down about cutting things out of your diet during an elimination phase, remind yourself that it's probably not forever.)

EXERCISE

Exercise is a cornerstone of a healthy lifestyle. It releases endorphins, improves mood and mental health, strengthens bones and muscles, helps prevent disease, and so much more. That said, exercise can be abused. Balance is important here as well. Over-exercising or not eating right or enough for how much you are exercising can lead to adrenal fatigue, among other problems. Your body needs rest between exercise sessions, and it's critical to be mindful of when it does. Every body is different, so what works for someone else may not work for you, or the exercise activity that someone else loves may not be the right fit for you. Find types of exercise that you enjoy, whether that means going on walks with your dog or your family, lifting weights, practicing yoga, doing cardio, or whatever else you take a liking to.

THINGS I DO: I switch up my exercise routine: I practice yoga, I try out various types of fitness classes, and I take walks and short hikes near my home.

how to use THIS BOOK

I am so excited for you to use this book as a practical resource for all of your day-to-day eating. Whether you're looking for recipes for on-the-go breakfasts or weekend brunches, for dinner party appetizers or weeknight slow cooker meals that everyone will love, or for desserts for a simple night in or to bring to a festive gathering, I think you'll find everything you want and more here (including a few cocktails for those special evenings, too)!

I've kept the recipes in this book, just like the recipes on my website, Lexiscleankitchen.com, as simple and practical as possible—meaning, I won't throw a totally random ingredient into a recipe that you'd buy to use just once. And, because I know you're busy, whenever possible I give the option to use clean, store-bought products for basic components, such as mayo, ketchup, and chicken broth. In the basics chapter (and in other chapters), I provide "Use In," "Use On," and "Serve With" ideas so that you don't end up with homemade sauces, condiments, and other recipe or meal components languishing in the back of the fridge.

I've also added some great resources, like how-to graphics, a handy conversion chart, a guide to seasonal produce, and so much more.

Feel free to get creative! Take a recipe and put your own spin on it. There's plenty of room for adaptations here.

HOW TO NAVIGATE *the recipes*

At the top of each recipe, you will find key information: yield or number of servings, prep and cook times, and allergen/eating protocol notes.

NUMBER OF SERVINGS: Because this is not a diet book, and because clean eating generally is not about calculating portion sizes or counting calories, the portions aren't meant to be small or restrictive. They are based on average eating habits and healthy appetites. The number of servings a recipe makes may vary based on serving size.

PREP AND COOK TIMES: I've included prep and cook times for each recipe (unless no cooking is involved, in which case you'll see only the prep time). The time to complete inactive prep tasks, such as marinating chicken overnight, are not included in the prep times but are noted, as reminders, right with the times.

Please remember that the time to make subrecipes, like my homemade BBQ sauce for BBQ Chicken Pizza (page 176), is not reflected in the prep or cook times for the recipe in which the subrecipe is used. So you will need to set aside some extra time to make any subrecipes that are called for in the recipes.

FOOD ALLERGEN AND EATING PROTOCOL NOTES: At the top of each recipe, you'll find notes about food allergens and eating protocols to help you know, at a glance, which recipes suit your dietary needs. All of the recipes in this book are gluten-free, and many of them fall within the categories listed below. When possible, I've included ingredient substitutions or omissions to make the recipes suitable for as many eating styles and dietary requirements as possible.

- Egg-Free
- Nut-Free
- Dairy-Free
- Paleo-Friendly (meaning gluten-free, grain-free, soy-free, refined sugar–free, and dairy-free, with the exception of ghee; see note below)
- Vegan

note: *Throughout this book, you'll find recipes that call for butter or ghee. Because the milk solids in butter are removed in the process of making ghee, many in the clean-eating and Paleo communities consider ghee to be dairy-free. For this reason, the recipes that use ghee are categorized as Paleo-friendly. Although many people who don't tolerate dairy well find that they can tolerate ghee, a percentage of dairy-intolerant people do have issues when consuming it. So, to err on the safe side, all of the recipes categorized as dairy-free in this book are completely free of all forms of dairy, including ghee.*

little TIDBITS

To keep you from getting bored and to make sure that you have options that appeal to everyone you are cooking for, I've included flavor variations for several of the recipes in this book.

Also, to help ensure that you get the best results, I've included helpful notes and tips throughout the recipes.

Finally, for all you visual learners out there, I'm especially excited about the visual graphics and photo illustrations sprinkled throughout this book. They are meant to be springboards to empower you to create your own dishes. These colorful, visual guides cover the how-tos of all sorts of food-making endeavors, from making grain-free pasta alternatives to preparing the best eggs at home, and from creating the ultimate soups and smoothies to building a juice at home that will impress.

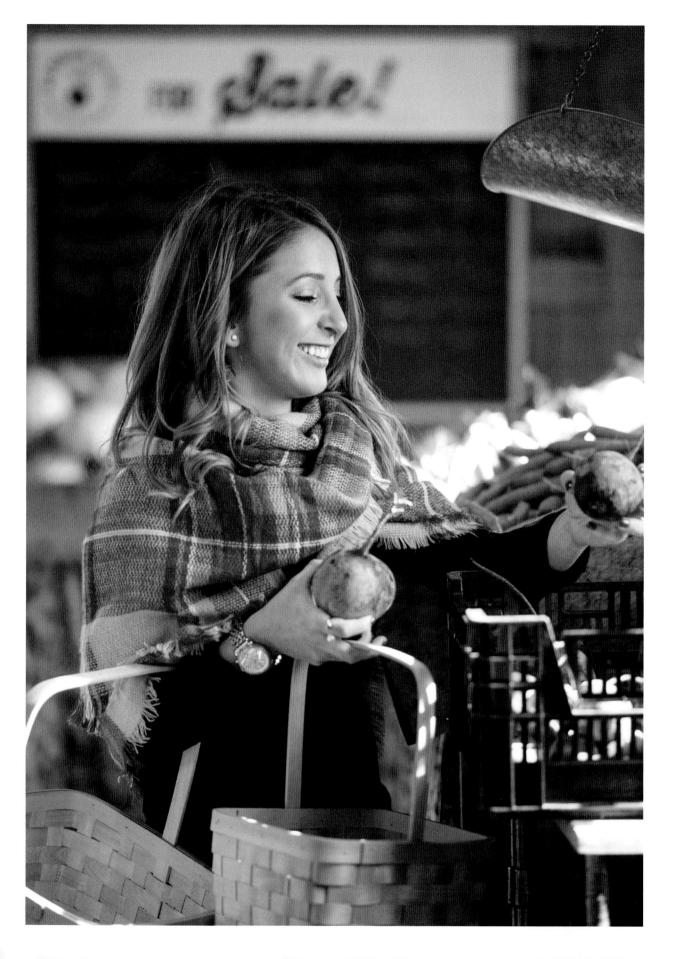

ingredients FOR A CLEAN KITCHEN

Aside from a few unique flours and condiments, I think you'll find that the ingredients you need for the recipes in this book are fairly straightforward. With that said, to get you on your way to stocking your own clean-eating pantry and fridge, I've included lists of the staples that I use most often and that you will find yourself reaching for when making these recipes.

While all of the items listed in this section are used in this book, don't feel that you need to stock every single one of them in your kitchen at all times. It takes a while to build a pantry! Also, when making recipes, feel free to switch things up and use what you have on hand. For example, if you don't have pine nuts for pesto, don't fret! Walnuts or many other nuts will work great.

Want a printable version of this list of pantry staples to take with you to the grocery store? Head to Lexiscleankitchen.com/cookbookpantrystaples.

....

PANTRY ITEMS

Chapter 9 includes recipes for several pantry staples, from homemade mayo and ketchup to broth, ghee, and more. But I realize that not everyone has the time to make every single thing from scratch (myself included!). Sometimes using a good-quality, clean store-bought equivalent is a perfectly acceptable option. To source clean products, simply read the ingredients! You'll be able to weed out what has junk added to it.

Note: Though most of the items in the following lists will keep fine for an extended period when stored at room temperature in the pantry or on the countertop, some, if not used relatively quickly—say, within a few weeks—should be stored in the fridge or freezer. These items are marked with an asterisk.)

....

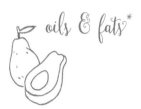 *oils & fats**

- Avocado oil
- Coconut oil
- Extra-virgin olive oil
- Toasted sesame oil
- White truffle oil

- Ghee (clarified butter)
- Palm shortening (Buy an organic, sustainably sourced, and non-hydrogenated brand such as Spectrum or Tropical Traditions.)

note: Organic grass-fed unsalted butter is another good eating and cooking fat, but because it is more perishable than the fats listed above, I keep my butter in the fridge. You will find it grouped with other dairy products under the "Fresh Items" heading on page 25.

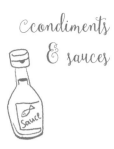

Condiments & sauces

- Coconut aminos (a soy sauce alternative)
- Fish sauce (I like Red Boat brand.)
- Hot sauce, such as Cholula, Frank's RedHot, or Tabasco
- Sriracha sauce
- Dijon mustard
- Whole-grain mustard
- Ketchup (I like Sir Kensington's or Muir Glen brand.)
- Mayonnaise, homemade or a store-bought product made with avocado oil (I like Chosen Foods, Primal Kitchen, or Sir Kensington's brand; be sure to read labels and avoid additives and seed oils.)
- Prepared horseradish

Vinegars

- Apple cider vinegar
- Balsamic vinegar
- Red wine vinegar
- Rice vinegar
- White vinegar
- White wine vinegar

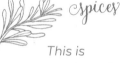

Sweeteners

- Organic raw honey
- Organic pure maple syrup
- Coconut palm sugar
- Granulated maple sugar
- Organic powdered sugar
- Blackstrap molasses
- Pitted Medjool dates

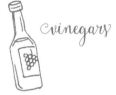

Spices

This is an overview of my spice drawer. If you buy only a few items, buy the bold ones.

- **Fine sea salt or pink Himalayan salt**
- **Black pepper** (Use peppercorns in a pepper mill for the best flavor, or buy ground pepper.)
- **Cayenne pepper**
- Celery seed
- **Chili powder**
- **Ground cinnamon**
- Cinnamon sticks
- Ground coriander
- **Ground cumin**
- Curry powder
- Dried basil
- Dried cilantro
- Dried dill
- Dried oregano
- Dried parsley
- Dried rosemary
- **Garlic granules/powder**
- **Italian seasoning**
- Nutmeg
- Minced onion
- **Onion powder/granules**
- **Paprika**
- **Red pepper flakes**
- Saffron
- Sesame seeds
- Smoked paprika
- **Turmeric powder**
- Za'atar spice blend

baking

- Aluminum-free baking powder
- Baking soda
- Unsweetened cocoa powder
- Unsweetened coconut flakes
- Dairy-free dark chocolate chips (I use chocolate with a 70% cacao content or higher. I love Guittard brand. For dairy-free and allergen-friendly chocolate, I like Enjoy Life Foods brand.)

- Organic pure vanilla extract
- Whole vanilla beans
- Ground flax meal*
- Chia seeds**

*Store ground flax meal in an airtight container in the fridge for the amount of time specified on the package.

**Store chia seeds in the pantry.

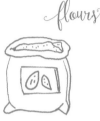

flours

- Blanched almond flour* (Be sure to purchase almond *flour*, not meal, which has a much coarser texture. I like Honeyville brand.)
- Arrowroot flour (aka arrowroot starch)
- Coconut flour
- Tapioca flour (aka tapioca starch)

*Store almond flour in an airtight container in the pantry for 2 to 3 months, in the fridge for up to 6 months, or in the freezer for up to a year.

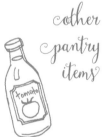

other pantry items

- Unsweetened applesauce (I use this ingredient often in baking.)
- Organic beef, chicken, and vegetable broth (I like Pacific Foods brand.)
- Canned full-fat coconut milk (I always keep one or two cans in the fridge for making dairy-free whipped cream; see page 282.)
- Collagen protein (I use this ingredient in smoothies, among other things, as an added source of health benefits. I like Vital Proteins brand.)
- Raw nuts and seeds*: almonds, hazelnuts, pine nuts, cashews, sunflower seeds, walnuts

- Nut butters (Read ingredient labels: buy products that are just nuts, no added sugars or oils.)
- Gluten-free oats
- Tomato paste, preferably organic with no salt added
- Tomato sauce, preferably organic with no salt added
- Diced tomatoes, preferably organic with no salt added (I like Muir Glen brand for jarred and Tuttorosso brand for canned.)
- White rice

*Store nuts and seeds in a closed container in the pantry for up to 3 months.

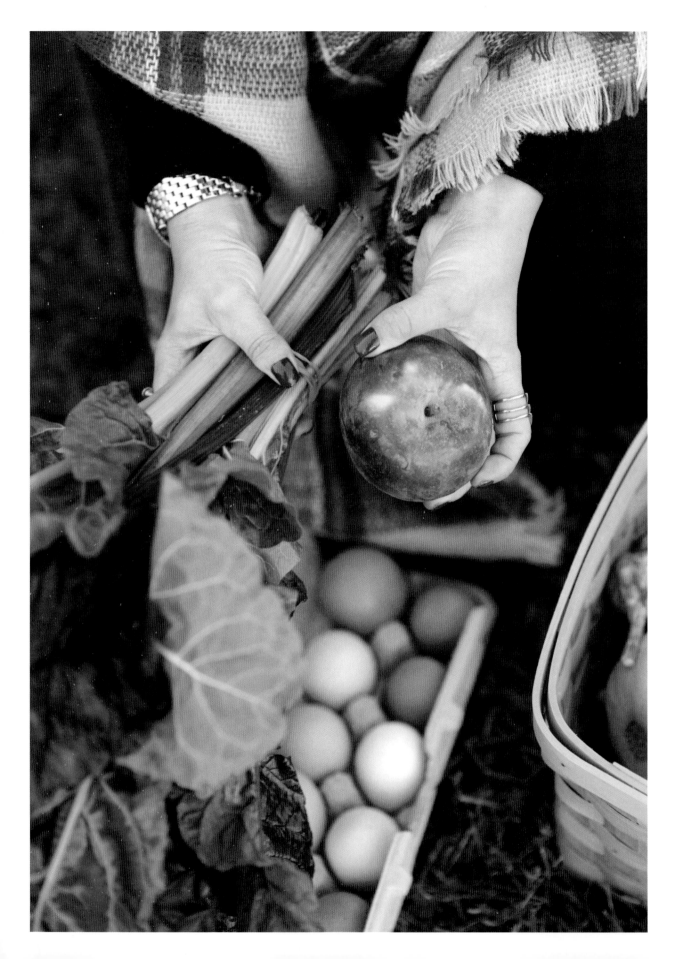

FRESH ITEMS

When sourcing fruit and veggies, buy organic and in-season. (See "What's in Season When" on pages 368 and 369.) For the best-tasting, most nutritious, and often least expensive produce, consider joining a CSA, shopping at local farmer's markets, or growing your own veggies.

MY GO-TO FRESH & PERISHABLE ITEMS:

fruit
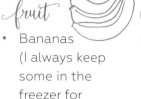

- Bananas (I always keep some in the freezer for smoothies.)
- Avocados
- Berries (fresh and frozen)
- Cherries
- Lemons
- Limes
- Oranges

veggies

- Leafy greens, braising greens, and salad greens (kale, spinach, and romaine lettuce)
- Bell peppers
- Broccoli
- Carrots
- Cauliflower
- Eggplant
- Scallions
- Sweet potatoes
- Tomatoes
- Zucchini

herbs

- Basil
- Cilantro
- Dill
- Parsley
- Thyme

aromatics

- Garlic
- Ginger
- Onions

dairy

- Grass-fed butter (I like Kerrygold.)
- Raw local cheeses, like cheddar and mozzarella
- Grass-fed yogurt

other

- Almond milk, homemade (page 266) or store-bought*

If buying, look for milk made with just almonds and water, and avoid sweetened milk. While sweetened almond milk may work in some recipes, it may not work in others.

MEAT, POULTRY, EGGS & SEAFOOD

When sourcing animal proteins and eggs, look for labels such as grass-fed, pasture-raised, non-GMO, organic, wild-caught, soy-free, sustainable, and locally sourced.

meat

- Beef
- Bison
- Lamb
- Pork
- Venison

Buy organic, grass-fed, pasture-raised meat. It is best to purchase from a local farmer or farmer's market!

poultry & eggs

- Chicken
- Duck
- Turkey
- Eggs

Buy organic, pasture-raised poultry and eggs from laying hens that are fed non-GMO and soy-free feed. It is best to purchase from a local farmer or farmer's market!

seafood

All varieties of fish and shellfish

Buy wild-caught and sustainably raised seafood; avoid farm-raised varieties.

tools & equipment:
YOUR BEST KITCHEN ASSISTANTS

I've kept the tools and equipment simple so that even with a basic kitchen setup, you can cook wonders from this book. Here's the equipment that I find essential for success in the kitchen:

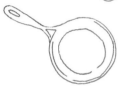

KNIVES. A good knife is a must! Find one that fits comfortably in your hand and keep it sharp. These are the knives that I use most often: chef's knife, paring knife, and serrated knife.

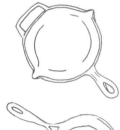

CAST-IRON SKILLET. I use my 6½-inch, 8-inch (probably the size that I use most often), and 10½-inch cast-iron skillets all the time. Cast-iron skillets are inexpensive and are wonderful for transferring from stovetop to oven.

POTS AND PANS. You'll want stainless-steel skillets (10-inch and 12-inch are good) and saucepans (2-quart and 4-quart are good sizes).

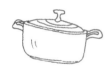

DUTCH OVEN. This large oven-safe pot is great for making slow-cooked dishes, soups, and more.

STOCKPOT AND STEAMER INSERT. I use a 16- to 20-quart stockpot for steaming veggies, making broths and soups, and making the perfect hard-boiled eggs. (See page 66 for my hard-boiled egg trick!)

SLOW COOKER. My 6-quart slow cooker is a favorite in my kitchen. Set it and forget it, and the perfect dinner awaits!

FOOD PROCESSOR. For making condiments, nut butters, and more. I used an 11-cup-capacity food processor for the recipes in this book.

BAKING SHEETS. I like to have two of each: rimmed and flat.

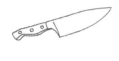

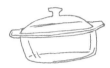

GLASS BAKING DISHES. For cooking, baking, marinating, and more. The sizes you will use most frequently to make the recipes in this book are 8-inch square, 8- or 9-inch round, and 9 by 13-inch rectangular.

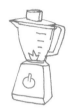

BLENDER, PREFERABLY HIGH-SPEED. For all things smoothie, soup, and so forth. A good blender, such as a Vitamix or Blendtec, is so worth the investment. A regular blender will accomplish many, but not all, of the same tasks, though less efficiently. A high-speed blender is required (or extremely helpful) to make almond milk (page 266), cashew cream (page 116), and No-Bake Sea Salt Cookie Dough Cups (page 284).

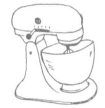

STAND MIXER. Great for making things like whipped cream, meringues, and frostings.

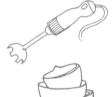

IMMERSION BLENDER. For pureeing soups directly in the pot!

MIXING BOWLS. Essential in all sizes. Bowls with spouts are useful for pouring batter into hot skillets, such as when making pancakes and crepes, and into baking dishes.

MEASURING TOOLS. You'll want dry measuring cups, liquid measuring cups, and measuring spoons.

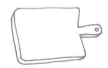

CUTTING BOARDS. I have an assortment of wood and plastic cutting boards in a variety of sizes. The more the better, in my opinion!

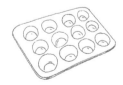

MUFFIN TINS WITH LINERS. I use a standard 12-cup metal muffin tin and line the cups with parchment paper liners or silicone liners.

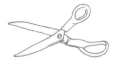

OTHER KEY ITEMS:

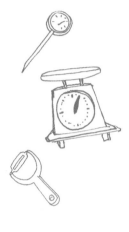

- Candy thermometer
- Colanders of various sizes
- Fine-mesh sieve (or cheesecloth for lining a colander)
- Handheld grater or box grater
- Kitchen scale
- Kitchen scissors
- Microplane zester
- Oven thermometer

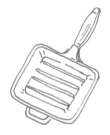

- Skewers for grilled foods
- Spatulas
- Spiral slicer or mandoline (for making veggie noodles)
- Tongs
- Vegetable peeler
- Whisks
- Wire racks for cooling
- Wooden spoons

EXTRAS:

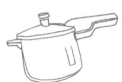

- Cast-iron grill pan
- Double boiler (for melting chocolate, basically!)
- Juicer

- Pressure cooker or multi-cooker
- Waffle maker

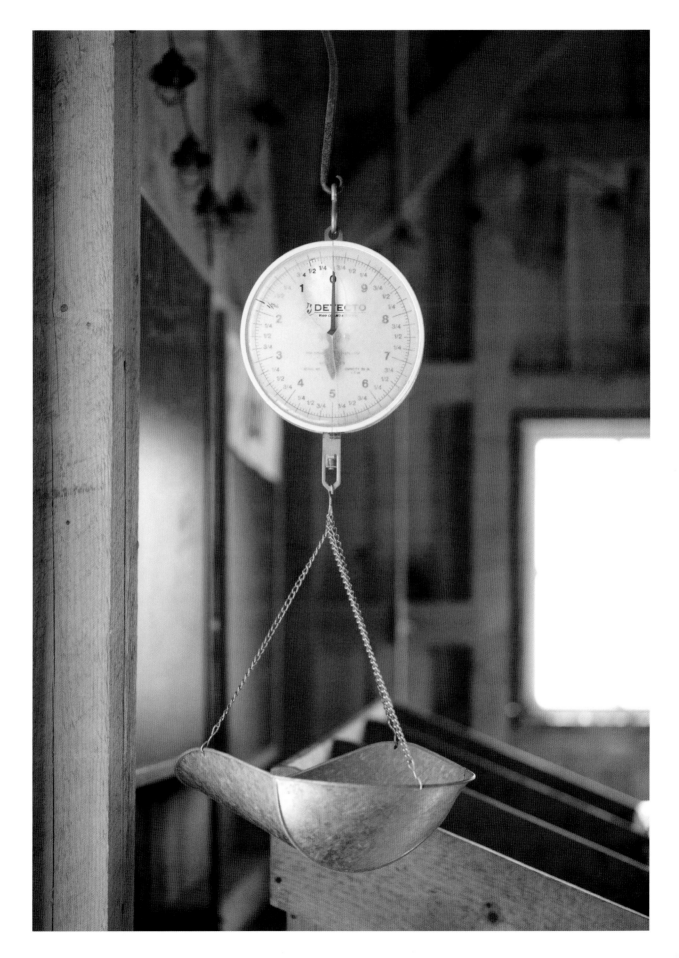

my cooking TIPS

Ready to start cooking? Me too! Here are a few last-minute tips before you dive in:

1. IT'S NOT AN ALL-OR-NOTHING *approach.*

Don't feel like you have to start cooking squeaky-clean from the very beginning. I encourage you to begin by working new recipes into your repertoire, perhaps trying a new one once a week, or getting used to using a new tool (like a spiral slicer), and focus on that for a while before attempting something like grain-free baking. As with so many things, it's about developing new habits and becoming comfortable working with new ingredients and techniques. Don't get overwhelmed or discouraged! Start slow, spend some time digging through your pantry and adding in cleaner products, and go from there.

2. PREP AHEAD *for success.*

Make up weekly menus (find a printable template here: Lexiscleankitchen.com/weeklymenuplanner), create shopping lists, and prepare for the week. You'll be less likely to opt for junk food if you have lunches, snacks, and grab-and-go eats readily available throughout the week.

3. READ THE ENTIRE RECIPE *before getting started.*

If you read through each step of a recipe before you begin, you'll be able to plan your kitchen time more efficiently and cut corners where possible. You'll also find out which recipe components, or subrecipes, you may need to make ahead (such as broth or mayonnaise), which tools you'll need to have out and ready to use, and so on.

4. pro tip: SEASON YOUR FOOD GENEROUSLY!

Seasoning meats, vegetables, and just about everything else with salt and pepper will make a world of difference, so don't be shy! The recipes in this book call for fine sea salt, or you can use Himalayan pink salt if you're feeling fancy. I prefer sea salt to standard table salt for its flavor and because it's a clean ingredient. (Standard table salt has iodine in it, which, though important to health, is something I prefer to source naturally by eating iodine-rich foods.) My recipes also call for freshly ground black pepper. Although you can buy your pepper preground if you like, I always prefer it freshly ground from a pepper mill.

5. have fun AND GET CREATIVE.

Not usually an all-star in the kitchen? Don't worry! I promise, you can make the recipes in this book, and they'll be wonderful. Put your fear aside and just *go for it.* I know you can do this!

Making a delicious dish is so rewarding. I love to get creative and adapt recipes to suit my own wants and needs, and I hope you'll do the same with my recipes! Get inspired and put your own spin on things—you can even swap in an ingredient that you received in your latest CSA haul. Dig through this book, have some fun and get messy, and feel great doing it!

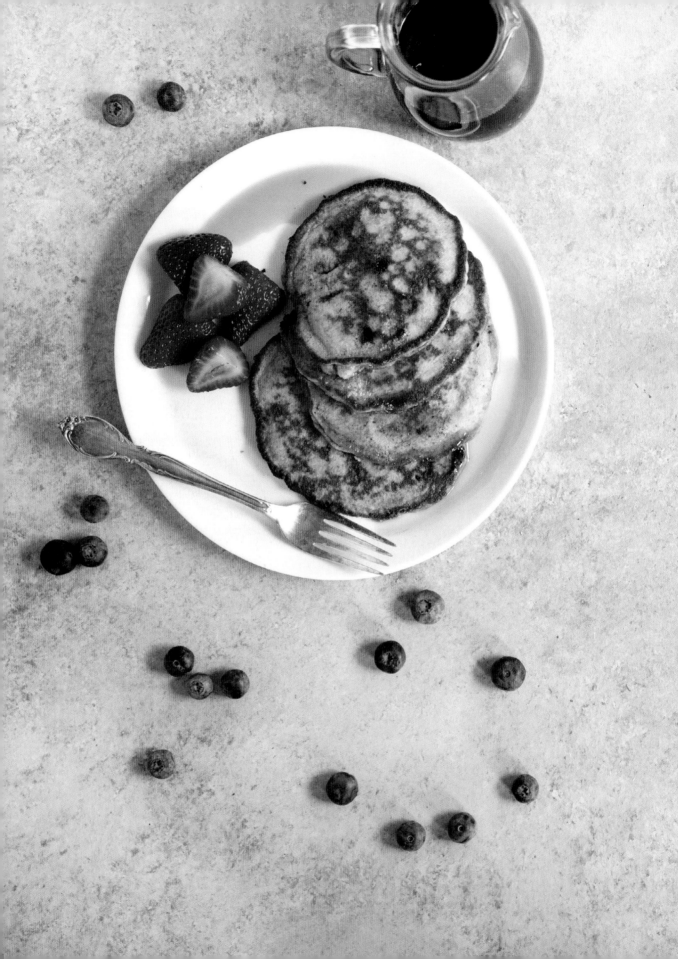

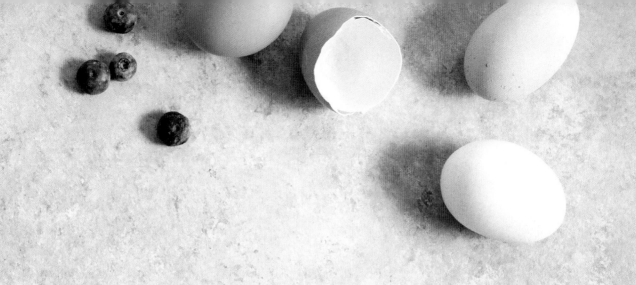

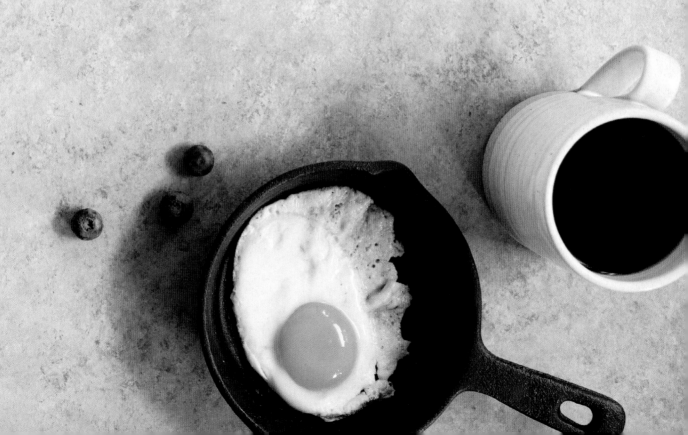

chapter 1

RISE & SHINE:
breakfasts to start your day off right

BEST-EVER FLUFFY PANCAKES

makes eight 3- to 4-inch pancakes *prep time* 5 minutes *cook time* 10 minutes

....

DAIRY-FREE OPTION: use coconut oil for the pan and serve with maple syrup only
PALEO-FRIENDLY OPTION: use ghee or coconut oil for the pan and serve with maple syrup only

....

I am a BIG-TIME brunch gal. I *love* hosting and putting out a nice big spread for family and friends. These pancakes are often included in that spread. They are the real deal, I promise you that. They've become not only a staple in our home, but also in the homes of our friends and family. In fact, I devised a pancake mix based on these pancakes, and it has become my most requested holiday gift! (See note below.)

ingredients:

½ cup blanched almond flour

½ cup tapioca flour

1 teaspoon baking powder

Pinch of fine sea salt

2 large eggs

¼ cup unsweetened applesauce

½ teaspoon vanilla extract

1 tablespoon unsalted butter, ghee (page 350), or coconut oil, for the pan

ADD-INS (OPTIONAL):

⅓ cup diced fresh fruit of choice (small berries can be left whole)

⅓ cup chocolate chips

⅓ cup chopped raw walnuts and ½ teaspoon ground cinnamon

FOR SERVING:

Butter

Pure maple syrup

directions:

1. Whisk together the almond flour, tapioca flour, baking powder, and salt in a mixing bowl, preferably one with a spout. Add the eggs, applesauce, and vanilla and mix well to combine.

2. Heat the butter in a large skillet over medium heat.

3. Stir the desired add-ins, if using, into the batter.

4. Pour the batter into the skillet to form 3- to 4-inch pancakes. Cook for 2 to 3 minutes, until bubbles begin to form on the top, then flip and cook for an additional 2 to 3 minutes, until the pancakes are fluffy and golden brown. Remove from the skillet, set aside, and repeat with the remaining batter.

5. Serve immediately with butter and maple syrup. Store leftover pancakes in the refrigerator for up to 1 week or in the freezer for up to 6 months.

note: To make a batch of convenient pancake and waffle mix, place 1 cup of blanched almond flour, 1 cup of tapioca flour, 2 teaspoons of baking powder, and 2 pinches of fine sea salt in a large mason jar. Screw the lid on tightly and shake to blend the ingredients. Store the mix in the pantry for up to 1 week or in the fridge for up to 1 month. (Don't forget to label and date the jar!) Shake the jar to reblend the mix, then wait about 30 seconds to let it settle before opening the jar. *Makes 2 cups (enough for two batches of pancakes or waffles).*

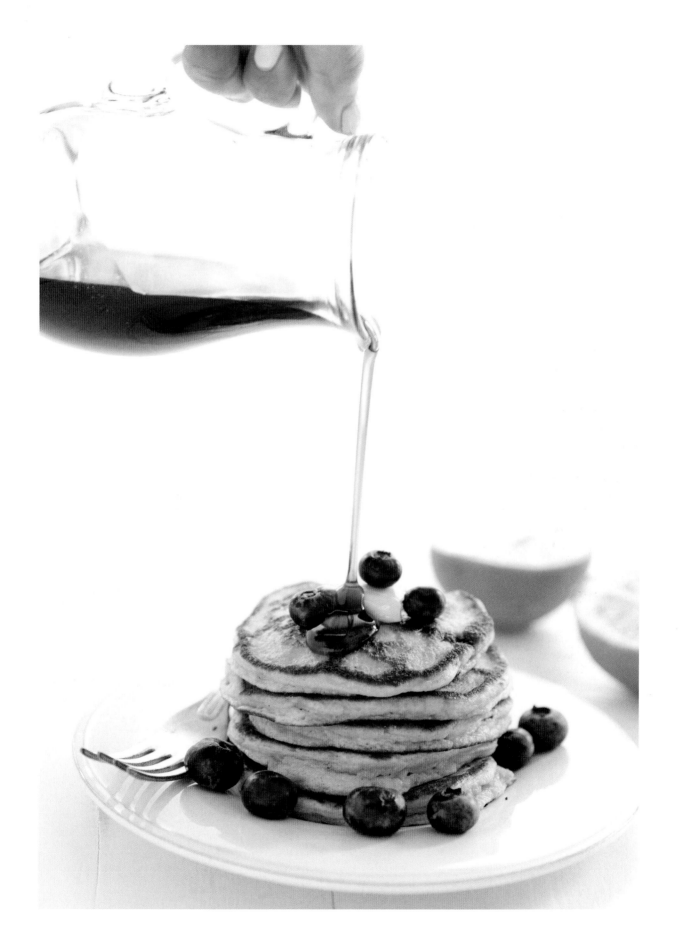

BEST-EVER FLUFFY WAFFLES

makes 2 waffles (8 individual pieces, or 2 servings) *prep time* 5 minutes *cook time* 10 to 15 minutes

DAIRY-FREE OPTION: grease waffle maker with avocado oil instead of butter and serve with maple syrup only / PALEO-FRIENDLY OPTION: grease waffle maker with avocado oil instead of butter and serve with maple syrup only

Waffles remind me of my childhood. I don't mean freshly made Belgian waffles topped with ice cream from a local shop; I mean the right-from-the-box frozen kind that you just pop in the toaster and carry out the door. While the convenience of those waffles is great, the ingredients are not. Plus, I like the smell of waffles cooking throughout the house! These waffles are delicious, fluffy, and customizable, and they freeze so *well*. They are perfect for running out the door on a busy morning or for a leisurely Sunday brunch.

ingredients:

1 tablespoon melted unsalted butter or avocado oil, for the waffle maker

½ cup blanched almond flour

½ cup tapioca flour

1 teaspoon baking powder

Pinch of fine sea salt

2 large eggs

¼ cup unsweetened applesauce

1½ teaspoons pure maple syrup

½ teaspoon vanilla extract

FOR SERVING:

Butter

Pure maple syrup

directions:

1. Preheat a waffle maker and brush it liberally with melted butter. Whisk together the almond flour, tapioca flour, baking powder, and salt in a mixing bowl, preferably one with a spout. Add the eggs, applesauce, maple syrup, and vanilla and mix to combine.

2. Following the directions for your waffle maker regarding batter quantity and cook time, pour in the batter and cook the waffle until done. Remove and transfer to a low oven to keep warm. Regrease the waffle iron and repeat with the remaining batter.

3. Serve the waffles hot with butter and maple syrup. Store leftovers in the refrigerator for up to 1 week or in the freezer for up to 6 months.

variations:

Chocolate Chip Waffles. Mix ⅓ cup of dark chocolate chips into the batter before cooking.

Chocolate Waffles. Add 2 tablespoons of cocoa powder to the dry ingredients in Step 1.

Fruit-Filled Waffles. Mix ⅓ cup of diced fresh fruit into the batter before cooking. (Small berries can be left whole.)

Pumpkin Waffles. Add ½ teaspoon of pumpkin pie spice and ½ teaspoon of ground cinnamon to the dry ingredients in Step 1. Substitute pumpkin puree for the applesauce.

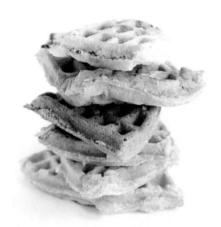

tip: They're freezer-friendly, too!

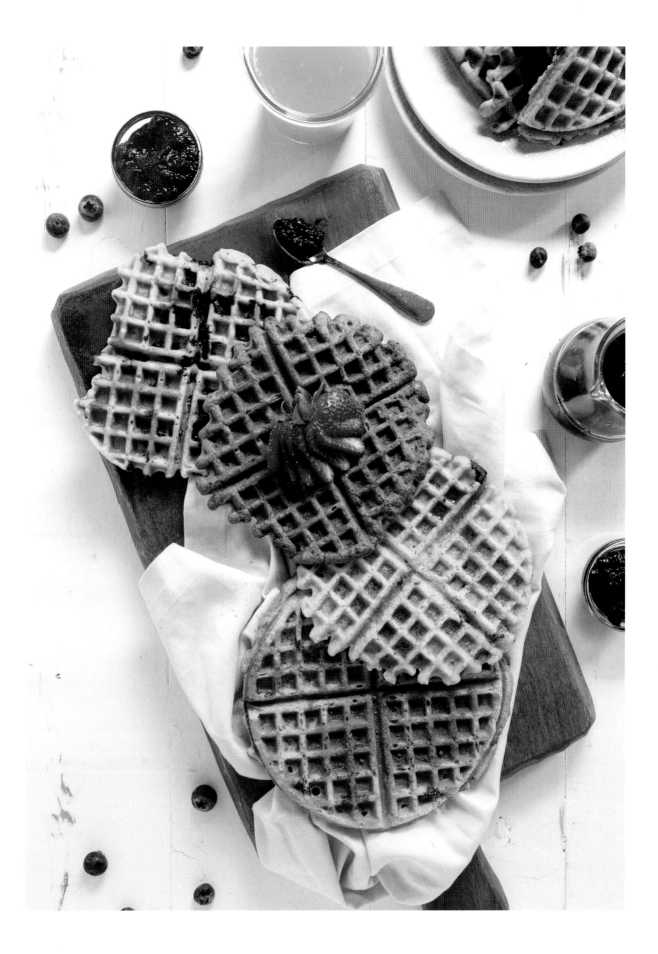

FRENCH TOAST STICKS

serves 4   *prep time* 10 minutes (not including bread)   *cook time* 12 to 20 minutes

DAIRY-FREE OPTION: use avocado oil for the pan
PALEO-FRIENDLY OPTION: use ghee or avocado oil for the pan and omit powdered sugar

We're having fun in the kitchen this morning, you guys! The best part is, you can make half of this recipe ahead of time and whip up a special breakfast with ease, any morning you wish! This recipe uses a batch of homemade sandwich bread. If you don't have a loaf on hand, remember to figure the time to make it into the preparation of this recipe.

ingredients:

1 batch All-Purpose Sandwich Bread (page 80), baked in an 8-inch square pan

2 large eggs

¼ cup unsweetened nondairy milk of choice, homemade (page 266) or store-bought

1 teaspoon vanilla extract

1 teaspoon ground cinnamon

2 tablespoons ghee (page 350), unsalted butter, or avocado oil, for the pan

Optional: 1 to 2 tablespoons powdered sugar, for serving

Pure maple syrup, for serving

directions:

1. Slice the bread into sticks.

2. In a large bowl, whisk together the eggs, milk, vanilla, and cinnamon. Add the bread sticks to the bowl and let sit for 5 minutes.

3. In a large skillet over medium heat, melt 1 tablespoon of ghee. Place as many coated bread sticks in the skillet as will comfortably fit without overcrowding and cook for 3 to 5 minutes on the top and bottom, until golden brown and no longer soft. Place the sticks on a plate and cover with foil to keep warm while you make the rest.

4. Repeat with the remaining bread sticks, adding more ghee to the pan between batches, until all of the sticks are cooked.

5. Dust immediately with powdered sugar, if using, and serve with maple syrup.

6. The French toast sticks will keep in a closed container in the refrigerator for up to 4 days or in the freezer for several months.

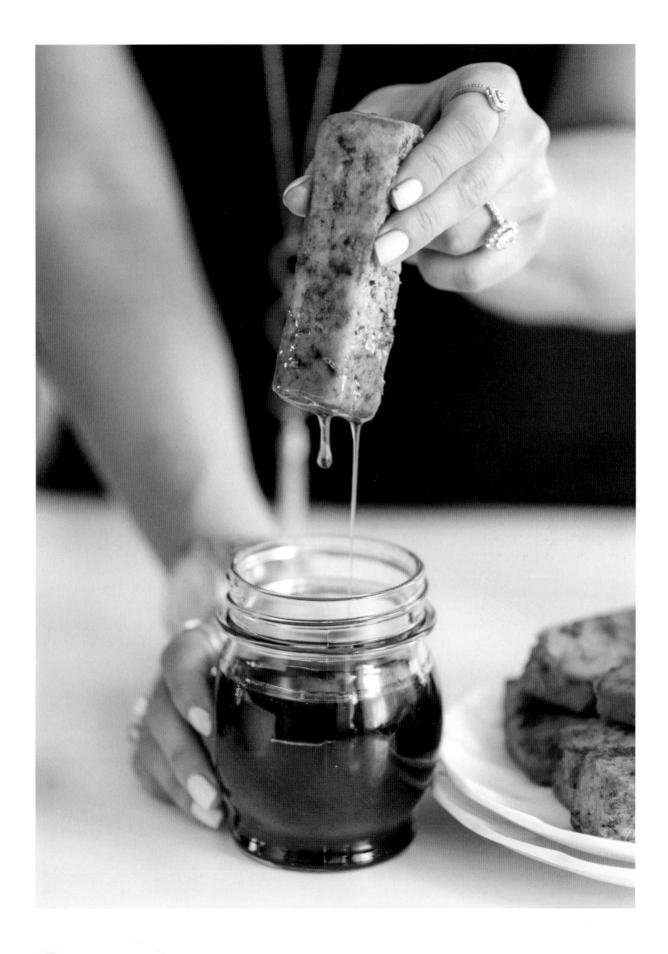

CREPES—SAVORY & SWEET

makes six 6-inch crepes *prep time* 10 minutes, plus filling *cook time* 10 minutes

....

NUT-FREE OPTION: use a nondairy milk that isn't made from nuts, such as coconut milk
DAIRY-FREE OPTION: use oil for cooking, and replace butter or ghee in batter with palm shortening
PALEO-FRIENDLY OPTION: use ghee

....

Crepes are wonderful for brunch or breakfast because they aren't too heavy and are totally customizable. In the mood for savory? Stuff them with scrambled eggs and bacon or chicken salad. In the mood for sweet? Let me suggest Homemade Chocolate Hazelnut Spread or All-Purpose Caramel Sauce and fresh fruit! And that's just a start. Use your imagination and the additional ideas I share below, and your crepe station will never be boring.

ingredients:

FOR THE CREPE BATTER:

½ cup tapioca flour

2 tablespoons coconut flour

1 teaspoon baking soda

¼ teaspoon fine sea salt

2 large eggs

½ cup unsweetened nondairy milk of choice, homemade (page 266) or store-bought

1 tablespoon melted unsalted butter or ghee (page 350)

Butter, ghee (page 350), or oil of choice, for cooking

ADDITIONAL INGREDIENTS FOR THE SWEET CREPE BATTER:

1 tablespoon pure maple syrup

½ teaspoon vanilla extract

SWEET FILLING IDEAS:

⅓ cup All-Purpose Caramel Sauce (page 360) with 1 cup diced fresh fruit

⅓ cup honey and Salted Vanilla Bean Whipped Cream (page 282) or store-bought Greek yogurt

Nut butter and banana slices

⅓ cup Quick & Easy Jam (page 330), 1 cup halved or quartered fresh berries (small berries can be left whole), and 1 cup homemade granola (page 44 or 46)

⅓ cup Homemade Chocolate Hazelnut Spread (page 358) with 1 cup diced fresh fruit

1 cup sliced apples, pears, or bananas sautéed in butter until caramelized

SAVORY FILLING IDEAS:

2 cups Chicken Salad (page 152)

Scrambled eggs and chopped cooked bacon (1 or 2 eggs and 2 slices bacon per crepe)

1 cup Caramelized Onions (page 332) and 3 cups spinach sautéed in butter until wilted (about 1 pound fresh spinach)

directions:

1. Make the filling of your choice for sweet or savory crepes and set aside.

2. Make the crepes: In a bowl, mix together the tapioca flour, coconut flour, baking soda, and salt until evenly blended. Add the eggs, milk, and melted butter. If you're making sweet crepes, add the maple syrup and vanilla as well. Whisk until no lumps remain. The mixture should resemble pancake batter.

3. Place a large sauté pan over medium heat and add enough butter to coat the pan. Pour about ¼ cup of the batter into the center of the pan to create a 6-inch crepe. Cook for 1 minute per side, until slightly golden.

4. Repeat with the remaining batter, adding more butter to the pan after making each crepe.

5. To fill the crepes, spread 2 to 3 tablespoons of filling along the center and fold up the sides.

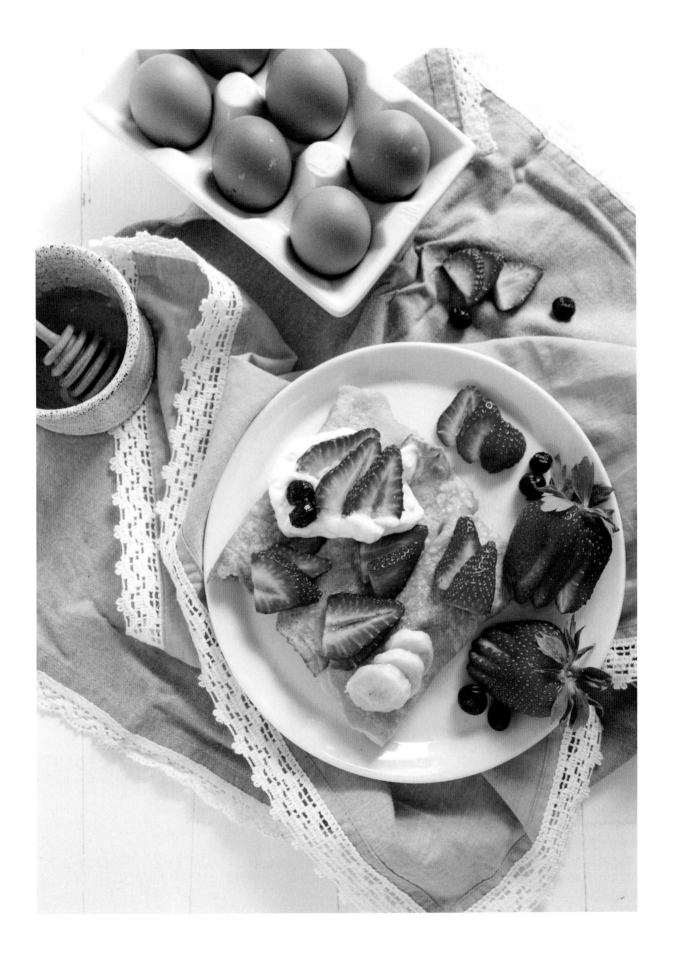

CLASSIC HOME FRIES

serves 4   *prep time* 10 minutes   *cook time* 45 minutes

EGG-FREE / NUT-FREE / DAIRY-FREE OPTION: cook home fries in oil
PALEO-FRIENDLY OPTION: cook home fries in ghee or oil / VEGAN OPTION: cook home fries in oil

Growing up in New York, my brother, Adam, and I had tons of weekend breakfasts out at diners, diners, and more diners (they're big in New York!). Every diner (and restaurant, for that matter) has its own unique way of making home fries. Out of all of our breakfast runs, and *lots* of home fries later, I've come to prefer mine cooked like this. Diced potatoes seasoned just right, with hints of onion and garlic, get their start on the stovetop and finish in the oven; the result is perfectly browned yet tender home fries every time. Serve with eggs any style (see page 66) and bacon for a crowd-pleasing brunch!

ingredients:

2 cloves garlic

1 large onion

1 green bell pepper

2 tablespoons ghee (page 350), unsalted butter, or oil of choice

4 medium russet potatoes

1 teaspoon garlic granules

1 teaspoon paprika

1 teaspoon fine sea salt

½ teaspoon freshly ground black pepper

Optional: ⅛ teaspoon cayenne pepper

Optional: 1 tablespoon chopped fresh flat-leaf parsley, for garnish

note: You can substitute sweet potatoes for the russet potatoes for an equally delicious dish!

directions:

1. Preheat the oven to 375°F.

2. Mince the garlic and finely dice the onion and bell pepper; set aside.

3. Heat the ghee in a large ovenproof skillet (such as cast iron) over medium heat until hot, about 5 minutes.

4. While the skillet is heating up, rinse and cut the potatoes into ½-inch dice and set aside.

5. Add the minced garlic, onion, and bell pepper to the hot skillet and cook, stirring often, until slightly soft, about 5 minutes.

6. Add the potatoes and cook for 10 minutes, stirring often to make sure they don't stick to the skillet (add more ghee if they do begin to stick).

7. In a small bowl, combine the garlic granules, paprika, salt, black pepper, and cayenne pepper, if using.

8. Sprinkle the seasonings over the potatoes, give them a good stir, and transfer the skillet to the oven. Bake for 25 minutes, or until the potatoes are soft, tender, and golden brown.

9. Garnish with the fresh parsley, if using, and serve hot with your favorite breakfast protein!

variation:

Pork Butt Home Fries. Cut ½ pound of pork butt into ½-inch dice and add it to the skillet with the potatoes in Step 6.

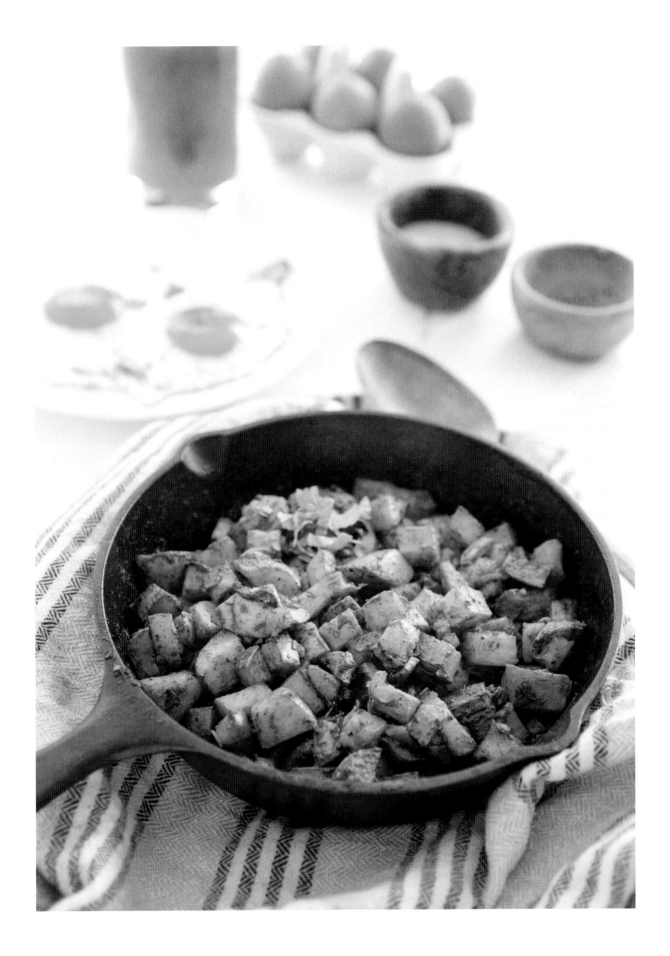

GLUTEN-FREE GRANOLA

makes about 5 cups   *prep time* 8 minutes   *cook time* 25 minutes

....

NUT-FREE OPTION: use seeds instead of nuts / DAIRY-FREE
VEGAN OPTION: replace honey with additional maple syrup

....

My original, classic granola recipe! It's sweetened just right, with all of the flavor and clusters you want in your granola. I batch it in jars for my mom and my nanny, and they absolutely adore it. Now, this granola uses gluten-free rolled oats, which some people can tolerate. If you avoid all grains, including oats, try my Paleo Granola on page 46 instead.

ingredients:

4 cups gluten-free rolled oats

1 cup mixed raw nuts and seeds, such as slivered or whole almonds, chopped walnuts, sunflower seeds, and pumpkin seeds

2 tablespoons coconut sugar or granulated maple sugar

1 tablespoon ground cinnamon

Pinch of fine sea salt

Optional: ½ cup whole or diced dried fruit of choice (see notes)

¼ cup coconut oil

¼ cup honey

3 tablespoons pure maple syrup

2 tablespoons molasses

1 teaspoon vanilla extract

1 large egg white, whisked

directions:

1. Preheat the oven to 350°F and line a rimmed baking sheet with parchment paper.

2. In a large bowl, combine the oats, nuts and seeds, sugar, cinnamon, and salt. If you will be consuming the granola within a week after baking it, add the dried fruit, if using.

3. In a small saucepan, heat the oil, honey, maple syrup, molasses, and vanilla until boiling. Once boiling, pour over the oat mixture and mix thoroughly.

4. Stir in the whisked egg white, making sure that it's mixed in well.

5. Spread out the mixture on the lined baking sheet and bake for 15 to 20 minutes, until golden brown. Watch the granola in the oven to avoid burning. Let cool completely in the pan.

6. Store in an airtight container for up to 1 month.

notes: When dried fruit is mixed into the oat and nut mixture and baked, the fruit gets hard after about a week. If you will be serving the granola within a week, feel free to add the dried fruit in Step 2. Another option is to add a small amount to each serving of granola when eating it. That's what I do.

For chunky clusters, let the granola cool *completely* before removing it from the pan.

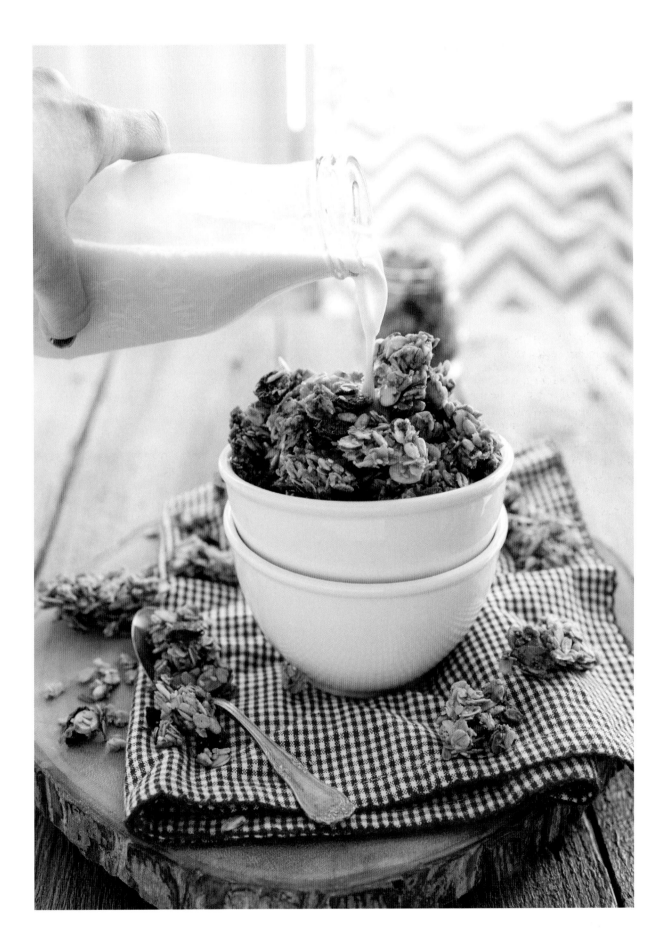

PALEO GRANOLA

makes about 4 cups *prep time* 8 minutes *cook time* 25 minutes

....

DAIRY-FREE / PALEO-FRIENDLY / VEGAN OPTION: **replace honey with additional maple syrup**

....

For those of you who avoid oats and want a classic granola, this is it! It has the greatest granola chunks and a wonderful flavor and texture. Did I mention how amazing your house will smell while it's baking? Mmm . . .

ingredients:

1 cup raw slivered almonds

1 cup raw pecans

1 cup raw walnuts

½ cup raw whole almonds

½ cup raw sunflower seeds

2 tablespoons coconut sugar or granulated maple sugar

1 tablespoon ground cinnamon

Pinch of fine sea salt

Optional: ½ cup whole or diced dried fruit of choice (see notes)

3 tablespoons honey

3 tablespoons pure maple syrup

2 tablespoons molasses

1 teaspoon vanilla extract

1 large egg white, whisked

directions:

1. Preheat the oven to 350°F and line a rimmed baking sheet with parchment paper.

2. In a food processor, chop the nuts and seeds into rice-sized pieces.

3. In a large bowl, combine the nuts, seeds, sugar, cinnamon, and salt. If you will be consuming the granola within a week after baking it, add the dried fruit, if using.

4. In a small saucepan, heat the honey, maple syrup, molasses, and vanilla until boiling. Once boiling, pour over the nut mixture and mix thoroughly.

5. Stir in the whisked egg white, making sure that it's mixed in well.

6. Spread out the mixture on the lined baking sheet and bake for 15 to 20 minutes, until golden brown. Watch the granola in the oven to avoid burning. Let cool completely in the pan.

7. Store in an airtight container for up to 1 month.

notes: When dried fruit is mixed into the nut and seed mixture and baked, the fruit gets hard after about a week. If you will be serving the granola within a week, feel free to add the dried fruit in Step 3. Another option is to add a small amount to each serving of granola when eating it. That's what I do.

For chunky clusters, let the granola cool *completely* before removing it from the pan.

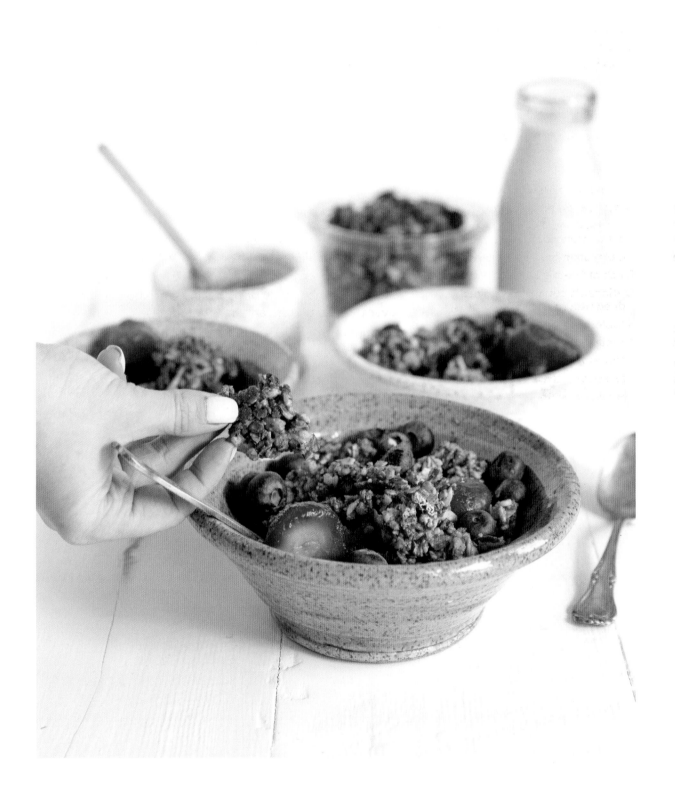

FRENCH VANILLA MUFFINS

makes 9 muffins *prep time* 10 minutes *cook time* 20 minutes

PALEO-FRIENDLY

Muffins are the perfect staple for a run-out-the-door kind of morning, a midday snack, or a weekend breakfast or brunch! This recipe is a classic—delicious as is or when used as a base for customizing with the add-in of your choice. My faves are chocolate chunks or blueberries. Add in your own favorite and devour! May I suggest slicing a muffin in half, toasting it, and slathering it with grass-fed butter? Delish!

ingredients:

2 cups sifted blanched almond flour

1 teaspoon baking soda

½ teaspoon baking powder

¼ teaspoon fine sea salt

3 large eggs

½ cup unsweetened applesauce

⅓ cup honey

2 tablespoons palm shortening

1 teaspoon vanilla extract

Seeds scraped from ½ vanilla bean

ADD-INS (OPTIONAL):

⅓ cup dark chocolate chunks

⅓ cup fresh blueberries

Optional: Coarse sugar, such as turbinado sugar or muscovado sugar, for sprinkling

directions:

1. Preheat the oven to 350°F and line 9 wells of a 12-cup muffin tin with parchment paper liners.

2. In a large bowl, whisk together the almond flour, baking soda, baking powder, and salt until well blended.

3. Add the eggs, applesauce, honey, shortening, vanilla extract, and vanilla bean seeds and mix to fully combine. Using a spatula, fold in the chocolate chunks or blueberries, if using.

4. Scoop the batter into the prepared muffin cups, filling each cup three-quarters full. Sprinkle coarse sugar on top, if desired.

5. Bake for 20 to 22 minutes, until a toothpick inserted in the middle of a muffin comes out clean.

6. Transfer the muffins to a wire rack to cool. Serve warm or at room temperature. The muffins will keep in a closed container at room temperature for up to 4 days or in the freezer for up to 1 month.

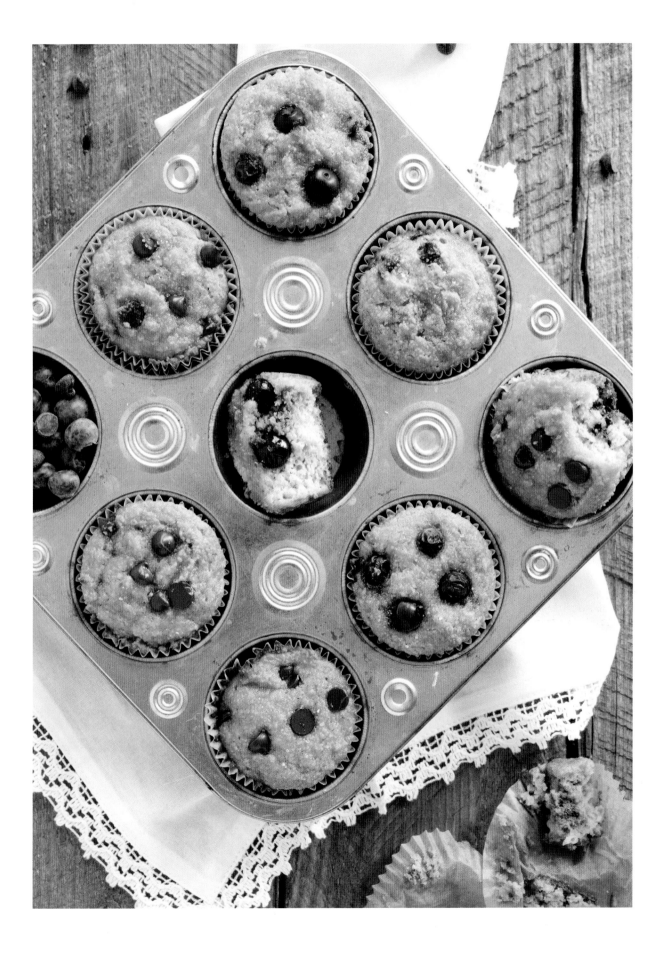

ORANGE CHOCOLATE CHUNK SCONES

makes 8 scones   *prep time* 10 minutes   *cook time* 30 minutes

....

DAIRY-FREE / PALEO-FRIENDLY OPTION: omit sprinkling of sugar and glaze

....

Scones are a wonderful breakfast treat—dessertlike, but totally acceptable for brunch. Right? Plus, you can ditch the orange and chocolate and go for any add-ins you like! (See the variations below for some ideas.)

ingredients:

2½ cups sifted blanched almond flour

1 teaspoon baking powder

½ teaspoon ground cinnamon

½ teaspoon fine sea salt

1 large egg

½ cup unsweetened applesauce

¼ cup pure maple syrup or honey

1 teaspoon vanilla extract

3 tablespoons grated orange zest

½ cup dark chocolate chunks

Optional: Coarse sugar, such as turbinado sugar or muscovado sugar, for sprinkling

FOR THE VANILLA GLAZE (OPTIONAL):

2 cups sifted powdered sugar, or more as needed

3 tablespoons almond milk, homemade (page 266) or store-bought, or more as needed

Seeds scraped from 1 vanilla bean

Pinch of fine sea salt

directions:

1. Preheat the oven to 350°F and line a baking sheet with parchment paper.

2. In a bowl, whisk the almond flour, baking powder, cinnamon, and salt until well blended.

3. Add the egg, applesauce, maple syrup, and vanilla extract and mix until a soft dough forms. Fold in the orange zest and chocolate chunks.

4. Using your hands, roll the dough into a ball and place it on the lined baking sheet. Gently flatten the dough into a disc about 1 inch high.

5. Using a pizza cutter or knife, slice the dough into 8 wedges. Gently separate the wedges slightly, but leave them in a circle. Sprinkle the scones with coarse sugar, if desired. If making the glaze, omit the coarse sugar.

6. Bake for 30 minutes, until golden and firm to the touch, with a crusty exterior. Transfer to a cooling rack to cool.

7. Make the vanilla glaze, if using: Whisk together all of the ingredients until smooth. Add more milk or powdered sugar as needed to create a smooth consistency that is thick but still pourable. Dunk the tops of the cooled scones into the glaze to coat.

8. Store leftover scones in an airtight container for up to 3 days or in the freezer for up to 3 months.

variations:

Cranberry Orange Scones. Replace the chocolate chunks with fresh or frozen cranberries.

Lemon Blueberry Scones. Replace the orange zest with lemon zest and the chocolate chunks with fresh or frozen blueberries. Bonus: Fold in 1 teaspoon of dried lavender buds in Step 3.

Pumpkin Chocolate Chunk Scones. Replace the applesauce with pumpkin puree, omit the orange zest, and add 2 teaspoons of pumpkin pie spice.

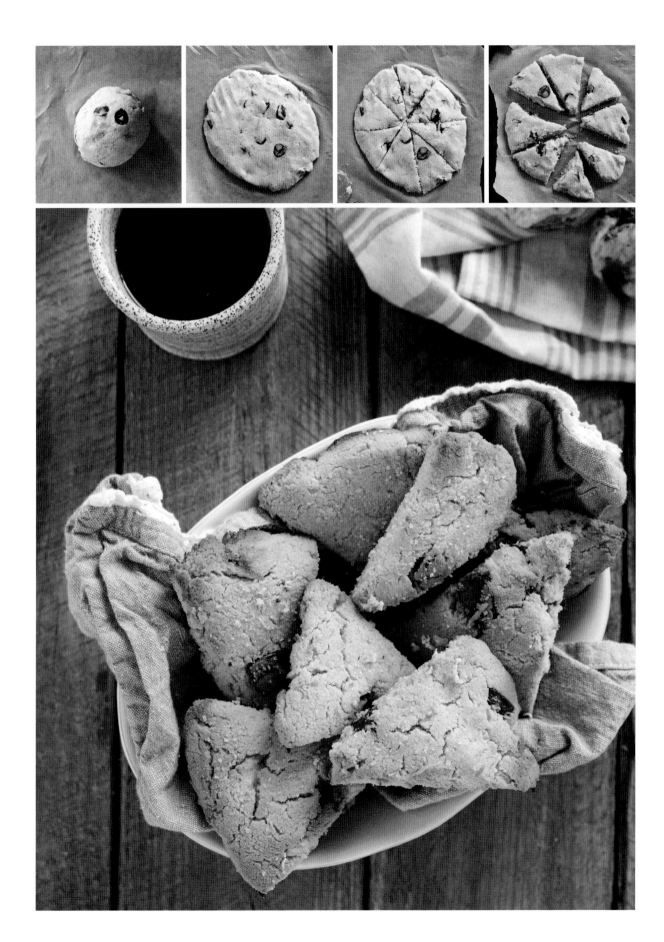

BREAKFAST GALETTE— SAVORY & SWEET

makes one 9 by 13-inch galette (serves 4)
prep time 20 minutes (not including tart crust dough)   *cook time* 40 minutes

Let me tell you about this galette: it's a flaky, buttery crust filled with all of the breakfast goodness you crave. It's customizable, it's delicious, and it is sure to impress your family and guests!

ingredients:

1 batch chilled tart crust dough (page 70)

1 large egg yolk, beaten, for brushing

FOR THE SAVORY GALETTE:

¼ cup ricotta cheese

1 cup cherry tomatoes, halved

1 small bunch asparagus, tough ends removed, cut into 2- to 3-inch lengths

½ red onion, sliced or roughly chopped

½ cup chopped cooked chorizo or crispy bacon

Pinch of fine sea salt

Pinch of freshly ground black pepper

2 or 3 large eggs

FOR THE SWEET GALETTE:

4 soft peaches or with give, peeled, halved, pitted, and cut into ¼ to ½-inch-thick wedges, about 3 cups

½ cup blueberries

⅓ cup granulated maple sugar or coconut palm sugar

2 tablespoons arrowroot flour

½ teaspoon ground cinnamon

directions:

1. Preheat the oven to 350°F.

2. Place the disc of chilled tart crust dough between two large sheets of parchment paper and roll it out into a 12-inch circle. Slide the rolled-out dough onto a baking sheet and remove the top piece of parchment paper.

3. *To make the savory galette:* Spread the ricotta cheese across the dough, leaving about an inch around the perimeter bare, then add the veggies and meat. Fold the outer edge of the crust up and over itself to create a nice border. Sprinkle the meat and veggies with the salt and pepper, then crack the eggs into the center. Brush the edges of the crust with the beaten egg yolk. Bake for 40 minutes, until the eggs are cooked and the crust is golden brown.

To make the sweet galette: In a bowl, combine the peaches, blueberries, sugar, arrowroot flour, and cinnamon. Pour the fruit mixture into the center of the crust, leaving about an inch around the perimeter bare. Fold the outer edge of the crust up and slightly over the fruit. Brush the edges of the crust with the beaten egg yolk. Bake for 40 minutes, until the fruit is bubbling and the crust is golden brown.

4. Slice with a pizza cutter or large knife and serve immediately.

notes: Any extra veggies you have on hand would be great additions to the savory galette!

Try adding any fresh fruit you have on hand to the sweet version.

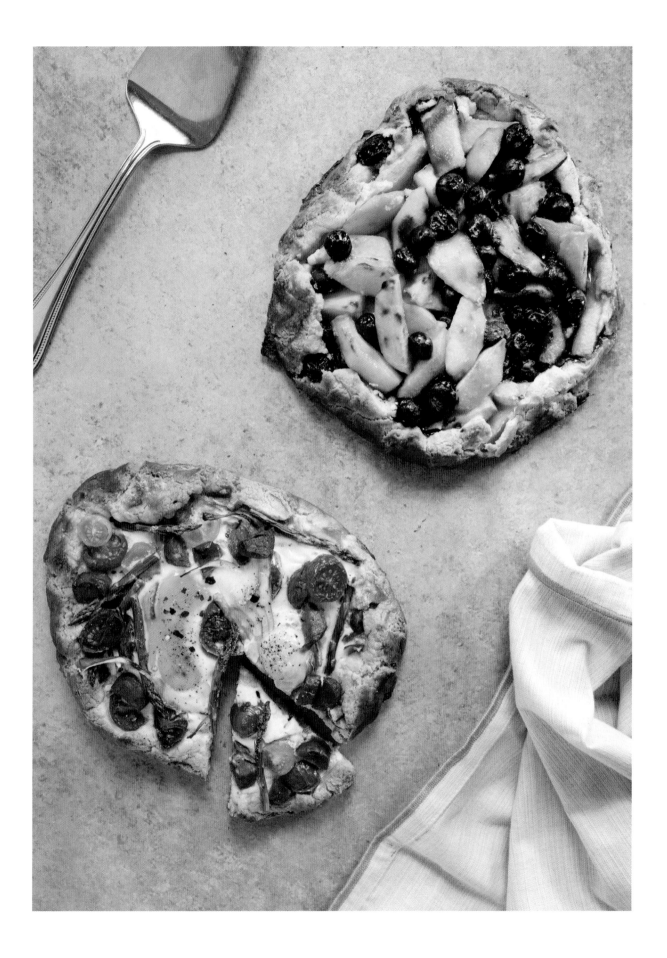

KITCHEN SINK FRITTATA

serves 4   *prep time* 10 minutes   *cook time* 30 minutes

NUT-FREE / DAIRY-FREE OPTION: **use oil instead of butter or ghee for the pan**
PALEO-FRIENDLY OPTION: **use ghee or oil instead of butter for the pan**

I love making a frittata for a leisurely weekend brunch or, when I know that I have a few busy days ahead of me, for "brinner" (aka breakfast for dinner). Frittatas are hearty, portable, and easy to make. For the best results, keep in mind these three tips: season the eggs well, use a heavy ovenproof skillet (cast iron is a great choice), and don't overbake. I love this combination of spicy chorizo, garlic, avocado, mushrooms, and broccoli, but don't feel limited to these add-ins—you can use just about anything you find in your fridge!

ingredients:

1 tablespoon unsalted butter, ghee (page 350), or oil of choice

1 onion, finely diced

1 large clove garlic, minced

2 links Mexican-style fresh (raw) chorizo, casings removed and meat crumbled

1 cup baby portabella mushrooms, finely chopped

1 cup finely chopped broccoli

½ avocado, peeled and cubed

10 large eggs

1 teaspoon paprika

1 teaspoon fine sea salt

½ teaspoon freshly ground black pepper

½ teaspoon garlic granules

note: If you tolerate dairy, ¼ cup of grated Parmesan or shredded cheddar cheese would be a great addition to this frittata. Sprinkle it over the chorizo-veggie mixture before pouring in the eggs. If using Parmesan cheese, decrease the amount of salt in the recipe to ¾ teaspoon.

directions:

1. Preheat the oven to 350°F.

2. Heat the butter in a medium ovenproof skillet over medium heat.

3. Add the onion and garlic and cook for 3 minutes, stirring often. Add the chorizo, mushrooms, broccoli, and avocado and cook for an additional 5 minutes, until the chorizo has cooked slightly, the broccoli has softened, and the mixture is fragrant.

4. In a bowl, whisk the eggs. Add the paprika, salt, pepper, and garlic granules and whisk to combine.

5. Pour the eggs over the chorizo-vegetable mixture and cook for 2 minutes, until the eggs are set on the bottom. Transfer the skillet to the oven and bake for 15 to 20 minutes, until the eggs are fully set and cooked through in the middle. To avoid overcooking, check the frittata after 15 minutes of baking. The eggs are done when they barely jiggle in the pan, without any liquidy egg visible.

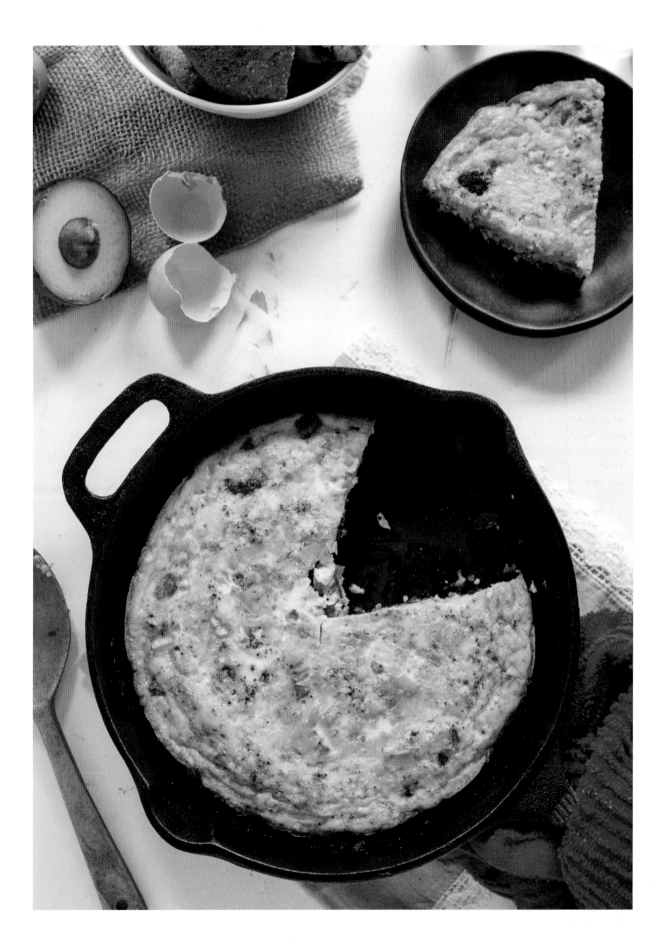

QUICHE

makes one 9-inch quiche (serves 4)   *prep time* 10 minutes (not including tart crust dough or caramelized onions)   *cook time* 35 minutes

I love eggs of all sorts—scrambled, poached, frittata-style, you name it! When it comes to a weekend brunch, though, I always bring this quiche. Made with a delicious buttery crust and filled with delicious add-ins, it's always a hit. But you don't need the excuse of a special event to make it; this is the perfect recipe to make an everyday breakfast a little more special! This quiche can be made in a tart pan or a pie pan; the only difference is that for a tart pan you chill the dough for 1 to 4 hours and press it directly into the pan by hand, and for a pie pan you chill the dough overnight before rolling it out with a rolling pin and placing it in the pan.

ingredients:

1 batch chilled tart crust dough (page 70)

8 large eggs

2 cloves garlic, minced

1 teaspoon fine sea salt

½ teaspoon freshly ground black pepper

Pinch of red pepper flakes, or more as desired

3 strips bacon, cooked and chopped

1 cup Caramelized Onions (page 332)

1 handful fresh spinach

1 tomato, thinly sliced

notes: If you tolerate dairy, you can add ⅓ cup of shredded cheddar cheese in Step 3.

Any other veggies you have on hand will be wonderful additions!

directions:

1. When the dough is sufficiently chilled (the chilling time depends on whether you are using a tart pan or a pie pan), preheat the oven to 350°F and remove the dough from the refrigerator. Grease a 9-inch tart pan or pie pan.

2. If making a tart, press the dough into the greased tart pan; if making a pie, roll out the dough between two sheets of parchment paper into a 13-inch circle and place in the pie pan. Par-bake the crust for 5 minutes.

3. While the crust is par-baking, whisk together the eggs, garlic, salt, black pepper, and red pepper flakes. Fold in the bacon, caramelized onions, and spinach.

4. Pour the egg mixture into the crust, then top with the tomato slices.

5. Bake for 25 to 30 minutes, until the eggs are fully cooked and no longer jiggly and the crust is golden. Serve immediately. Store leftovers in the refrigerator for up to 3 days. To reheat, place in the oven for a few minutes, until warm.

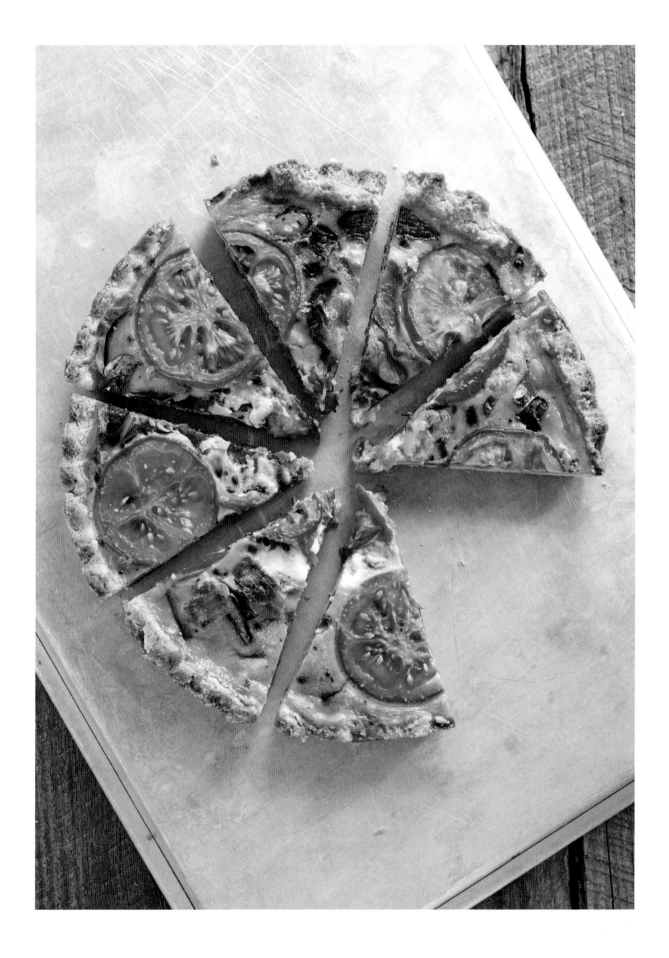

AVOCADO TOAST

serves 4   *prep time* 10 minutes (not including bread or "buns" or glaze, if using)
cook time depends on choice of toast and toppings

EGG-FREE OPTION: omit eggs and use sweet potato "buns"
NUT-FREE OPTION: use sweet potato "buns" / DAIRY-FREE / PALEO-FRIENDLY
VEGAN OPTION: omit eggs and bacon and use sweet potato "buns"

Avocado toast is trendy right now, and I definitely understand why. I mean, it's absolutely delicious! The thing is, I want it to be so much more than just smashed avocado on toast. So I made you the greatest (in my opinion) avocado spread that has the most fantastic flavor! Serve this spread on my sandwich bread, or ditch the bread entirely and go with sweet potato "buns" instead. Top with the desired toppings and devour.

ingredients:

4 to 6 slices All-Purpose Sandwich Bread (page 80) and/or Sweet Potato "Buns" (recipe follows)

FOR THE AVOCADO SPREAD:

2 tablespoons avocado oil or extra-virgin olive oil

1 shallot, finely diced

1 clove garlic, minced

2 teaspoons ground cumin

1 teaspoon paprika

Pinch of fine sea salt

Pinch of freshly ground black pepper

2 avocados

3 tablespoons lemon juice (about 1 lemon)

Optional: Red pepper flakes, to taste

TOPPING IDEAS:

Poached eggs (page 66)

Chopped crispy bacon

Chopped scallions

Roughly chopped fresh flat-leaf parsley or cilantro

Balsamic Glaze (page 334) or balsamic vinegar

Sriracha sauce

Red pepper flakes

Coarse sea salt

Lime wedges

directions:

1. If using sandwich bread, toast the slices, then set them aside. If making sweet potato "buns," make them following the recipe below.

2. Prepare the spread: Warm the oil in a large skillet over medium heat. Add the shallot and garlic and cook for 3 to 5 minutes, until fragrant and translucent.

3. Season the shallot mixture with the cumin, paprika, salt, and black pepper and mix to combine. Cook, stirring, for 30 seconds, then remove from the heat and set aside.

4. Peel and pit and avocados, then mash the flesh in a large bowl. Add the cooled shallot mixture, along with the lemon juice and red pepper flakes, if using, and mix well to combine. Taste and add additional lemon juice, cumin, salt, and/or black or red pepper, if desired.

5. Serve immediately on the toasted bread or sweet potato "buns," with the desired toppings.

SWEET POTATO "BUNS"

1 large sweet potato, sliced crosswise into 1-inch-thick rounds

1 tablespoon avocado oil or extra-virgin olive oil

1 teaspoon fine sea salt

1. Preheat the oven to 400°F and grease a rimmed baking sheet.

2. Toss the sweet potato rounds with the oil and salt. Lay the "buns" on the baking sheet and bake for 20 minutes, then flip over and bake for another 20 minutes, until tender and golden brown. Let cool slightly before using.

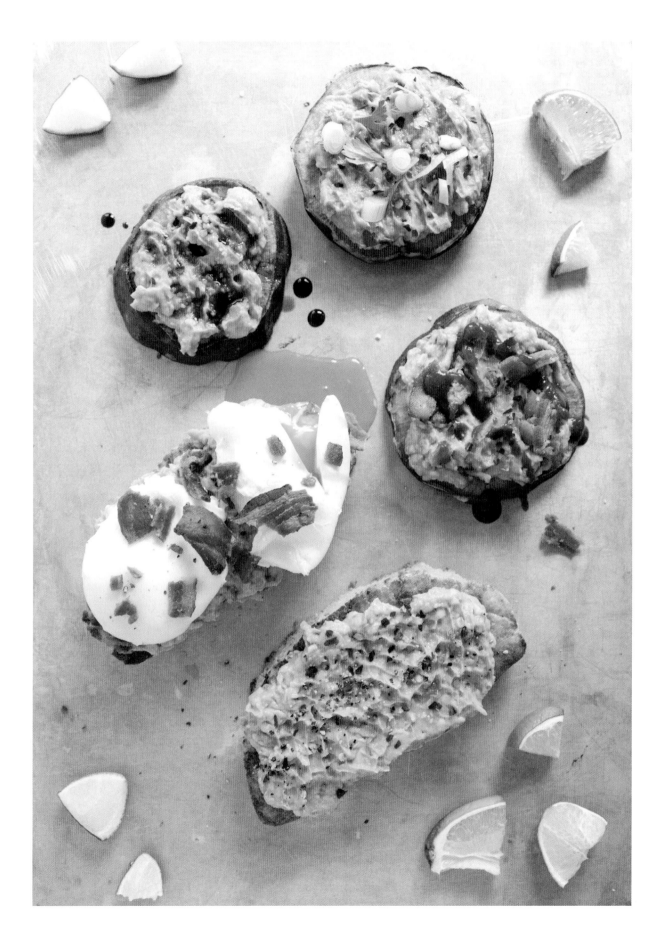

CHIA PUDDING EVERY WHICH WAY

serves 2 *prep time* 5 minutes, plus at least 3 hours to chill

EGG-FREE / NUT-FREE OPTION: use a nondairy milk that isn't made from nuts, such as coconut milk
DAIRY-FREE / PALEO-FRIENDLY / VEGAN OPTION: use maple syrup instead of honey

Chia pudding is one of my favorite non-egg breakfasts. It is packed with nutrients, has the texture of pudding (yes, please!), and is totally customizable to whatever flavor you are in the mood for! This plain version and its three variations below will give you a taste of what's possible.

ingredients:

1 cup nondairy milk of choice, homemade (page 266) or store-bought

¼ cup chia seeds

2 teaspoons honey or pure maple syrup

1 cup diced or sliced fresh fruit of choice (small berries can be left whole), for serving

directions:

1. In a container, stir together the milk, chia seeds, and honey to combine.

2. Place the chia seed mixture in the refrigerator for a minimum of 3 hours or up to 24 hours, until it has the thick texture of pudding.

3. When ready to serve, remove the pudding from the refrigerator, taste, and add more sweetener, if desired, keeping in mind the sweetness of the fruit topping. Divide the pudding between two serving cups or glasses and serve immediately, topped with the fresh fruit.

variations:

Apple Pie Pudding. In a skillet over medium heat, add 1 peeled and finely diced apple, 1½ teaspoons of water, ½ teaspoon of honey, and ¼ teaspoon of ground cinnamon and mix to combine. Cook for 5 minutes, until the apples begin to soften, then add 2 tablespoons of golden raisins and stir to combine. Remove from the heat and let cool for 5 minutes. Layer the apple pie topping with the chia pudding and serve.

Bananas Foster Pudding. In a skillet over medium heat, melt 2 tablespoons of ghee (page 350) or unsalted butter. Add ¼ cup of coconut sugar and whisk until dissolved, then add 1 teaspoon of vanilla extract and 2 sliced bananas. Cook for 2 to 4 minutes, gently stirring, then add 1 tablespoon of dark rum and/or ¼ cup of chopped raw walnuts, if desired. Cook for an additional 3 to 4 minutes, then remove from the heat and let cool for 5 minutes. Layer the banana topping with the chia pudding and serve.

Chocolate Turtle Pudding. Add 1 tablespoon of cocoa powder to the mixture in Step 1. When ready to serve, drizzle with 1 to 2 tablespoons of All-Purpose Caramel Sauce (page 360) and ¼ cup of chopped raw pecans.

notes: If you don't have time to wait, place the chia seeds, milk, and honey in a container with a lid and shake vigorously until the pudding thickens, about 5 minutes.

For a prettier presentation, try layering the pudding and fruit.

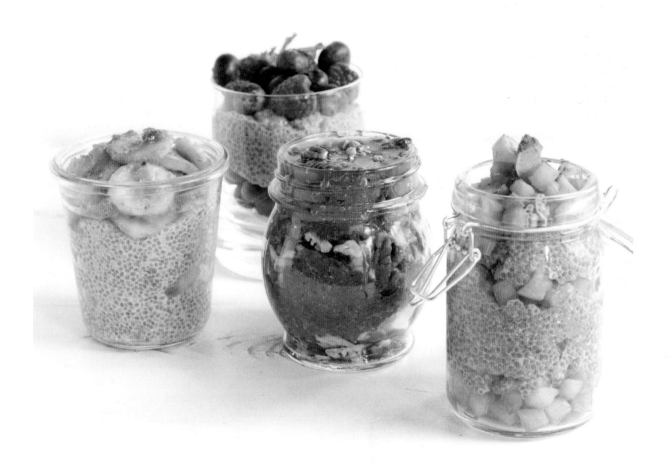

HEALING TROPICAL SMOOTHIE BOWL

serves 1 *prep time* 5 minutes

EGG-FREE / NUT-FREE OPTION: use coconut water instead of almond milk and use nut-free toppings
DAIRY-FREE / PALEO-FRIENDLY

Smoothie bowls are all the rage, and for good reason: they are heartier than the average smoothie and fun to eat. Plus, you can get creative with the toppings, using whatever you are in the mood for that day! To make this smoothie bowl extra healing, make sure to use raw honey, which has antibacterial, anti-inflammatory, and antifungal properties. A high-speed blender is ideal for making this super-thick smoothie.

ingredients:

FOR THE SMOOTHIE:

¾ cup coconut water or almond milk, homemade (page 266) or store-bought

1 cup frozen mango chunks

½ cup frozen pineapple chunks

½ banana, cut into chunks and frozen

1 tablespoon honey

1 tablespoon ground flaxseed

1 teaspoon chia seeds

Pinch of ginger powder or 1 teaspoon grated fresh ginger

Pinch of ground cinnamon

Pinch of turmeric powder

Pinch of fine sea salt

Optional: 1 scoop protein powder

TOPPING OPTIONS:

Banana slices

Bee pollen

Berries

Cacao nibs

Chia seeds

Coconut flakes

Gluten-Free Granola (page 44) or Paleo Granola (page 46)

Pepitas or other seeds of choice

Slivered almonds

directions:

1. Place all of the ingredients for the smoothie in a blender and blend until completely smooth and thick, about 30 seconds.

2. Pour the smoothie mixture into a bowl, top with the toppings of your choice, and serve immediately.

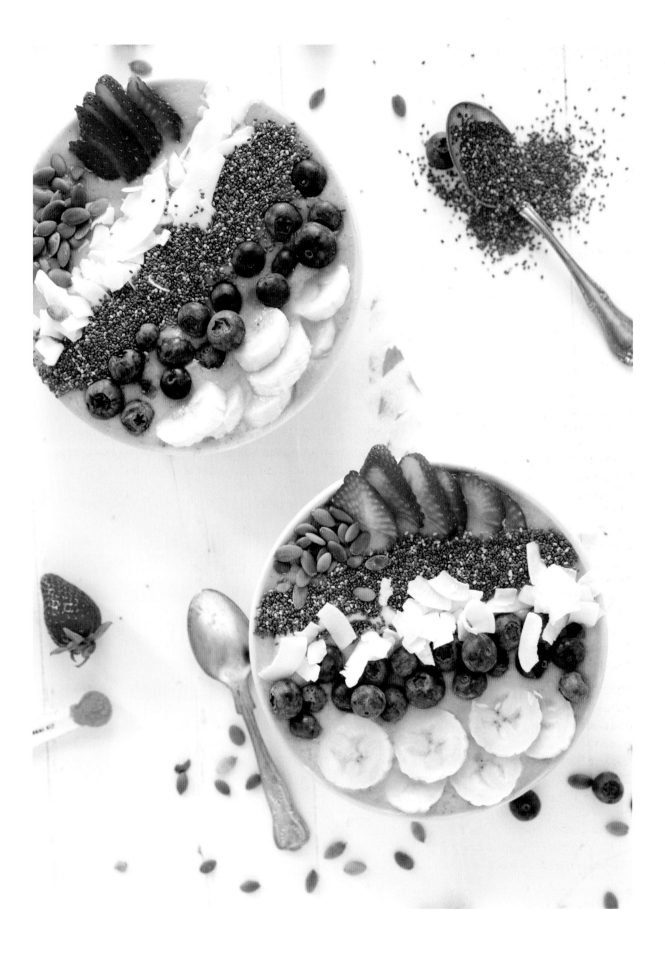

SHAKSHUKA

serves 2   *prep time* 8 minutes   *cook time* 15 minutes

NUT-FREE / DAIRY-FREE OPTION: use olive oil for the pan
PALEO-FRIENDLY OPTION: **use olive oil for the pan**

Shakshuka is one of my favorite hearty, flavor-packed breakfasts. With eggs, tomato sauce, and tons of Moroccan-inspired flavor, this dish is perfect for breakfast for dinner or a weekend brunch!

ingredients:

1 tablespoon unsalted butter or extra-virgin olive oil

1 onion, sliced

1 clove garlic, minced

1 small red bell pepper, sliced

1 packed cup fresh spinach

1 (14½-ounce) can diced tomatoes

1 teaspoon chili powder

½ teaspoon ground cumin

½ teaspoon paprika

Optional: ¼ teaspoon cayenne pepper, or more to taste

Optional: ¼ teaspoon turmeric powder

Pinch of freshly ground black pepper

½ teaspoon fine sea salt

4 large eggs

FOR GARNISH:

Chopped fresh flat-leaf parsley

Cracked black pepper

Red pepper flakes

directions:

1. Heat the butter in a large skillet over medium heat. Add the onion, garlic, and bell pepper and cook for 5 minutes, until the mixture is fragrant and the onion and pepper have begun to soften.

2. Add the spinach and sauté for 1 minute, until wilted. Add the tomatoes, spices, and salt and mix to combine.

3. Gently create four small wells in the sauce mixture and crack the eggs into the wells. Cook until the whites are opaque and the yolks reach your desired doneness. For quicker cooking, cover the skillet for 2 to 3 minutes, until the eggs are set.

4. Garnish with chopped parsley, cracked black pepper, and red pepper flakes and serve.

variation:

Meaty Shakshuka. Add 2 cooked and chopped spicy chicken sausages along with the spinach in Step 2.

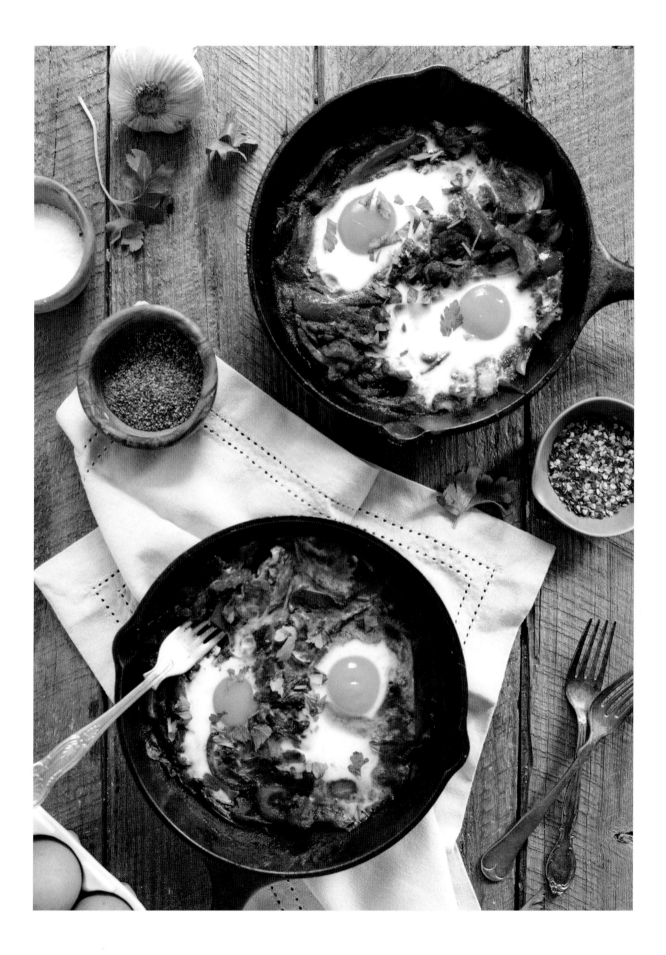

EGGS ALL THE WAYS

POACHED

directions:

1. Bring about 4 inches (or 2 cups) of water to a simmer in a medium-sized saucepan or pot and add 1 tablespoon of white vinegar.

2. Crack an egg into a small bowl or ramekin.

3. Using a spoon, stir the water in a circular motion until you create a whirlpool effect in the center. Gently slide the egg into the center of that whirlpool.

4. Gently cook the egg for 5 to 6 minutes, then use a slotted spoon to remove it to a plate. Repeat with additional eggs as desired.

HARD-BOILED

These should really be called "hard-cooked" rather than "hard-boiled" because the eggs are steamed. I prefer this cooking method because it ensures even, gentle cooking. The eggs come out perfect, without rubbery whites, and a quick plunge in an ice bath makes peeling easier.

directions:

1. Place 1 inch of water in a large pot. Place a steamer basket in the pot. Cover the pot and bring the water to a boil.

2. Once boiling, add eggs to the steamer basket, cover, and let steam for 11 minutes.

3. Remove the eggs and place them directly in a bowl of ice water. When chilled, peel and enjoy!

variation: **Soft-Cooked Eggs.** Follow the instructions above, but reduce the steaming time to 6 minutes.

SCRAMBLED

directions:

1. In a bowl, whisk the eggs with a pinch of salt and pepper until blended.

2. For 3 to 5 eggs, heat 1 tablespoon of butter in a medium-sized skillet over medium heat until hot.

3. Pour in the eggs. As they begin to set, gently pull the eggs across the pan with a spatula to form large, soft clumps or curds. Reduce the heat to low and fold the curds over on themselves.

4. When there is no more liquidy egg left in the pan, transfer the eggs to a plate and serve.

FRIED, SUNNY-SIDE UP

directions:

1. Heat 1 tablespoon of butter in a skillet (preferably a well-seasoned cast-iron one) over medium heat and swirl it around to coat until somewhat hot.

2. Crack in an egg and reduce the heat to medium-low. After about 30 seconds, cover the skillet to cook the top of the egg. Remove it from the pan when the yolk is cooked to your liking.

3. Transfer to a plate and enjoy.

OMELET

directions:

1. If making a filled omelet, have 1 cup of filling prepared and at the ready before beginning to make the omelet.

2. Heat 1 tablespoon of butter in a medium-sized skillet over medium heat until hot.

3. In a bowl, whisk 3 eggs with a pinch each of salt and pepper until blended.

4. Pour in the eggs. They should begin to set immediately.

5. Using a rubber spatula, gently lift the cooked sections of egg along the edge of the skillet, then tilt the skillet to allow uncooked, liquidy egg to run underneath the lifted section and reach the hot skillet.

6. When the top of the eggs has thickened and set but is still creamy, spread your filling of choice across half of the omelet.

7. Using the spatula or a turner, lift and fold the unfilled side over the filled side of the omelet, then slide onto a plate and serve.

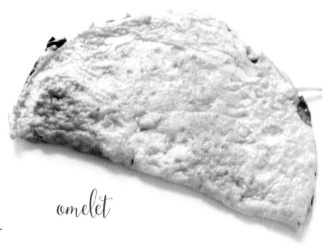

omelet

hard-boiled egg

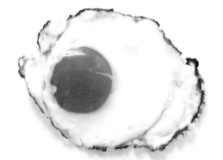

fried egg

scrambled eggs

poached egg

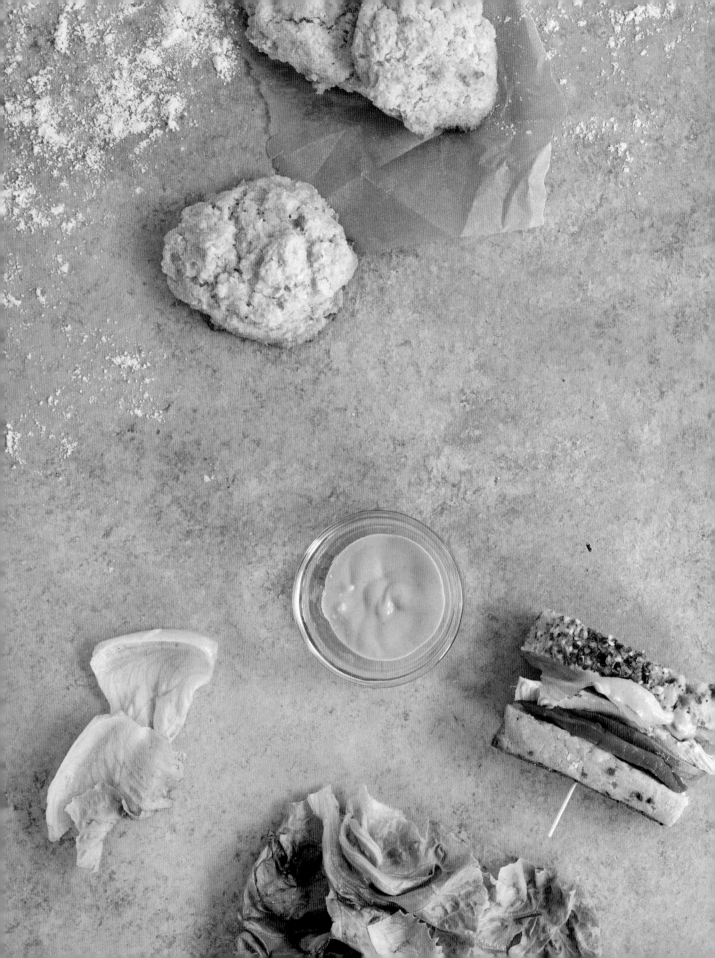

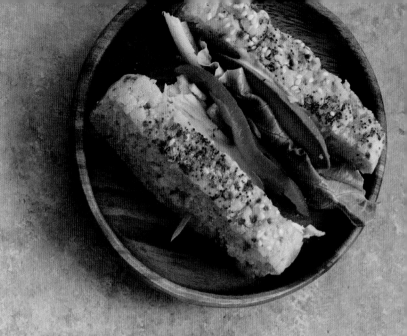

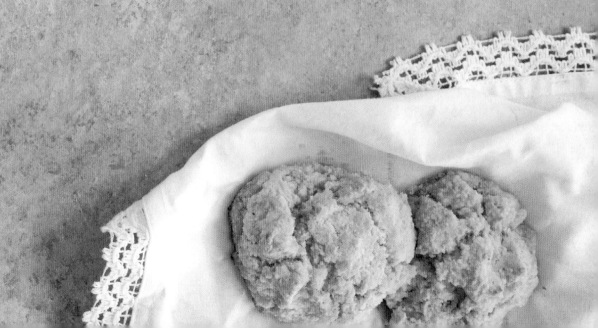

chapter 2

BREADS, CRUSTS
& CRACKERS

TART CRUST

makes one 9-inch tart crust, four 4½-inch tart crusts, or one 9-inch single pie crust
prep time 15 minutes, plus time to chill dough *cook time* 10 minutes

This all-purpose crust can be used for everything from savory galettes and quiches to dessert tarts and pies. It's versatile, buttery, and delicious!

ingredients:

1 cup blanched almond flour
1 cup tapioca flour
½ teaspoon fine sea salt
½ cup (1 stick) cold unsalted butter, cubed
1 large egg
1 teaspoon honey

note: Do not freeze the dough. Store it in the refrigerator for up to 5 days until ready to use.

directions:

1. In a food processor, pulse the almond flour, tapioca flour, and salt. Add the cubed cold butter and pulse until it starts to meld with the flour and form a dough. Add the egg and honey and pulse until a ball of dough forms. It will be slightly sticky.

2. Pat the dough ball into a thick disc, wrap it in plastic wrap, and place it in the refrigerator to chill. If making a tart or galette, leave the dough in the fridge for a minimum of 1 hour; if making a pie, let it chill overnight.

3. When ready to use the dough, preheat the oven to 350°F and remove the dough from the refrigerator. If making a tart, press the dough into a greased 9-inch tart pan or divide the dough into 4 equal portions and press them into 4 greased small tart pans; if making a pie, roll out the dough between two sheets of parchment paper into a circle about 13 inches in diameter and press it into a 9-inch pie pan.

4. Par-bake the crust(s) for 10 minutes before adding the desired fillings.

use in:

52
Breakfast Galette

56
Quiche

290
Pear Tartlets

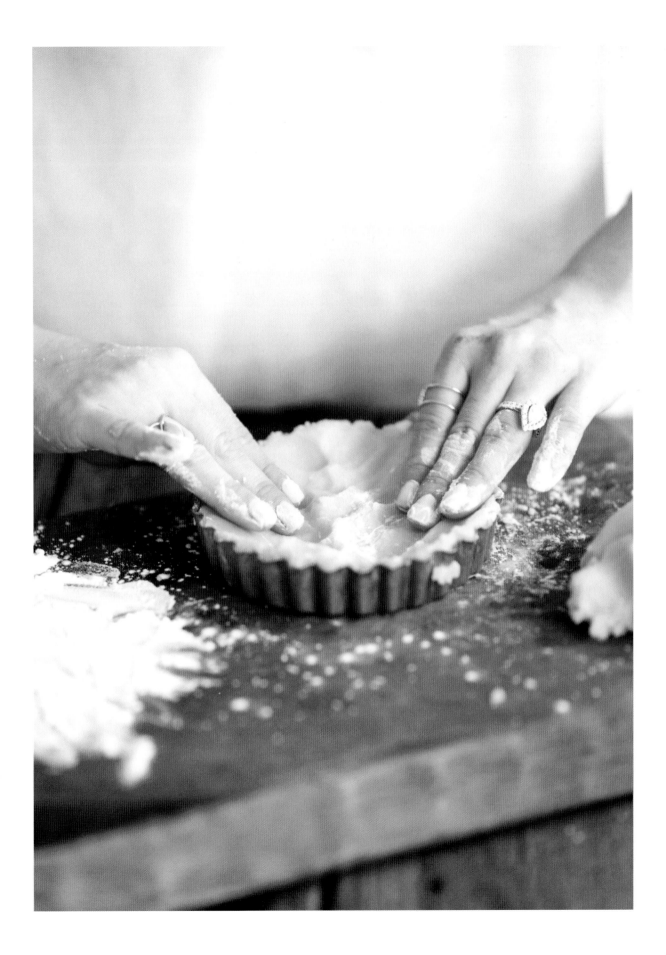

TORTILLAS

makes six 6-inch tortillas   *prep time* 5 minutes   *cook time* 12 minutes

....

NUT-FREE OPTION: use a nondairy milk that isn't made from nuts, such as coconut milk
PALEO-FRIENDLY OPTION: use ghee instead of butter

....

I am a *huge* fan of Mexican cuisine and all things tortilla, so it was important to me to create wonderful tortillas that would meet all of your needs. Tacos, enchiladas, crepes, tostadas . . . you name it, these tortillas can do it!

ingredients:

½ cup tapioca flour

2 tablespoons coconut flour

1 teaspoon baking soda

¼ teaspoon fine sea salt

2 large eggs

½ cup unsweetened, unflavored nondairy milk of choice, home-made (page 266) or store-bought

1 tablespoon unsalted butter or ghee (page 350), melted, plus more for the pan

directions:

1. In a bowl, mix together the tapioca flour, coconut flour, baking soda, and salt until well blended. Add the eggs, milk, and melted butter and whisk until no lumps remain. The mixture should resemble pancake batter.

2. Place a large sauté pan over medium heat and add enough butter to coat the pan. Pour about 3 tablespoons of the batter into the center of the pan to create a 6-inch tortilla. Cook for 1 minute per side, until slightly golden. Repeat with the remaining batter, adding more butter to the pan after making each tortilla.

3. The tortillas are best if eaten right away, but will keep for up to 2 days in the refrigerator or longer in the freezer. Reheat in a skillet before using.

variations:

Taco Shells. Remove a rack from the oven. Preheat the oven to 375°F. After removing the tortillas from the skillet in Step 2, drape them over two of the metal grates of the oven rack so they hang downward, then place the rack in the center of the heated oven. Bake for 10 to 15 minutes, until the shells are golden brown and hold their shape. They are best if eaten right away, but will keep for up to 2 days. To reheat, warm in the oven for 5 minutes.

Tostadas. Preheat the oven to 375°F. After removing the tortillas from the skillet in Step 2, place them on a parchment paper–lined baking sheet and bake for 10 minutes, then flip them over and continue to bake until toasted and crispy, about 10 more minutes. They are best if eaten right away, but will keep for up to 2 days. To reheat, warm in the oven for 5 minutes.

use in:

Crepes

Chicken Enchiladas

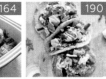

Fish Tacos

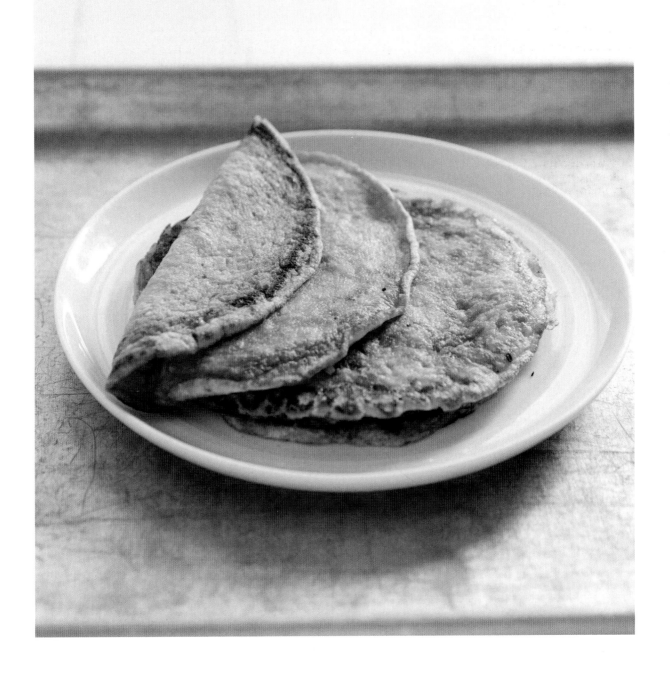

BUTTERY DROP BISCUITS

makes 6 biscuits   *prep time* 10 minutes   *cook time* 15 minutes

Say hello to the ultimate brunch, lunch, or dinner biscuit that has all of the flaky, buttery goodness you would want!

ingredients:

1 cup sifted blanched almond flour

½ cup tapioca flour

2 tablespoons coconut flour

1 teaspoon baking powder

¼ teaspoon fine sea salt

3 tablespoons cold unsalted butter

¼ cup unsweetened applesauce

1 large egg

directions:

1. Preheat the oven to 350°F and grease a baking sheet.

2. In a bowl, stir together the almond flour, tapioca flour, coconut flour, baking powder, and salt until well blended.

3. Add the butter and mix until the butter is well combined with the flour mixture. Add the applesauce and egg and mix until a smooth dough forms.

4. Using your hands, roll the dough into 6 balls, each about 2½ inches in diameter. Place the dough balls on the baking sheet, about 1 inch apart. Bake for 15 minutes, or until golden and crusty all around and firm to the touch, with no soft dough remaining in the center.

5. Store leftover biscuits in the refrigerator for up to 5 days. Reheat in the oven or toaster oven for 5 minutes.

variations:

Bit of Honey Biscuits. For slightly sweet biscuits, add 2 teaspoons of honey along with the applesauce and egg in Step 3.

Pumpkin Biscuits. Substitute pumpkin puree for the applesauce.

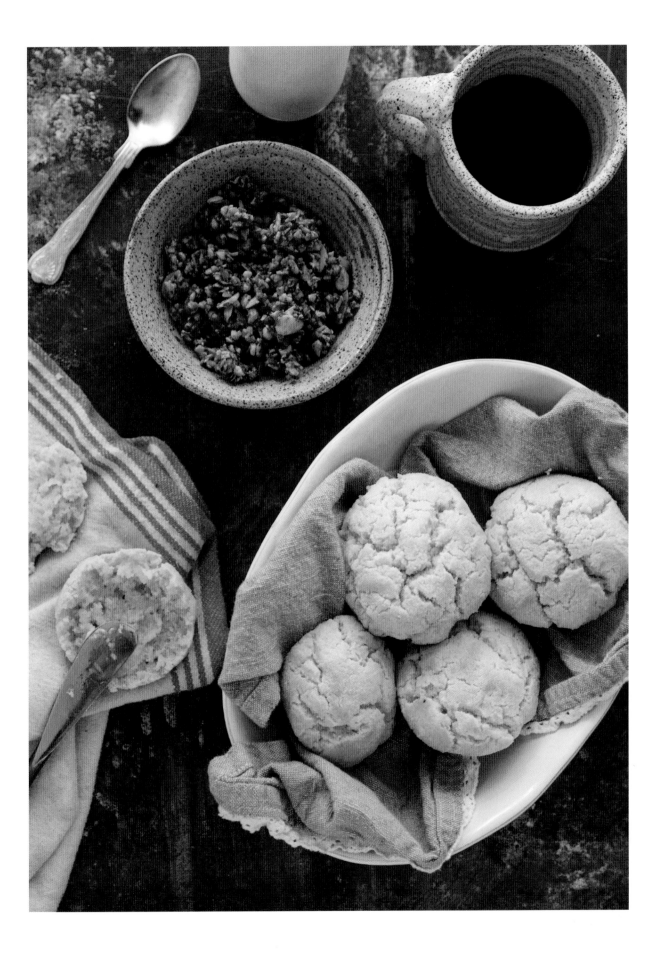

PIZZA CRUST

makes one thicker-crust pizza, about 9 by 12 inches, or one thin-crust pizza, about 10 by 14 inches
prep time 10 minutes   *cook time* 10 minutes to par-bake, 20 minutes to fully bake

....

NUT-FREE / DAIRY-FREE / PALEO-FRIENDLY

....

I made you a pizza crust that is ideal for any pizza party! Whether that means a Friday night dinner for two, a family pizza night, or a get-together with friends, this crust is your answer. You see, it can be made Chicago deep-dish style, New York thin-crust style, or even as a flatbread appetizer!

ingredients:

1 cup tapioca flour

3 tablespoons coconut flour

3 tablespoons ground flax meal

1 teaspoon baking powder

½ teaspoon fine sea salt

1 large egg

⅓ cup palm shortening

⅓ cup warm water

variations:

Mini Deep-Dish Pizzas. Grease 10 wells of a standard 12-cup muffin tin. After completing Step 4, use your hands to separate the dough into ten 1½-inch balls. Press the dough balls into the bottoms of the greased muffin cups. Par-bake for 10 minutes, then add sauce and toppings and bake for an additional 7 to 10 minutes, until golden brown. *Makes 10 mini pizzas.*

Flatbread. In Step 5, roll the dough into a very thin rectangle, ¼ to ⅓ inch thick. Remove the top piece of parchment paper and bake for 5 minutes. Then add sauce and toppings and bake for an additional 10 minutes, until golden brown. *Makes one 12 by 6-inch flatbread.*

directions:

1. Preheat the oven to 350°F and line a baking sheet with parchment paper.

2. In a bowl, combine the tapioca flour, coconut flour, flax meal, baking powder, and salt until well blended.

3. Add the egg and shortening and mix with a wooden spoon to combine. Add the warm water and mix until the dough is smooth but somewhat sticky.

4. Form the dough into a ball. If it's too sticky, wet your hands with water or a touch of oil first. (If not using the dough right away, wrap it in plastic wrap and store it in the refrigerator for up to 3 days.)

5. Place the ball of dough on the lined baking sheet and cover it with an additional piece of parchment paper. Using a rolling pin, gently roll out the dough into a circle or rectangle that is between ½ and ¾ inch thick for a thicker-crust pizza or between ⅓ and ½ inch thick for a thin-crust pizza. (Don't go thinner than ⅓ inch; if you roll it out too thin, it'll be crunchy like flatbread.)

6. Remove the top piece of parchment paper and par-bake for 10 minutes for a thicker crust or 8 minutes for a thin crust. Remove from the oven, add the sauce and toppings of your choice, and then return the pizza to the oven to bake for an additional 10 minutes, until golden brown.

use in:

176
BBQ Chicken Pizza

102
Prosciutto Flatbread with Grilled Peaches & Caramelized Onions

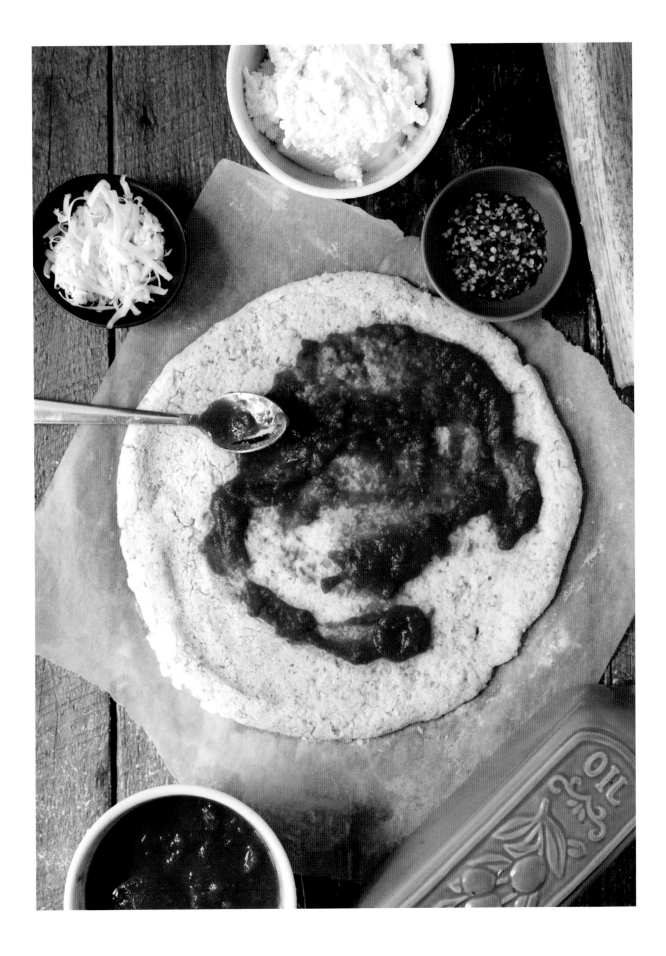

CRACKERS

makes about 30 crackers   *prep time* 5 minutes   *cook time* 20 minutes

....

DAIRY-FREE OPTION: **use oil instead of butter or ghee**
PALEO-FRIENDLY OPTION: **use ghee or oil instead of butter**

....

These easy-breezy homemade crackers can be made in different flavors to suit any occasion—see variations below!

ingredients:

1 cup blanched almond flour

¼ cup ground flax meal

1 teaspoon fine sea salt

1 large egg

2 tablespoons unsalted butter, ghee (page 350), or oil of choice

directions:

1. Preheat the oven to 300°F and position an oven rack in the center of the oven. Line a baking sheet with parchment paper.

2. In a mixing bowl, combine all of the ingredients and mix until completely combined. Form the dough into a ball.

3. Place the ball of dough in the center of the lined baking sheet and cover with a second piece of parchment paper. Using a rolling pin, roll out the dough into a rectangle that's approximately ⅛ inch thick.

4. Using a pizza cutter, slice the dough into squares. If you end up with leftover scraps of dough, gather them up and repeat Steps 3 and 4.

5. Bake for 15 to 20 minutes, until golden brown and crispy, watching to avoid burning. Store the crackers in a resealable plastic bag or sealed container in the pantry for up to 3 days.

variations:

Sea Salt Crackers. Before baking, sprinkle the crackers with 1 teaspoon of coarse sea salt.

Garlic and Herb Crackers. In Step 2, mix in 1 teaspoon of garlic powder, ½ teaspoon of dried Italian seasoning, and ½ teaspoon of dried rosemary leaves. Before baking, top the crackers with additional rosemary.

Everything Crackers. Before baking, sprinkle the crackers with 1 teaspoon of coarse sea salt, 1 teaspoon of sesame seeds, ½ teaspoon of garlic granules, and ½ teaspoon of onion granules.

Graham Crackers. In Step 2, omit the salt, replace the butter with 2 tablespoons of honey, and mix in 1 tablespoon of coconut sugar and 1 teaspoon of ground cinnamon. Before baking, sprinkle the crackers with additional coconut sugar and cinnamon.

To make **graham cracker crumbs** for use in S'mores Pots de Crème (page 280) or Caribbean Dessert Parfaits (page 282), let the crackers cool completely, then pulse a few times in a food processor or blender, until fine. Add 2 teaspoons of coconut sugar to the crumbs and mix to combine. *Makes about 1 cup of graham cracker crumbs.*

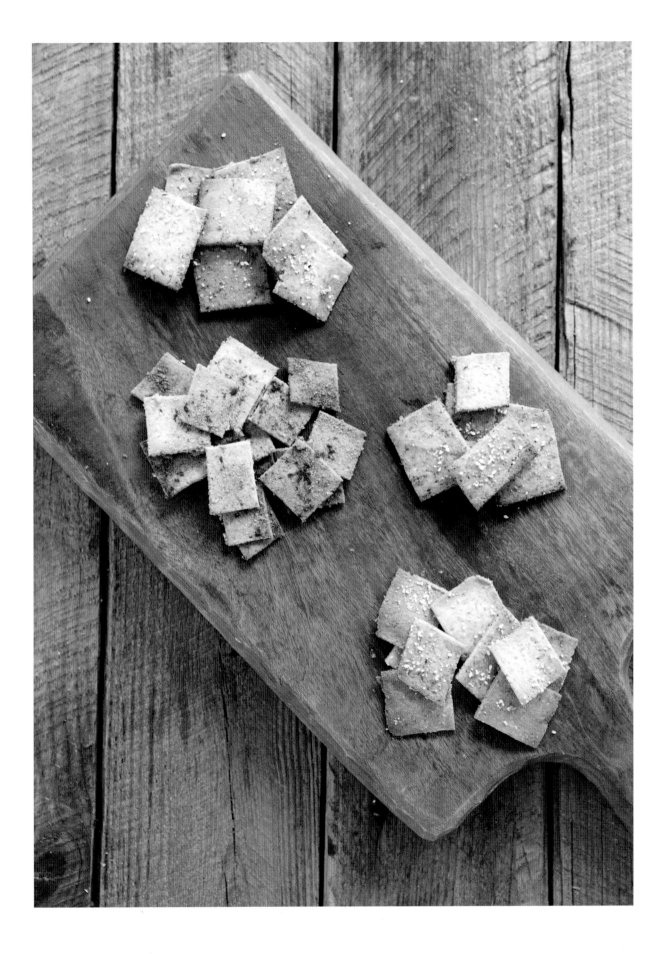

ALL-PURPOSE SANDWICH BREAD

makes one 8½ by 4½-inch loaf, 8 buns, or one 8-inch square pan of focaccia-style sandwich bread *prep time* 5 minutes *cook time* 25 minutes

DAIRY-FREE / PALEO-FRIENDLY

This sandwich bread is loved by tons of my readers across the Internet! It really has the perfect texture, and one that you wouldn't expect from a gluten-free, grain-free, and yeast-free bread. It is perfect for a sandwich or a burger or a slice of toast with nut butter and jam (page 330)—simply anything and everything!

ingredients:

1 cup sifted blanched almond flour
1 cup tapioca flour
1 teaspoon baking powder
½ teaspoon fine sea salt
4 large eggs
½ cup unsweetened applesauce

SPECIAL EQUIPMENT
(OPTIONAL, FOR MAKING BUNS):
Baking ring molds

variation:

"Everything" Bread. Before baking, sprinkle the top with 1 teaspoon of dried minced onion, 1 teaspoon of dried minced garlic, ½ teaspoon of white sesame seeds, ½ teaspoon of black sesame seeds, ½ teaspoon of poppy seeds, and a pinch of coarse sea salt.

directions:

1. Preheat the oven to 350°F.

2. In a bowl, combine the almond flour, tapioca flour, baking powder, and salt until well blended.

3. Mix in the eggs and applesauce and whisk until no clumps remain. The batter will be thick.

4. *To make a loaf*, pour the batter into a greased 8½ by 4½-inch loaf pan.

   To make buns, line a baking sheet with parchment paper. Grease the insides of eight 3½-inch baking ring molds and place them on the baking sheet. Pour the batter evenly into the molds.

   To make focaccia-style sandwich bread, pour the batter into a greased 8-inch square baking pan.

5. Bake for 25 to 30 minutes, until the top is golden and a toothpick inserted in the middle comes out clean.

6. Let cool in the pan, then slice and serve. Store leftover bread in the refrigerator for up to 4 days or in the freezer for up to several months.

use in:

Croutons
82

French Toast Sticks
38

Avocado Toast
58

New England Lobster Rolls
196

All-American Burgers
198

notes: This bread rises about two-thirds of the way up in the loaf pan, resulting in slices that are about two-thirds as tall as standard-size slices of sandwich bread. When I make this bread focaccia-style in an 8-inch square pan, I cut it into squares and then cut the squares horizontally through the middle to create a "top" and a "bottom" for a sandwich.

If you don't have baking ring molds, you can make buns using mason jar lids.

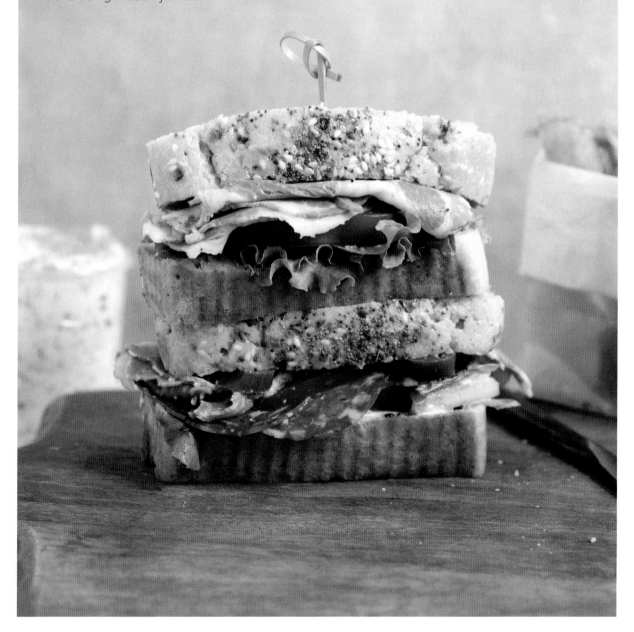

CROUTONS

makes 2 cups *prep time* 5 minutes (not including bread) *cook time* 50 minutes

DAIRY-FREE / PALEO-FRIENDLY

Croutons are the salad topping that I missed oh-so-much when I cleaned up my diet. No more missing croutons now, though! These crispy, easy-to-make beauties are the real deal. And they will transform your next Caesar salad.

ingredients:

1 batch All-Purpose Sandwich Bread (page 80), cut into cubes

directions:

1. Preheat the oven to 225°F.

2. Place the bread cubes on a rimmed baking sheet and bake for 45 to 50 minutes, until golden brown, dried out, and completely hard.

3. Store the croutons in a sealed container in the pantry for up to 2 days or in the refrigerator for up to 1 week.

variation:

Garlic Croutons. In a small saucepan over medium heat, heat 1 tablespoon of butter with 2 cloves of minced garlic and ½ teaspoon of fine sea salt. Cook for 1 minute, then add the bread cubes and toss to coat. Continue with Step 1.

use in:

Curry Butternut Squash Soup

Kale Caesar Salad

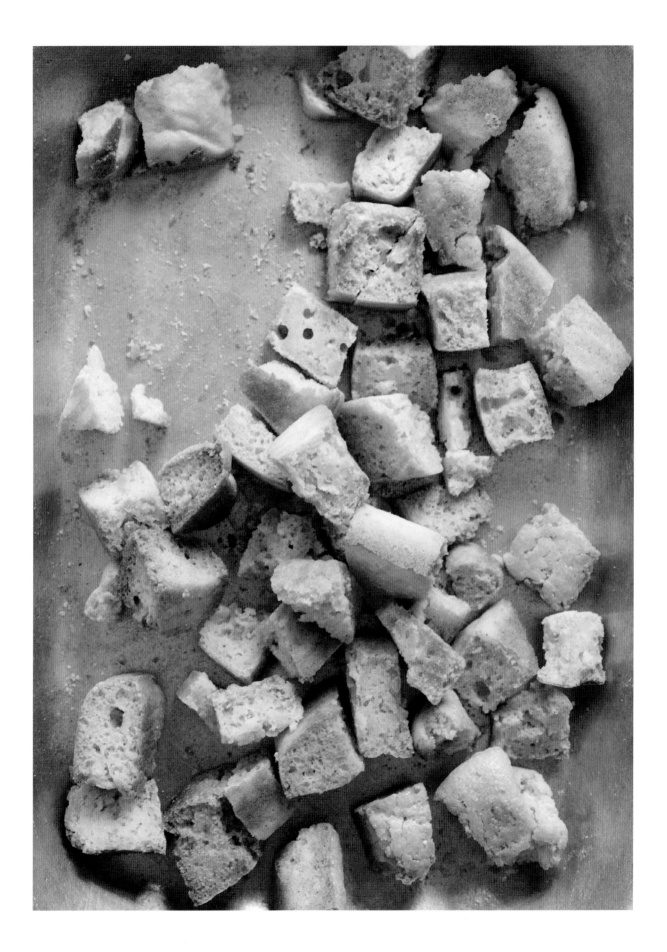

CLASSIC FOCACCIA

makes one 8-inch square pan (9 to 12 slices)   *prep time* 10 minutes
cook time 25 minutes

DAIRY-FREE / PALEO-FRIENDLY

Growing up, the bread basket was one of my favorite parts of a dinner out—especially when the basket was filled with warm, flavorful focaccia. In fact, when I decided to change my diet, my husband, Mike, was in awe that I was able to resist the good ol' bread basket! Now I can make my very own delicious focaccia using my sandwich bread recipe as the base and not worry about how I'll feel afterward.

ingredients:

1 cup sifted blanched almond flour

1 cup tapioca flour

1 teaspoon baking powder

½ teaspoon fine sea salt

4 large eggs

½ cup unsweetened applesauce

FOR THE TOPPINGS:

3 cloves garlic, minced

½ small white onion, sliced thin

⅓ cup crushed tomatoes or finely diced fresh tomatoes

1 tablespoon extra-virgin olive oil

1 teaspoon Italian seasoning

1 teaspoon dried rosemary leaves

1 teaspoon fine sea salt

Pinch of red pepper flakes, or more as desired

directions:

1. Preheat the oven to 350°F. Grease an 8-inch square baking pan.

2. In a bowl, combine the almond flour, tapioca flour, baking powder, and salt until well blended. Whisk in the eggs and applesauce until no clumps remain. You will have a thick batter.

3. Pour the batter into the greased baking pan and smooth the top. Sprinkle on the toppings, evenly distributing them across the top of the batter.

4. Bake for 25 minutes, or until the bread is golden brown and the onions on top are cooked down and shriveled. Cut into squares and serve hot. Store leftovers in the refrigerator for up to 3 days.

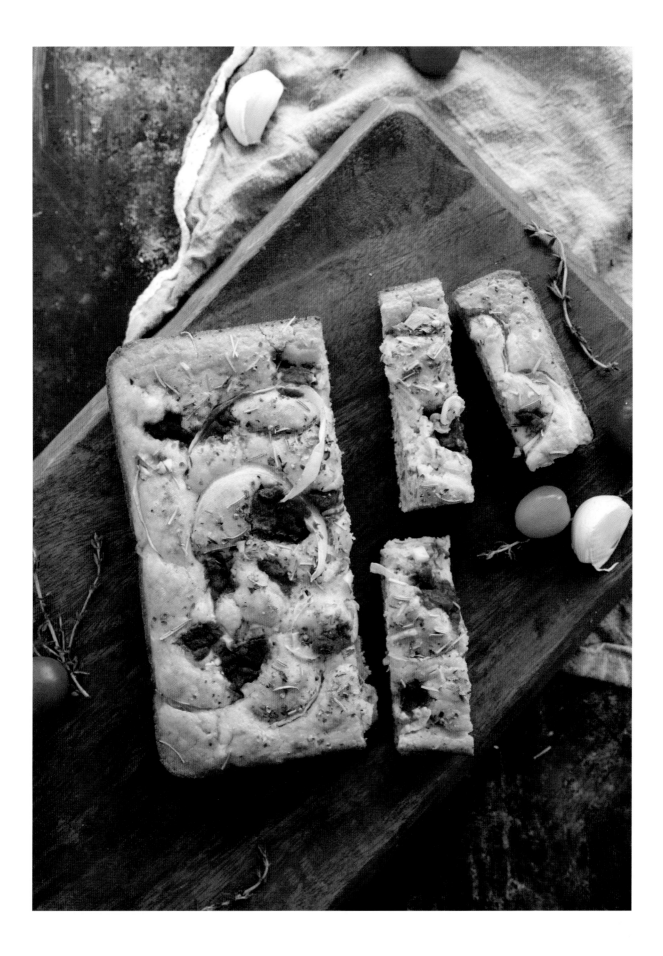

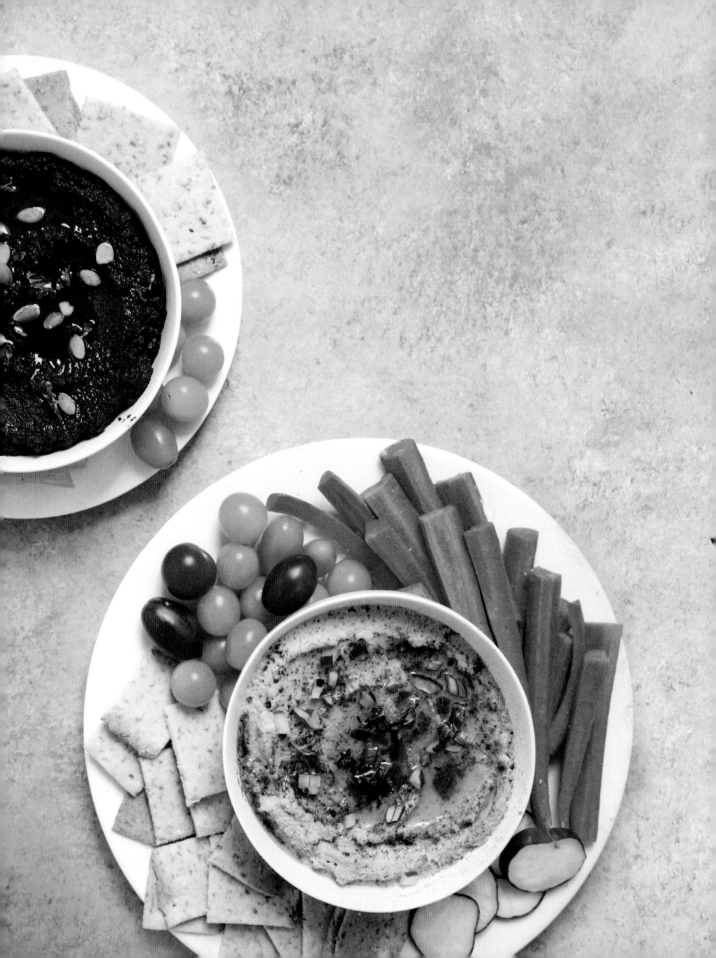

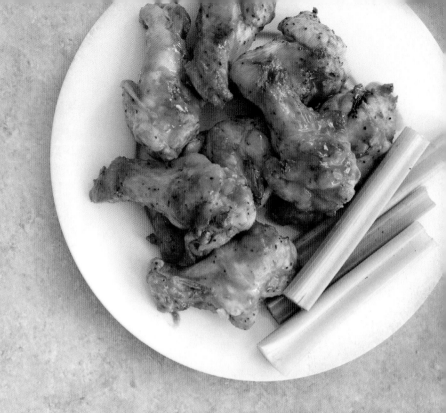

chapter 3

LITTLE BITES:
appetizers for every gathering

LEXI'S BEST GUACAMOLE

serves 4 to 6 | *prep time* 10 minutes

EGG-FREE / NUT-FREE / DAIRY-FREE / PALEO-FRIENDLY / VEGAN

If you have followed my blog for some time, then you know it's no secret that I love Mexican cuisine. I love it all, but I *really* love guacamole—as a dip and on salads, fajitas, tacos . . . anything! I felt it was my duty to share with you in this book two of my favorite simple guacamole recipes—a classic version and a pineapple jalapeño version—since both go down pretty regularly in my home.

ingredients:

4 ripe avocados

¼ cup chopped cilantro leaves

1 tablespoon lime juice

½ teaspoon garlic powder

½ teaspoon fine sea salt

Optional: ¼ cup finely chopped red onion

Optional: ¼ cup chopped cherry tomatoes

Optional: Pinch of red pepper flakes

directions:

1. Cut the avocados in half and remove the pits, then scrape the flesh into a large bowl.

2. Mash the avocados roughly with a fork, then add the cilantro, lime juice, garlic powder, and salt. If desired, add the optional red onion, cherry tomatoes, and/or red pepper flakes. Mash until the guacamole reaches your desired texture—make it smooth or leave it a little chunky. Taste and add more salt, if desired.

3. Serve immediately. If storing leftovers, they will keep for up to 1 day. To minimize browning, sprinkle with additional lime juice and cover tightly with plastic wrap, placing the wrap directly on the surface of the guacamole. Mix before serving.

variation:

Pineapple Jalapeño Guacamole. After you've given the avocados an initial mash in Step 2, mix in ⅓ cup of finely chopped fresh pineapple and 1 finely chopped jalapeño pepper. If you like your guac a tad less spicy, remove and discard some of the seeds from the jalapeño before chopping it.

serve with:

Chicken Fajita Salad

Homemade Crackers

Fresh vegetable slices

Plantain chips

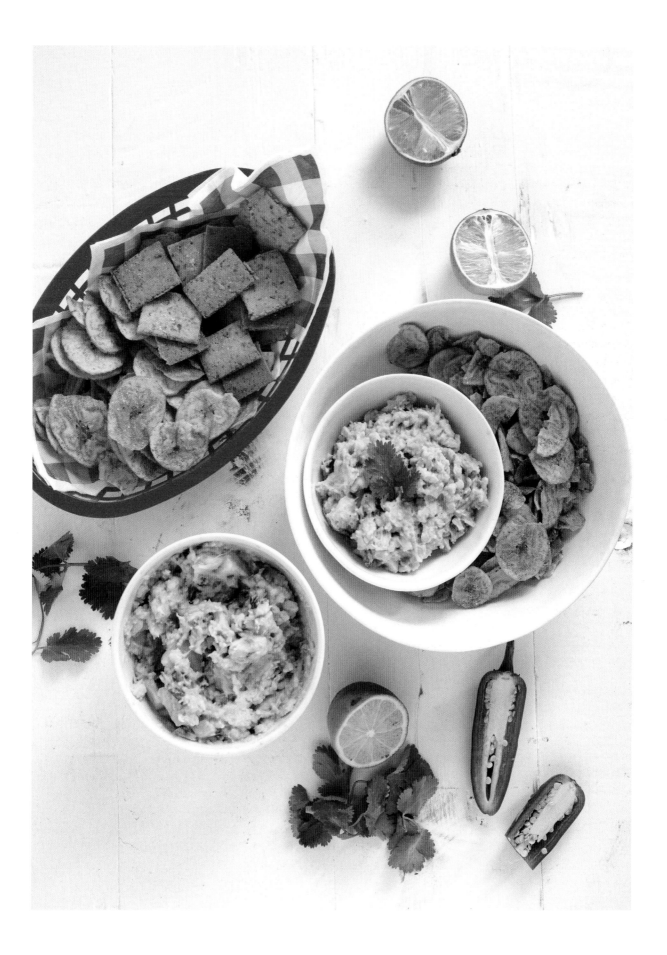

GARLIC ROASTED CAULIFLOWER NO-BEAN HUMMUS

serves 4 *prep time* 20 minutes *cook time* 40 minutes

EGG-FREE / NUT-FREE / DAIRY-FREE / PALEO-FRIENDLY / VEGAN

ingredients:

5 to 6 cups cauliflower florets
(1 medium head cauliflower)

2 tablespoons extra-virgin olive oil,
divided, plus more for garnish

¼ cup tahini

Juice of ½ lemon

1 small clove garlic, roughly chopped

½ teaspoon fine sea salt

Pinch of black pepper

FOR GARNISH:

Chopped fresh flat-leaf parsley

Chopped red onion

Paprika

Coarse sea salt

directions:

1. Preheat the oven to 375°F. Line a rimmed baking sheet with parchment paper.

2. Toss the cauliflower florets with 1 tablespoon of the olive oil and spread out on the prepared baking sheet. Roast until fork-tender, about 40 minutes.

3. Put the roasted cauliflower in a food processor or high-speed blender. Add the remaining tablespoon of olive oil along with the rest of the hummus ingredients. Pulse until smooth, 2 to 3 minutes, scraping down the sides as needed. Taste and add more salt, if desired.

4. Garnish as desired and serve with homemade crackers (page 78) and/or sliced veggies.

SWEET BEET NO-BEAN HUMMUS

serves 4 *prep time* 10 minutes *cook time* 45 minutes to 1 hour

EGG-FREE / NUT-FREE / DAIRY-FREE / PALEO-FRIENDLY / VEGAN OPTION: use maple syrup instead of honey

ingredients:

5 medium beets (about 1 pound),
preferably with greens

¼ cup tahini

1½ tablespoons honey

1 tablespoon extra-virgin olive oil

1 tablespoon water

½ teaspoon fine sea salt

Pinch of black pepper

FOR GARNISH:

Extra-virgin olive oil

Raw or roasted pepitas

Optional: Finely chopped beet
greens (reserved from above)

directions:

1. Preheat the oven to 375°F.

2. Cut off the bottoms and tops of the beets, then peel and dice the beets. If they came with greens, reserve them for garnish, if desired. Place the beets in an 8-inch square baking dish. Add 2 tablespoons of water, cover with foil, and bake for 45 minutes to 1 hour, until fork-tender.

3. Remove the beets with a slotted spoon, allowing the excess water to drip back into the pan, and place in a food processor or high-speed blender. Add the rest of the hummus ingredients and pulse until smooth, about 3 minutes, scraping down the sides as needed. Taste and add more salt, if desired.

4. Garnish as desired and serve with homemade crackers (page 78) and/or sliced veggies.

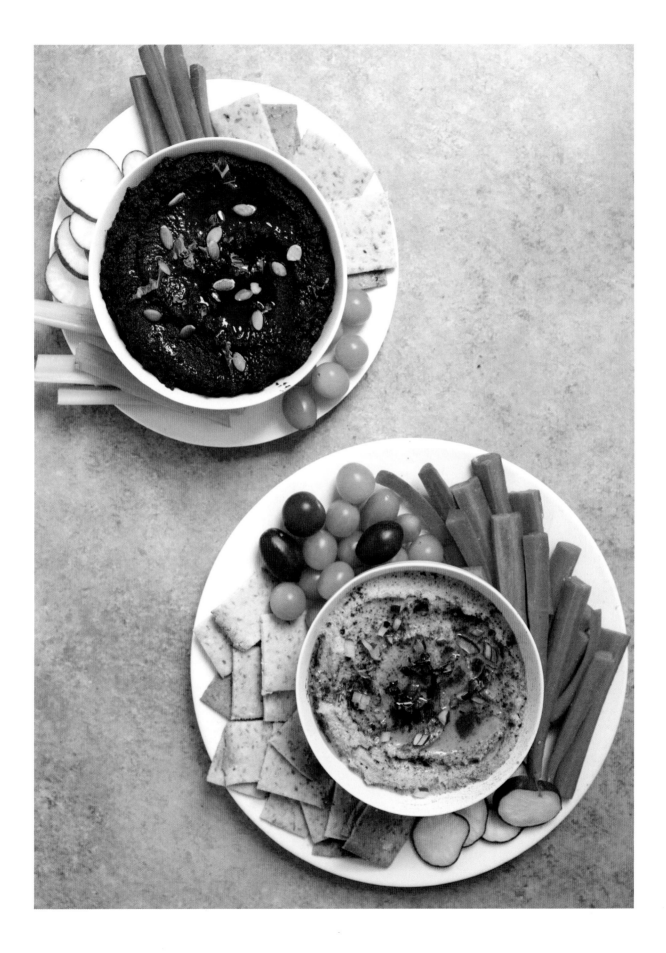

THE BEST SHRIMP COCKTAIL

serves 4 to 6   *prep time* 15 minutes   *cook time* 3 minutes

EGG-FREE / NUT-FREE / DAIRY-FREE / PALEO-FRIENDLY

This delicious go-to appetizer can seem both simple and daunting: simple because it contains just a few ingredients and requires little or no cooking, and daunting because it's difficult to re-create restaurant-quality shrimp cocktail at home. Or at least it used to be! Using my easy method, you can have restaurant-style shrimp cocktail any night of the week.

ingredients:

FOR THE COCKTAIL SAUCE (MAKES ABOUT ¾ CUP):

½ cup ketchup, homemade (page 342) or store-bought

¼ cup prepared horseradish, homemade (page 346) or store-bought

2 teaspoons lemon juice

Optional: 1 teaspoon chili paste

½ teaspoon Tabasco sauce or hot sauce of choice, or more as desired

¼ teaspoon freshly ground black pepper, or more as desired

Juice of 1 lemon

2 bay leaves

1 tablespoon whole black peppercorns

1 teaspoon fine sea salt

1 pound large shrimp, deveined (leave shells on) (see notes)

1 lemon, sliced into wedges, for serving

directions:

1.   Make the cocktail sauce: Stir together all of the sauce ingredients in a bowl. Taste and season with more black pepper and/or hot sauce, if desired. Store in an airtight container in the refrigerator until ready to serve.

2.   Prepare the shrimp: Fill a large pot with cold water. Add the lemon juice, bay leaves, peppercorns, and salt and bring to a boil over high heat. Drop the shrimp into the boiling water and turn off the heat. Cook the shrimp, stirring occasionally, until they turn pink and curl, 2 to 3 minutes.

3.   Drain the shrimp and place in a bowl of ice-cold water to cool to room temperature, then drain and peel them. Serve right away or refrigerate until ready to serve. If made ahead, remove the shrimp from the refrigerator 20 minutes before serving to bring them to room temperature.

4.   To serve: Place the cocktail sauce in a small bowl in the center of a large plate or bowl and arrange the shrimp around it. Serve with lemon wedges.

notes: You can make the cocktail sauce and shrimp up to 1 day ahead.

To devein shrimp with their peels on before cooking, hold a shrimp between your thumb and forefinger with the rounded, or convex, side of the shrimp facing upward. Place the pointed end of a wooden skewer or toothpick at the junction of the second and third segments of the shell, about ⅛ inch down from the top. Gently push the skewer through the shell at a right angle to and under the vein, then lift up to remove the vein.

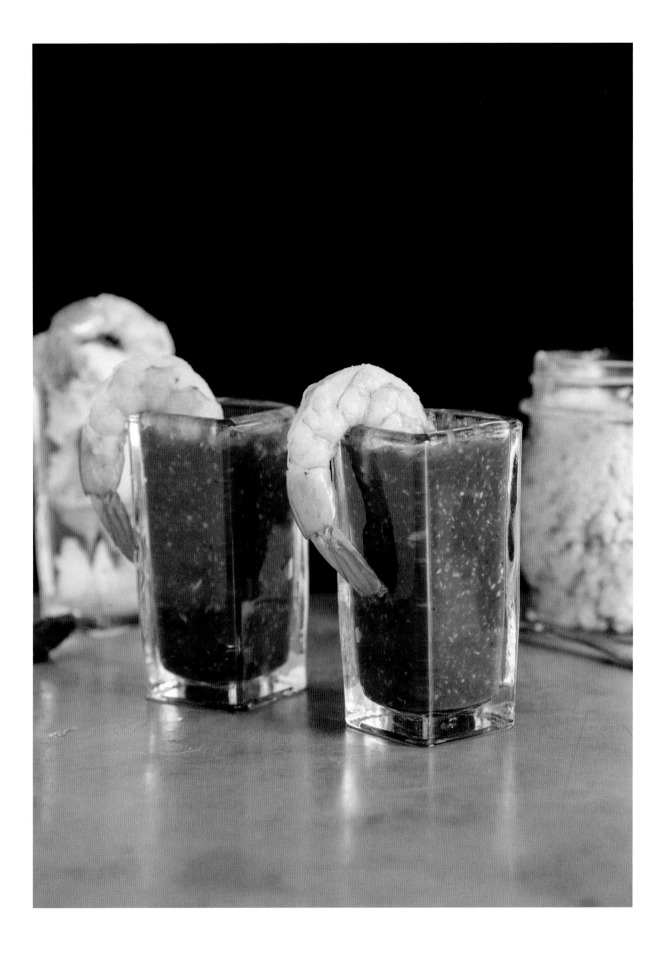

THE ULTIMATE MEAT & CHEESE BOARD

serves 6 to 8   *prep time* 20 minutes

EGG-FREE / NUT-FREE OPTION: omit nuts and crackers and bread made with nut flour

Even though I mostly stay away from cheese, I rarely host a party without a meat and cheese board on the table. Everyone goes crazy for it! I customize it based on how many people we are hosting, and it's a delicious, easy, and attractive appetizer to serve. Bonus: You probably have fun platters, bowls, and other items around the house that you can use to make your own meat and cheese board the ultimate!

Platters & Props:

Grab one or two platters, depending on the number of guests. You may already have things to use at home! A small chalkboard and individual cheese markers are fun additions: use them to identify the various cheeses included on your platter.

- Wooden boards or wood cutting boards
- Marble slabs
- Slate cheese boards
- Small chalkboard or individual cheese markers and/or flags

Cheese: (APPROXIMATELY 3 OUNCES PER PERSON)

Pick a variety of three or more cheeses. Provide a separate knife for each cheese. Try different styles—from fresh to semi-soft to aged and firm—as well as different milks (cow, goat, and sheep). These are my favorites:

- **Aged:** Cheddar, Gouda
- **Creamy Blue:** Danish blue, Gorgonzola
- **Firm:** Manchego
- **Soft:** Brie, chèvre or other goat cheese, Fromager d'Affinois, Humboldt Fog Grande

Crackers & Breads:

I like an assortment that can work for anyone and everyone, whether they're eating gluten- and grain-free or not.

- Gluten-free crackers, homemade (page 78) or store-bought
- Regular crackers
- Gluten-free bread, homemade (page 80) or store-bought
- Sliced baguette
- Breadsticks

Meats:

Cured meats are great additions to a cheese platter. Here are my favorites:

- Pepperoni
- Prosciutto
- Salami

Nuts:

Candied nuts, roasted and salted nuts, or raw nuts are great accompaniments. Try these:

- Raw almonds
- Marcona almonds
- Candied pecans or walnuts
- Pistachios

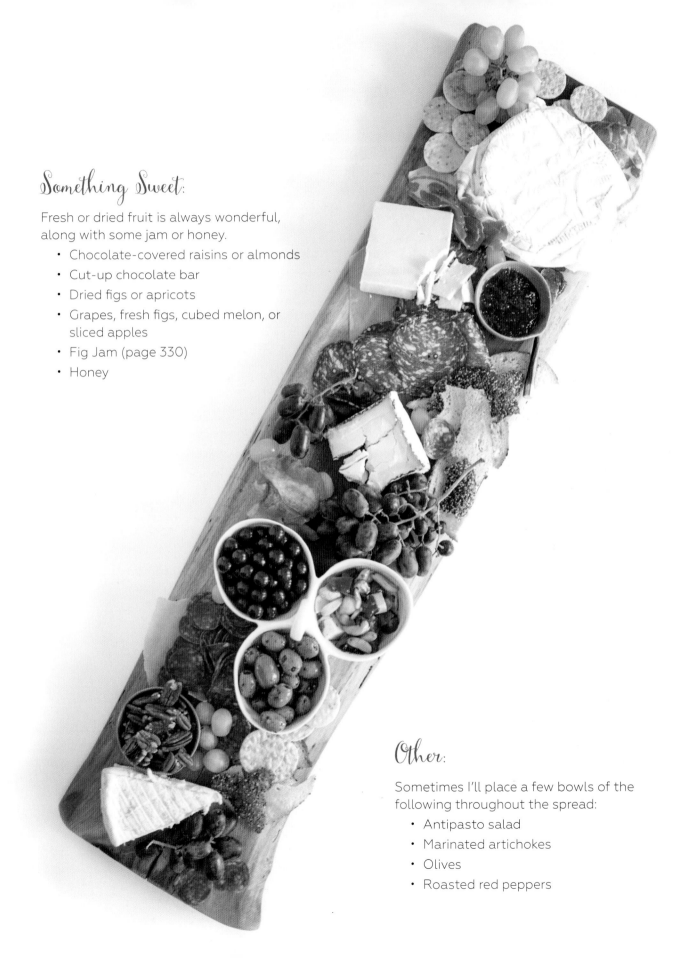

Something Sweet:

Fresh or dried fruit is always wonderful, along with some jam or honey.

- Chocolate-covered raisins or almonds
- Cut-up chocolate bar
- Dried figs or apricots
- Grapes, fresh figs, cubed melon, or sliced apples
- Fig Jam (page 330)
- Honey

Other:

Sometimes I'll place a few bowls of the following throughout the spread:

- Antipasto salad
- Marinated artichokes
- Olives
- Roasted red peppers

BRUSCHETTA BITES WITH BALSAMIC GLAZE

makes 8 to 10 bites   *prep time* 10 minutes (not including bread or glaze)
cook time 25 minutes

EGG-FREE / DAIRY-FREE / PALEO-FRIENDLY

Bruschetta on fresh, crusty bread was something I used to miss constantly after I cleaned up my diet. But with my delicious homemade grain-free bread and this perfect bruschetta mix, I never miss classic bruschetta, and you won't, either. And with a balsamic glaze on top? Bring it on! Make the bread in advance to throw together this easy app in a flash.

ingredients:

1 batch All-Purpose Sandwich Bread (page 80), baked in an 8½ by 4½-inch loaf pan

FOR THE BRUSCHETTA:

5 medium Roma tomatoes, finely diced

1 small red onion, finely diced (⅓ to ½ cup)

1 clove garlic, minced

1 teaspoon extra-virgin olive oil

1 teaspoon fine sea salt

1 teaspoon freshly ground black pepper

Leaves from 2 sprigs fresh basil (about 10 leaves), roughly chopped, plus more for garnish

1 batch Balsamic Glaze (page 334)

note: Try this bruschetta on grilled chicken! Marinate 2 boneless, skinless chicken breast halves in ¼ cup of balsamic vinegar, 2 tablespoons of extra-virgin olive oil, 1 teaspoon of fine sea salt, and ½ teaspoon of freshly ground black pepper in the refrigerator for 30 minutes or up to overnight. Grill the chicken until done, then top it with the bruschetta.

directions:

1. Slice the bread into 8 to 10 slices; set aside.

2. Make the bruschetta: Toss the tomatoes, onion, and garlic together in a large bowl. Add the olive oil, salt, pepper, and basil and mix to combine. Set aside.

3. Just before serving, place an oven rack in the top position and preheat the broiler to high. Place the bread slices directly on the oven rack and toast until golden and slightly crispy, 5 to 7 minutes, watching them closely to avoid burning. Remove from the oven and let cool.

4. To assemble the bites: Place the toasted bread slices on a plate. Top each slice with a heaping spoonful of bruschetta and drizzle with balsamic glaze. Serve immediately, garnished with additional basil.

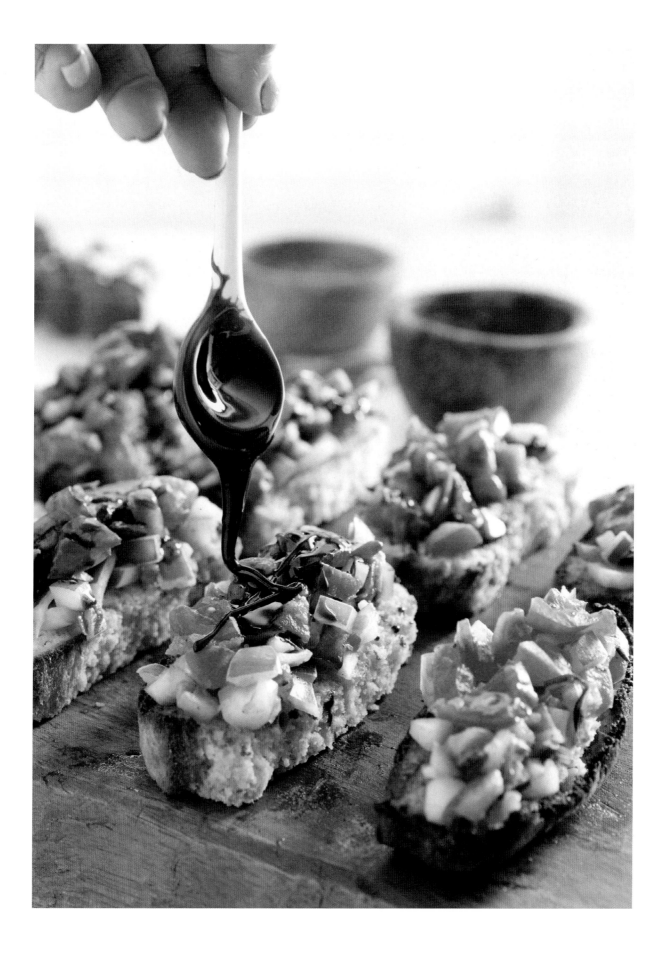

AHI TUNA BITES

serves 2 to 4   *prep time* 15 minutes, plus time to marinate tuna

NUT-FREE / DAIRY-FREE / PALEO-FRIENDLY

I love, love, love ahi tuna. I love topping salads with it, like my Sesame Seared Ahi Tuna Salad with Ginger Dressing (page 150), and I love making it the star of a fun appetizer, as here. These bites are so tasty, and you have multiple options for serving them: serve them on plantain chips or cucumber slices for two equally delicious yet very different bites!

ingredients:

1 pound sushi-grade ahi tuna, cubed

2 tablespoons chopped scallions, plus more for garnish

1 tablespoon coconut aminos

½ teaspoon fish sauce

Optional: ½ jalapeño pepper, minced

FOR SERVING:

Plantain chips or ½-inch-thick cucumber slices (or a combination)

1 avocado, sliced

Optional: Finely shredded daikon radish

⅓ cup Spicy Mayo (page 312) (see notes)

White and black sesame seeds, for garnish

directions:

1. In a bowl, toss the cubed ahi tuna with the scallions, coconut aminos, fish sauce, and minced jalapeño, if using, to evenly coat. Cover with plastic wrap and place in the refrigerator to marinate for 20 minutes or up to 1 hour.

2. When ready to serve, line a plate with plantain chips and/or cucumber slices. Top with avocado slices, shredded daikon (if using), and the marinated tuna, then drizzle with the spicy mayo. Garnish with sesame seeds and additional chopped scallions. The assembled bites can be refrigerated for up to 4 hours, although they are best if served immediately.

notes: If you don't want to make homemade spicy mayo, add 1 teaspoon of Sriracha sauce to ½ cup of your favorite store-bought, clean-ingredient mayo and stir to combine.

Ahi tuna isn't the only fish that I love raw; in fact, I love *all* fish raw! Sushi-grade salmon is another good option for this recipe.

Try garnishing the bites with some crumbled dried seaweed for a little extra texture!

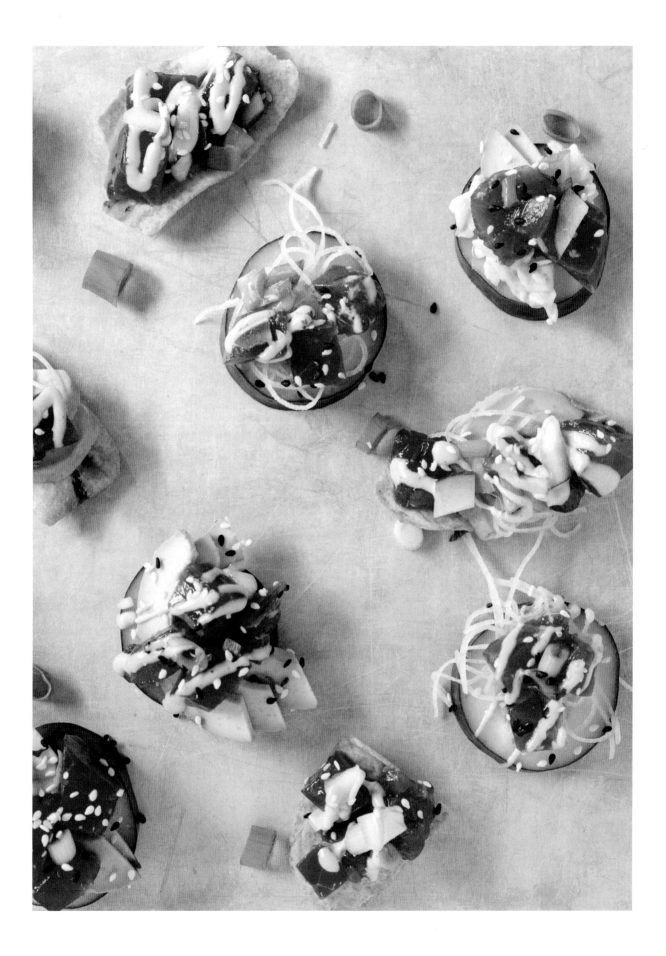

BACON-WRAPPED SCALLOPS WITH BALSAMIC GLAZE

serves 6 to 8 *prep time* 5 minutes (not including glaze) *cook time* 15 minutes

EGG-FREE / NUT-FREE / DAIRY-FREE / PALEO-FRIENDLY

Simply put, these bacon-wrapped scallops are a real crowd-pleaser!

ingredients:

1½ pounds large sea scallops

1 (12-ounce) package bacon (*not* thick-cut)

Pinch of fine sea salt

Pinch of freshly ground black pepper

1 batch Balsamic Glaze (page 334)

note: Serve with a side of Spicy Mayo (page 312)!

directions:

1. Place an oven rack in the top position and preheat the broiler to low.

2. Wrap each scallop in a piece of bacon and secure with a toothpick.

3. Place the bacon-wrapped scallops on a rimmed baking sheet and season with the salt and pepper. Broil for about 15 minutes, flipping them over halfway through cooking, until the bacon is cooked through and slightly crispy.

4. Arrange the scallops on a serving dish, drizzle with balsamic glaze, and serve immediately.

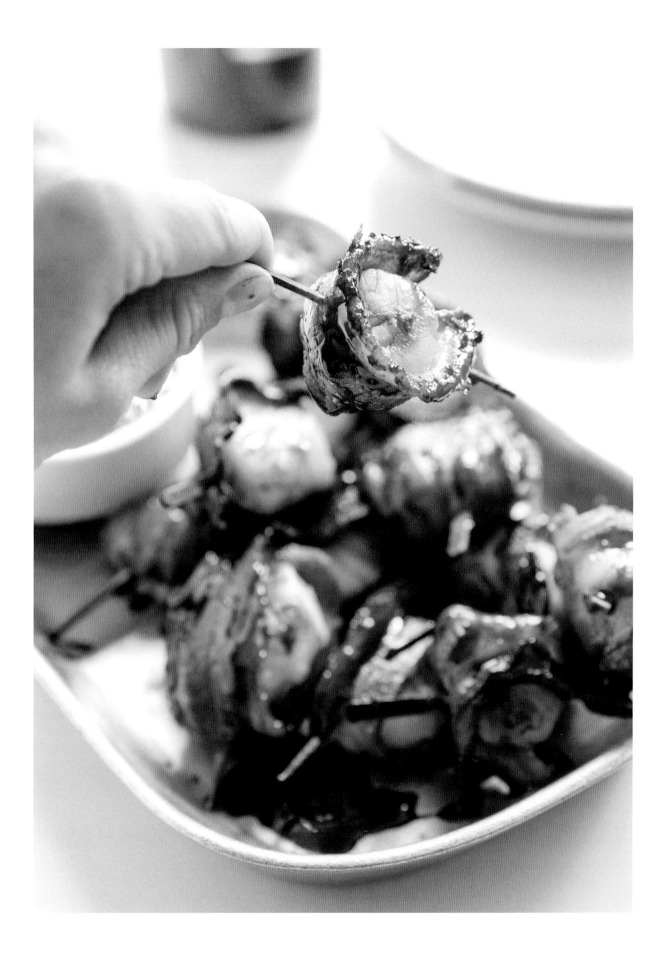

PROSCIUTTO FLATBREAD WITH GRILLED PEACHES & CARAMELIZED ONIONS

makes one 12 by 6-inch flatbread (4 to 6 servings)   *prep time* 10 minutes (not including flatbread or caramelized onions)   *cook time* 20 minutes

....

DAIRY-FREE OPTION: use olive oil instead of butter and omit cheese
PALEO-FRIENDLY OPTION: use olive oil instead of butter and omit cheese

....

Grilled peaches, crispy prosciutto, caramelized onions, garlic, and olive oil on fresh flatbread—need I say more? This is a delicious appetizer to whip up!

ingredients:

2 peaches, sliced about ½ inch thick

2 tablespoons extra-virgin olive oil or melted unsalted butter

2 cloves garlic, minced

1 par-baked Flatbread (page 76)

Optional: 1 cup shredded or cubed mozzarella or ricotta cheese

12 to 15 pieces thinly sliced prosciutto

1 cup Caramelized Onions (page 332)

Fine sea salt and freshly ground black pepper

FOR THE ARUGULA TOPPING:

1 cup arugula

1 tablespoon extra-virgin olive oil

1 teaspoon lemon juice

notes: The caramelized onions can be made a day ahead.

Don't have a grill or grill pan? Roast your peaches instead! Line a rimmed baking sheet with parchment paper and roast the peaches at 350°F for 10 minutes.

directions:

1. Preheat the oven to 350°F and a grill or grill pan to medium-high heat.

2. Oil the hot grill grate. Brush the peach slices with olive oil and grill for just long enough to give them grill marks on both sides (they will finish cooking in the oven).

3. In a small bowl, whisk together the olive oil and minced garlic. Brush the mixture onto the par-baked flatbread. If adding cheese, sprinkle it on the flatbread, then lay the prosciutto, caramelized onions, and grilled peaches on top. Sprinkle with salt and pepper.

4. Place the flatbread on a rimmed baking sheet. Bake for 10 minutes, until the peaches are soft and the crust is golden.

5. When ready to serve, make the arugula topping: Toss the arugula with the olive oil and lemon juice and place on top of the flatbread. Serve immediately.

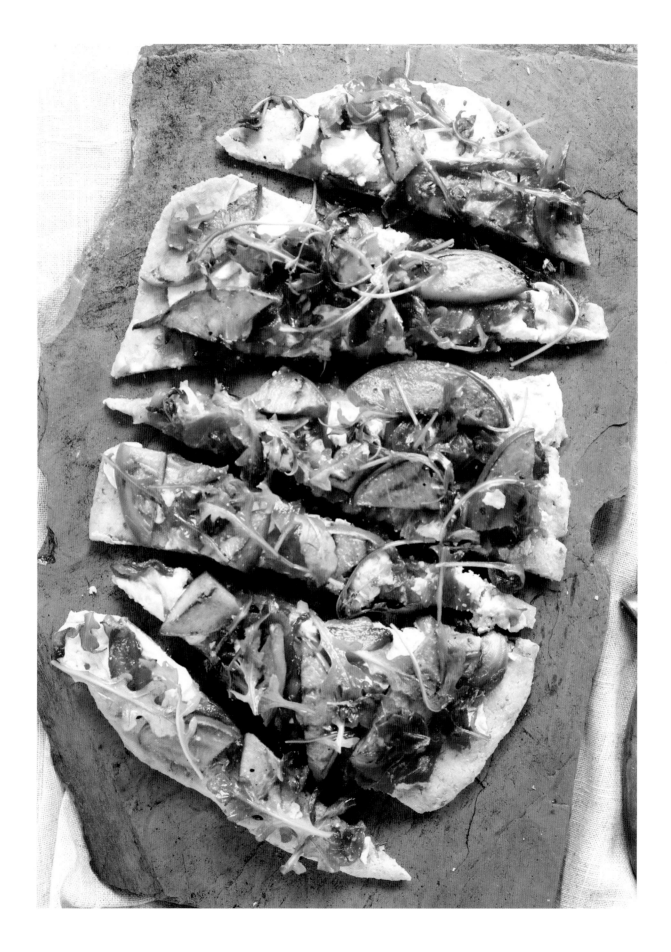

WINGS THREE WAYS: BUFFALO, SRIRACHA HONEY & HERB RUB

serves 4 to 6   *prep time* 10 minutes, plus 30 minutes to marinate Buffalo or Sriracha Honey wings
cook time 30 minutes

EGG-FREE OPTION: omit ranch and spicy mayo dipping sauces / NUT-FREE
DAIRY-FREE OPTION: replace ghee/butter with oil
PALEO-FRIENDLY OPTION: use ghee instead of butter

These wings are my favorite—all three versions! Make them as an appetizer, for a game-day snack, or even for dinner with some sides. They are seriously so delicious. Bonus: The wings can be cooked on the grill or in the oven!

ingredients:

FOR ALL VERSIONS:

2½ to 3 pounds chicken wings and/or drumsticks

1 teaspoon fine sea salt

½ teaspoon freshly ground black pepper

Celery sticks, for serving

FOR BUFFALO WINGS:

⅓ cup Buffalo sauce

2 tablespoons ghee (page 350) or unsalted butter, melted

1 teaspoon fine sea salt

1 teaspoon freshly ground black pepper

⅓ cup Ranch Dressing (page 318), for dipping

FOR SRIRACHA HONEY WINGS:

⅓ cup Sriracha sauce

3 tablespoons honey

Pinch of fine sea salt

FOR HERB RUB WINGS:

3 tablespoons extra-virgin olive oil

1 teaspoon chili powder

1 teaspoon dried ground oregano

1 teaspoon dried rosemary leaves

1 teaspoon fine sea salt

½ teaspoon garlic powder

½ teaspoon onion powder

Pinch of cayenne pepper

Sliced scallions, for garnish

Sesame seeds, for garnish

⅓ cup Spicy Mayo (page 312), for dipping

directions:

1. If making oven-baked wings, place an oven rack in the top position, preheat the oven to 400°F, and line a rimmed baking sheet with foil. If making grilled wings, preheat a grill to high heat (400°F).

2. Season the wings with the 1 teaspoon of salt and the ½ teaspoon of pepper and set aside.

3. *To make Buffalo or Sriracha Honey Wings:* Whisk together the ingredients for the flavor of your choice in a bowl. (If desired, reserve some of the marinade for later; see tip.) Place the seasoned wings in a glass dish or a resealable plastic bag, then pour the Buffalo or Sriracha Honey marinade over the wings and mix to combine. Marinate the wings for 30 minutes at room temperature or up to 8 hours in the fridge.

   To make Herb Rub Wings: Combine the oil and seasonings in a bowl, then press the herb rub all over the seasoned wings. (The Herb Rub Wings do not need to marinate.)

4. *To grill the wings:* Grease the hot grill grate and place the wings on the grill. Close the lid and grill for 7 minutes on each side.

   To bake the wings: Place the wings on the lined baking sheet and bake for 10 minutes on each side. To get them crispy, broil on high for 5 minutes, watching to avoid burning.

5. Place the wings on a plate and serve hot, with celery sticks and dipping sauce on the side.

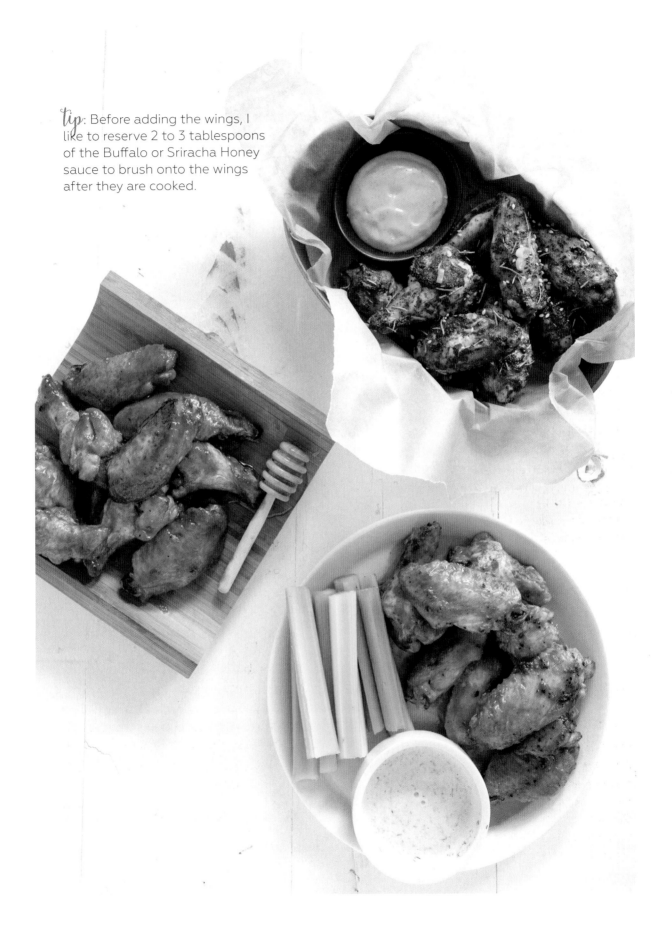

tip: Before adding the wings, I like to reserve 2 to 3 tablespoons of the Buffalo or Sriracha Honey sauce to brush onto the wings after they are cooked.

CHICKEN SATAY SKEWERS WITH DIPPING SAUCE

serves 4 to 6   *prep time* 10 minutes, plus time to marinate chicken   *cook time* 15 minutes

EGG-FREE / DAIRY-FREE / PALEO-FRIENDLY

Chicken satay is a popular Indonesian dish of seasoned, skewered meat served with a dipping sauce. My chicken satay skewers are jam-packed with flavor and perfect year-round!

ingredients:

1 pound boneless, skinless chicken breasts

FOR THE MARINADE:

¼ cup coconut aminos

1 tablespoon chili paste

1 teaspoon toasted sesame oil

1 teaspoon lime juice

½ teaspoon turmeric powder

½ teaspoon coconut sugar or granulated maple sugar

Pinch of fine sea salt

Pinch of freshly ground black pepper

FOR THE DIPPING SAUCE:

⅓ cup unsweetened creamy almond butter

2 to 4 tablespoons hot water, as needed

1 clove garlic, crushed to a paste

1 (1-inch) chunk fresh ginger, peeled and grated

1 teaspoon honey

1 teaspoon toasted sesame oil

Pinch of red pepper flakes

Pinch of fine sea salt

OPTIONAL GARNISHES:

Chopped fresh flat-leaf parsley

Lime wedges

SPECIAL EQUIPMENT:

Metal or soaked wooden skewers

directions:

1. Slice the chicken into strips, about 1 inch by 5 inches. Thread the chicken strips lengthwise onto skewers, working the stick through the middle of the chicken. Place the skewers in a shallow dish large enough to hold the skewers in one layer, such as a rectangular baking dish.

2. In a bowl, whisk together the marinade ingredients. Pour the marinade over the chicken and turn the skewers to coat. Marinate for 30 minutes at room temperature or up to 6 hours in the fridge.

3. In a small bowl, whisk together the dipping sauce ingredients and set aside. You may need to whisk in additional hot water before serving to get the right consistency.

4. Preheat a grill to medium heat. Grease the hot grill grate and place the skewers on the grill. Cook for 5 to 7 minutes on each side, depending on the thickness of the chicken, until no pink remains.

5. Serve hot with the dipping sauce. Garnish with parsley and lime wedges, if desired.

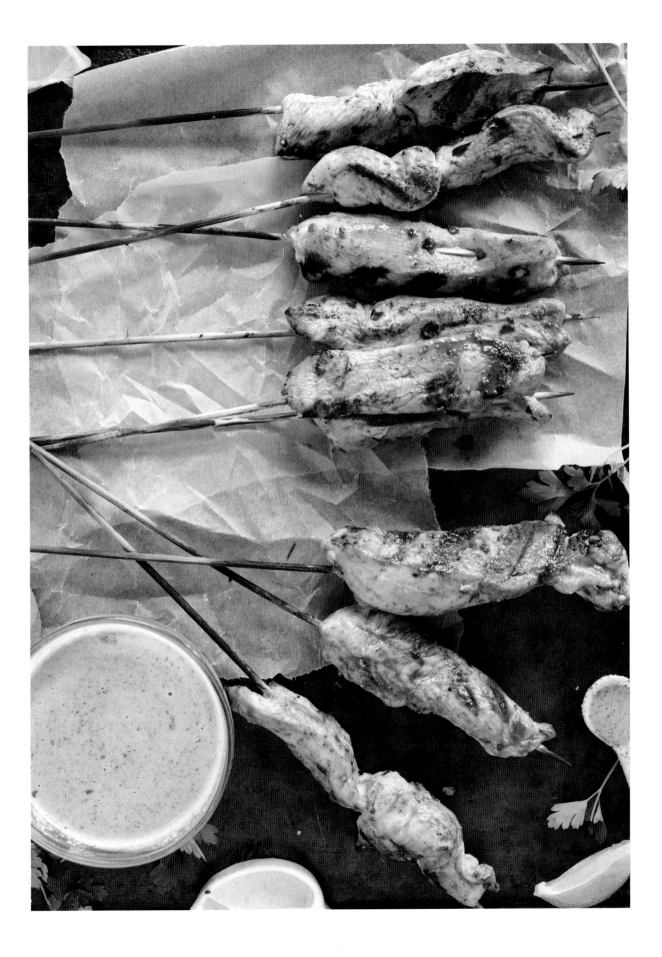

PATATAS BRAVAS TWO WAYS

serves 4 (when both versions are served)
prep time 15 minutes (not including spicy mayo or avocado crema) *cook time* 50 minutes

....

EGG-FREE OPTION: omit mayo from classic version / NUT-FREE
DAIRY-FREE OPTION: omit cheese / PALEO-FRIENDLY OPTION: omit cheese

....

Two of my favorite restaurants serve up patatas bravas in two different ways
that I am head over heels for. The first is a classic Spanish style made with white
potatoes and served with a red sauce and a white sauce; the second is a sweet-
and-spicy sweet potato version that caramelizes in the oven and melts in your
mouth. Whenever I crave potatoes, I crave these two dishes (and my Classic
Home Fries on page 42, but that's another story!).

ingredients:

CLASSIC PATATAS BRAVAS

1 teaspoon paprika

½ teaspoon smoked paprika

1 teaspoon garlic granules

1 teaspoon fine sea salt

½ teaspoon freshly ground black pepper

Optional: ⅛ teaspoon cayenne pepper

4 medium russet potatoes, cubed

2 tablespoons extra-virgin olive oil or avocado oil

FOR THE RED SAUCE (FOR SERVING):

1 cup crushed tomatoes

½ small onion, sliced

2 cloves garlic, minced

1 teaspoon coconut sugar or granulated maple
  sugar

½ teaspoon paprika

½ teaspoon smoked paprika

½ teaspoon fine sea salt, more to taste

½ teaspoon ground white pepper, more to taste

¼ teaspoon ground cumin

2 tablespoons Spicy Mayo (page 312), for serving

Chopped fresh flat-leaf parsley, for garnish

SWEET-AND-SPICY PATATAS BRAVAS

1 large sweet potato, cubed

2 tablespoons extra-virgin olive oil or avocado oil

2 teaspoons honey

2 teaspoons Sriracha sauce

½ teaspoon ground cinnamon

½ teaspoon fine sea salt

1 batch Avocado Crema (page 344), for serving

Chopped fresh flat-leaf parsley, for garnish

Optional: ⅓ cup crumbled feta cheese, for garnish

directions:

1. Preheat the oven to 375°F and line a rimmed baking sheet with parchment paper.

2. *To make Classic Patatas Bravas:* In a small bowl, combine the paprika, smoked paprika, garlic granules, salt, black pepper, and cayenne pepper, if using. Toss the potatoes with the oil and seasoning mixture.

3. *To make Sweet-and-Spicy Patatas Bravas:* In a large bowl, toss the cubed sweet potatoes with the oil, honey, Sriracha, cinnamon, and salt to evenly coat.

4. Spread out the seasoned potatoes on the lined baking sheet. Bake for 40 minutes, until fork-tender. When done, the white potatoes for the Classic Patatas Bravas will be crispy on the edges and golden; the sweet potatoes will be caramelized.

5. While the potatoes are baking, prepare the red sauce for the Classic Patatas Bravas: In a medium-sized saucepan over medium heat, whisk together the sauce ingredients and bring to a boil. Reduce the heat and simmer for 5 minutes. Taste and adjust the spices and seasoning as desired.

6. *To serve Classic Patatas Bravas:* Place the potatoes in a dish, drizzle with red sauce and spicy mayo, and garnish with parsley. Serve immediately.

7. *To serve Sweet-and-Spicy Patatas Bravas:* Place the sweet potatoes in a dish, top with a dollop of avocado crema, and sprinkle with chopped parsley and crumbled feta cheese, if using. Serve immediately.

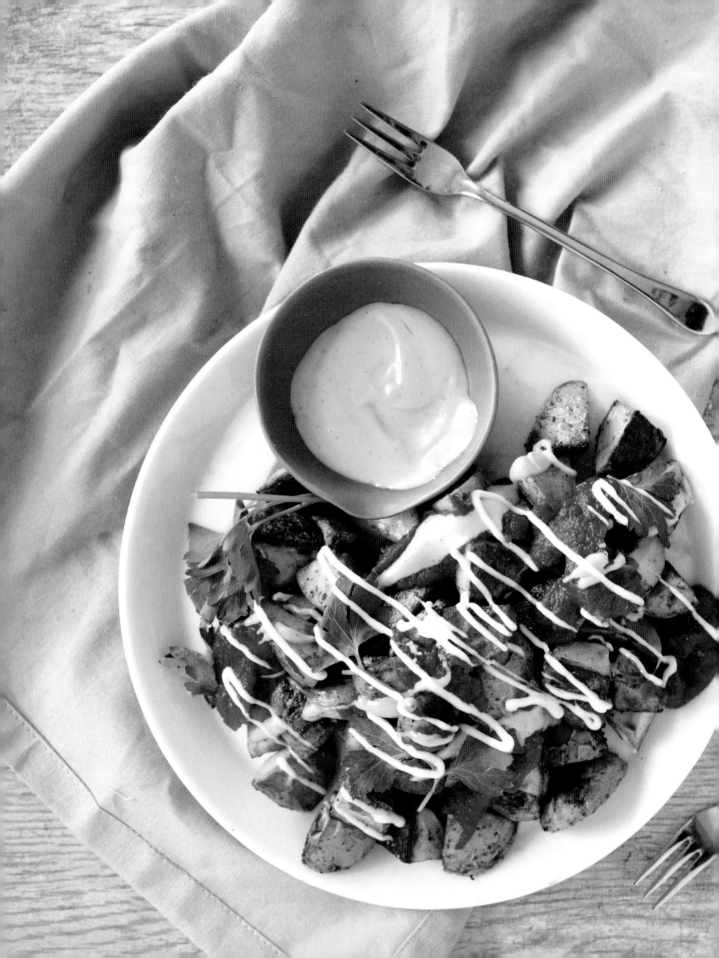

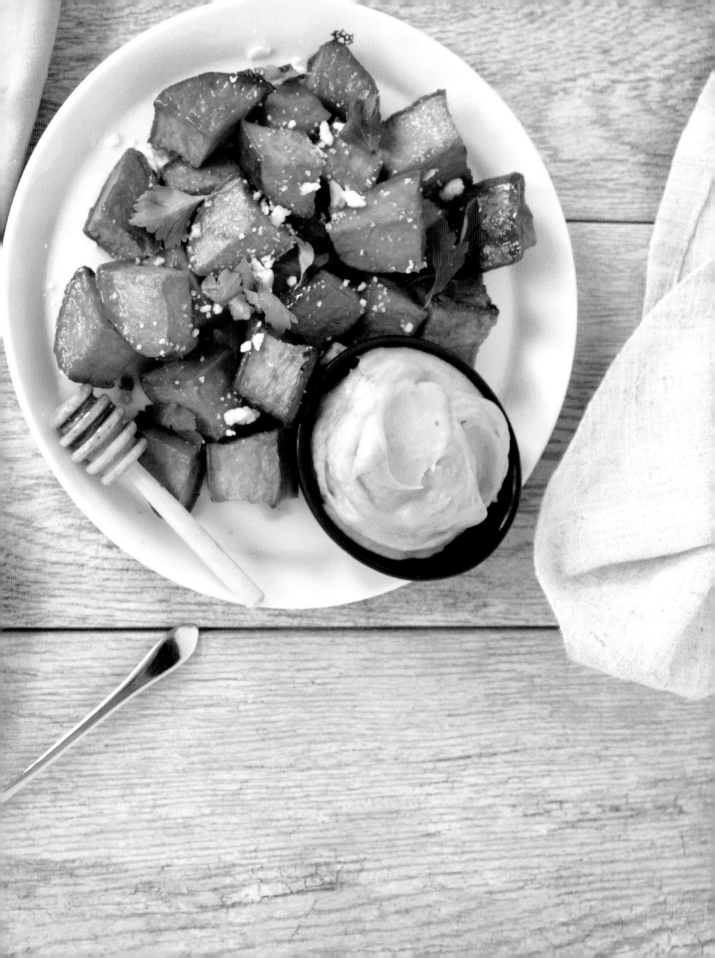

BUFFALO CHICKEN BITES

serves 4   *prep time* 15 minutes (not including dressing)   *cook time* 15 minutes

NUT-FREE / PALEO-FRIENDLY OPTION: use ghee instead of butter

Crispy fried chicken bites that are guilt-free. How can that be?! These also work great for a dinner for two!

ingredients:

FOR THE BATTER:

½ cup tapioca flour

2 large eggs

1 teaspoon medium-hot hot sauce, such as Frank's RedHot

½ teaspoon fine sea salt

½ teaspoon freshly ground black pepper

1 pound boneless, skinless chicken breasts, cubed

¼ cup avocado oil or extra-virgin olive oil, for frying

FOR THE SAUCE:

⅓ cup plus 2 tablespoons medium-hot hot sauce

2 tablespoons ghee (page 350) or unsalted butter

½ teaspoon freshly ground black pepper

FOR SERVING:

⅓ cup Ranch Dressing (page 318)

Optional: Celery sticks and/or carrot sticks

directions:

1. In a bowl, whisk together the batter ingredients until smooth.

2. Place the cubed chicken in the batter and toss to coat thoroughly. Let sit for 5 minutes.

3. Meanwhile, heat the oil in a large skillet over medium heat. Splash a drop of water on it; if it sizzles, it's ready to go.

4. Carefully place the chicken in the hot skillet and fry for 5 minutes on each side, until the outside is golden and no pink remains in the center. Remove to a plate lined with paper towels.

5. Make the sauce: In the same skillet, heat the hot sauce, ghee, and pepper over low heat until melted and combined. Add the chicken and gently toss to coat with the sauce.

6. If you want your chicken extra-crispy, transfer it to a rimmed baking sheet lined with foil and broil for 3 minutes on each side, watching carefully to avoid burning.

7. Serve the chicken bites with ranch dressing and celery or carrot sticks, if desired.

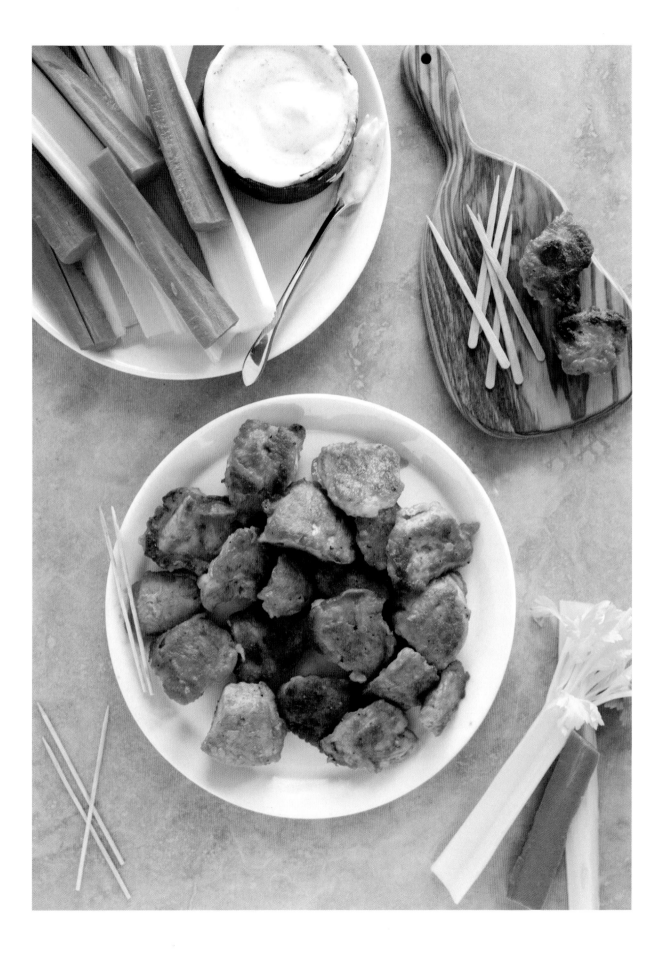

MEXICAN MEATBALLS

serves 4 to 6   *prep time* 10 minutes (not including guacamole)   *cook time* 12 minutes

EGG-FREE / NUT-FREE / DAIRY-FREE OPTION: **omit cheese**
PALEO-FRIENDLY OPTION: **omit cheese**

These meatballs are a fun and inexpensive appetizer to throw together in a pinch. Put them on a plate with toothpicks, along with some salsa and guacamole, for wonderful, flavorful little bites.

ingredients:

FOR THE MEATBALLS:

1 pound ground chicken or turkey

¼ cup chopped scallions

2 cloves garlic, minced

1 tablespoon extra-virgin olive oil or avocado oil

1 tablespoon chili powder

1 teaspoon fine sea salt

½ teaspoon ground cumin

½ teaspoon paprika

¼ teaspoon freshly ground black pepper

Optional: ¼ cup shredded cheddar cheese

FOR SERVING:

1 cup salsa, homemade (page 336) or store-bought

1 cup Lexi's Best Guacamole (page 88)

directions:

1. Preheat the oven to 350°F. Line a rimmed baking sheet with foil and grease the foil with the oil of your choice.

2. Place the ingredients for the meatballs in a mixing bowl. Using your hands, mix the ingredients together until evenly combined. Form the mixture into 12 to 15 meatballs and place on the lined baking sheet.

3. Bake for 12 to 15 minutes, until golden and fully cooked through.

4. Serve immediately with salsa and guacamole.

note: Try these meatballs on top of a salad!

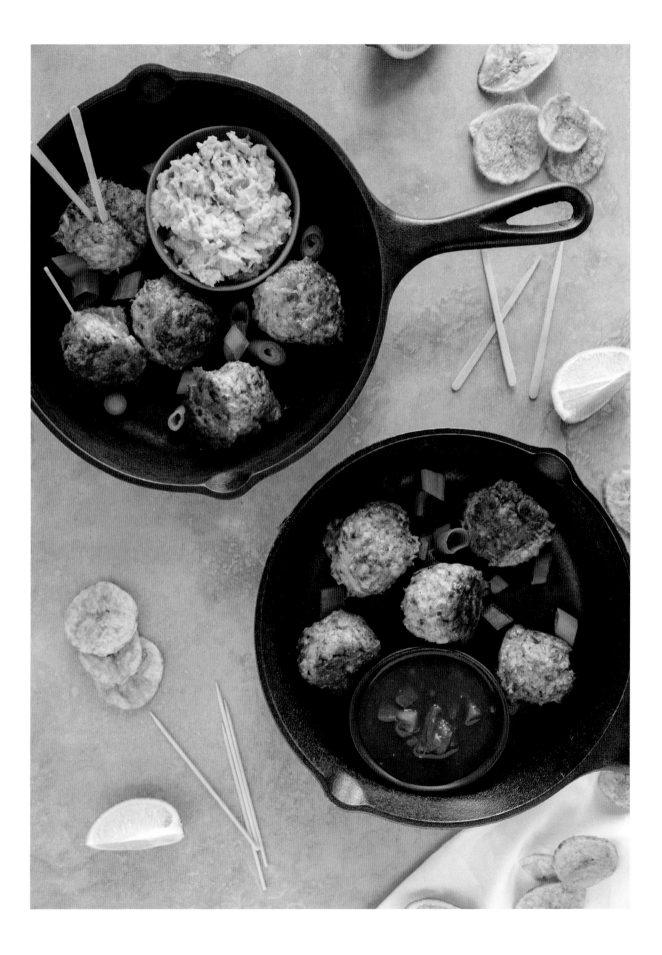

SPINACH DIP STUFFED MUSHROOMS

serves 6   *prep time* 10 minutes, plus time to soak cashews   *cook time* 30 minutes

EGG-FREE / DAIRY-FREE OPTION: use olive oil and omit cheese
PALEO-FRIENDLY OPTION: use ghee or olive oil and omit cheese
VEGAN OPTION: use olive oil and omit cheese

These, oh these . . . I am seriously in love with these. Spinach dip was my favorite way back when. This recipe nails that exact spinach dip flavor that I love, but is made with healthier ingredients and is transformed into delightfully handy pass-around appetizers.

ingredients:

FOR THE CASHEW CREAM:

1 cup raw cashews

1 teaspoon extra-virgin olive oil

½ teaspoon fine sea salt

FOR THE SPINACH DIP:

2 tablespoons ghee (page 350), unsalted butter, or extra-virgin olive oil

½ onion, minced

1 shallot, minced

1 clove garlic, minced

3 packed cups fresh spinach

Fine sea salt

Red pepper flakes

1 pound cremini mushrooms, cleaned and destemmed

Optional: ½ cup shredded cheddar cheese

Leftover Cashew Cream:

Make my No-Bake Cookie Dough Cups on page 284!

directions:

1. Soak the cashews in a bowl of water for at least 1 hour or up to 8 hours.

2. Preheat the oven to 375°F. Line a rimmed baking sheet with parchment paper.

3. Heat the ghee in a large skillet over medium heat. Add the onion, shallot, and garlic and cook until soft, about 3 minutes. Fold in the spinach and cook, stirring occasionally, until the spinach is wilted. Add salt and red pepper flakes to taste and set aside.

4. Make the cashew cream: Drain the soaked cashews and place them in a small food processor or high-speed blender. Add the 1 teaspoon of olive oil and ½ teaspoon of salt and puree until smooth, adding more oil if needed. Fold ½ cup of the cashew cream into the spinach mixture until evenly combined.

5. Arrange the mushroom caps on the lined baking sheet and brush the outsides of the caps lightly with olive oil. Scoop a large spoonful of the spinach mixture into each cap. Top with the cheese, if using.

6. Bake for 15 to 20 minutes, until the mushrooms are soft and the cheese has begun to brown. Serve warm or at room temperature.

variation:

Hot Spinach Dip. Egg-free and dairy-free (if the cheese is omitted), this is a hot, creamy party dip that everyone can enjoy. Make the spinach dip as described above, following Steps 1 through 4. Place the dip in an oven-safe bowl, top with shredded cheddar cheese, if desired, and bake in a preheated 350°F oven until the cheese is golden. Use homemade crackers (page 78), veggies, or plantain chips for dipping. *Serves 6.*

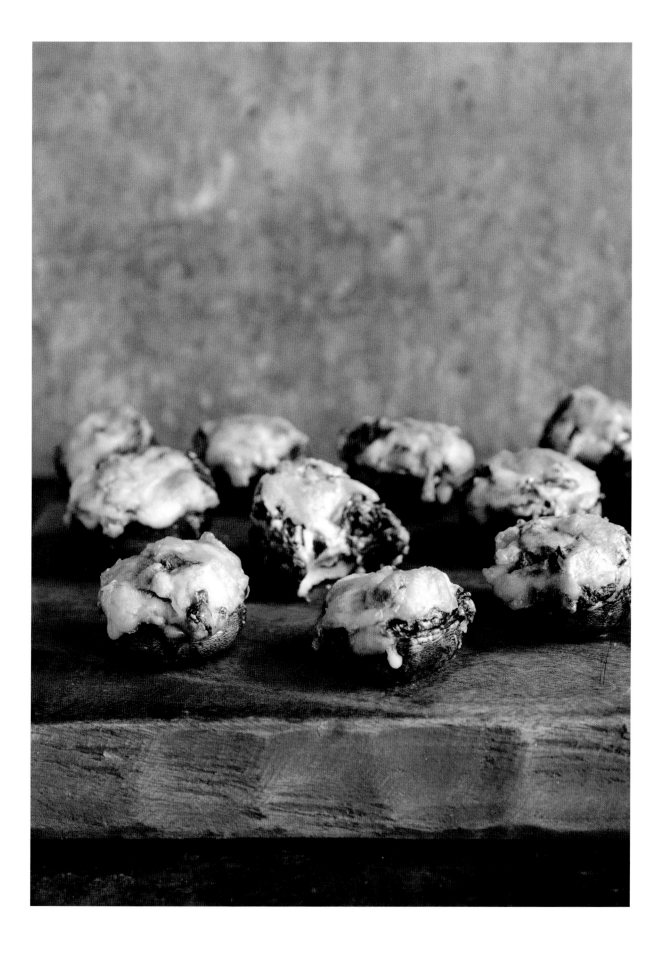

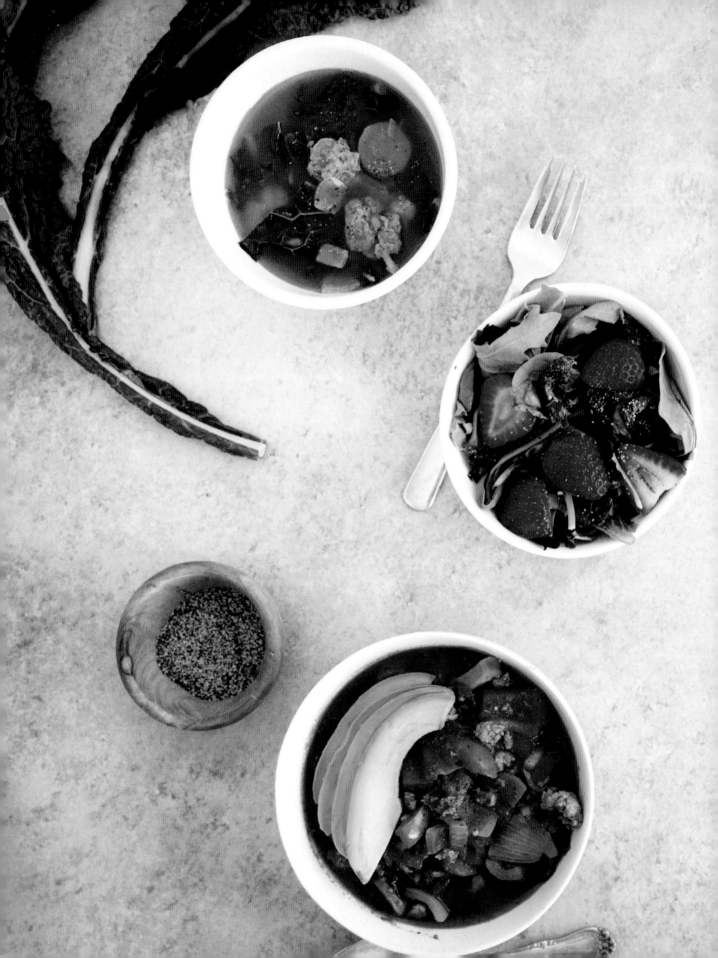

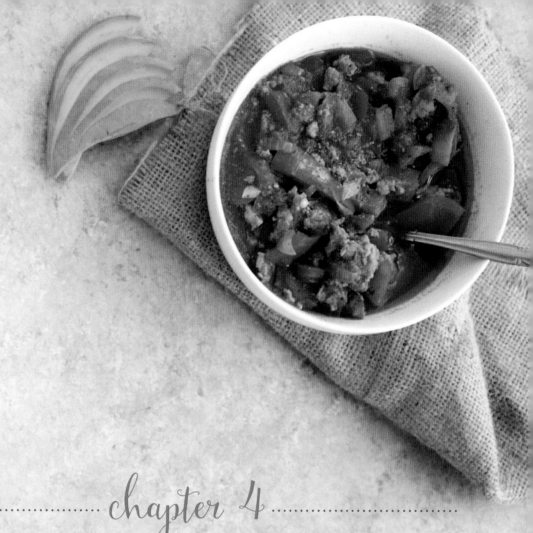

chapter 4

DELICIOUS SOUPS
& HEARTY SALADS

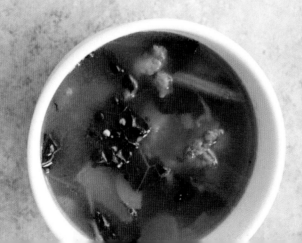

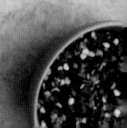

CLASSIC CHILI

serves 6 to 8   *prep time* 20 minutes   *cook time* about 3½ hours

EGG-FREE / NUT-FREE / DAIRY-FREE OPTION: omit cheese topping
PALEO-FRIENDLY OPTION: omit beans and cheese topping

This is my go-to classic chili recipe all fall and winter long. I call it "healthy comfort food in a bowl" because it's hearty and satisfying for those chilly days. It is perfect for a big gathering, like Sunday football festivities, and it's a good weekly meal prep option since the recipe makes tons of leftovers! The best part? You can customize this chili to your liking. Some days I'll add more veggies based on what is in season. I've also perfected this chili to be equally delicious with or without the beans.

ingredients:

1 tablespoon extra-virgin olive oil

3 cloves garlic, minced

2 medium onions, diced

2 bell peppers (any color), chopped

2 large carrots, chopped

2 stalks celery, chopped

Optional: 1 medium sweet potato, peeled and cubed

2 pounds ground turkey or beef

2 cups water, more as needed

1 (15-ounce) can tomato sauce

1 (14½-ounce) can diced tomatoes

1 teaspoon fine sea salt, or more to taste

3 tablespoons chili powder

1 tablespoon cayenne pepper, or more to taste

1 tablespoon ground cumin

1 tablespoon paprika

2 teaspoons celery seed

½ teaspoon freshly ground black pepper, or more to taste

Pinch of red pepper flakes

Optional: 1 (15-ounce) can black beans

Optional: 1 (15-ounce) can kidney beans

Optional: 1 small jalapeño pepper, finely chopped

OPTIONAL TOPPINGS:

Fresh cilantro leaves

Shredded cheese

Sliced avocado

Sliced scallions

directions:

1. Heat the oil in a soup pot over medium heat. Add the garlic, onions, bell peppers, carrots, celery, and sweet potato, if using, and sauté for 5 to 7 minutes, until soft.

2. Add the meat and cook until browned, 5 to 7 minutes, stirring often to break up the chunks.

3. Once the meat is browned, add the water, tomato sauce, diced tomatoes, salt, and spices. Mix well to combine. If you are adding the beans and jalapeño, add them to the pot now, rinsing and draining the beans first.

4. Bring to a boil, then reduce the heat and simmer, uncovered, until the chili is nice and thick, about 3 hours. Add additional water during cooking if you want your chili to be more souplike. Toward the end of the cooking time, taste and adjust the seasonings as desired. Add more cayenne pepper for an extra kick and more salt and pepper as needed.

5. Serve with your favorite chili toppings, if desired. Store the chili in the refrigerator for up to 1 week, or freeze it for later use.

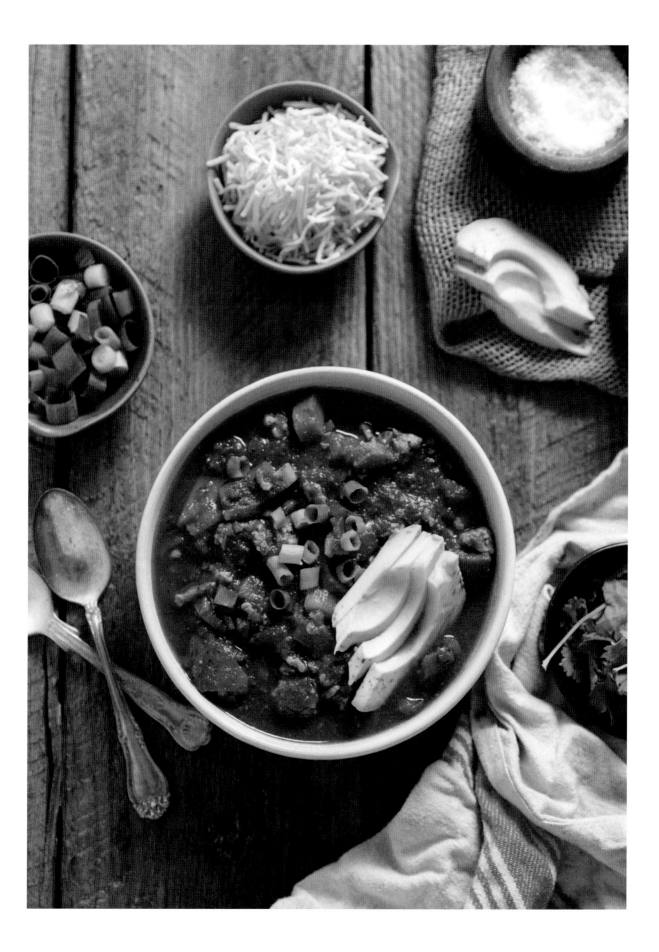

SLOW COOKER SPICY CHICKEN SOUP

serves 6 to 8   *prep time* 15 minutes   *cook time* 3 to 4 hours or 6 to 8 hours

EGG-FREE / NUT-FREE / DAIRY-FREE OPTION: **omit cheese garnish**
PALEO-FRIENDLY OPTION: **omit cheese garnish**

I absolutely L-O-V-E my slow cooker. Throw some ingredients in, set it, *forget it* (like get-up-and-leave-the-house forget it), and BOOM—a delicious soup is waiting for you to devour. This soup is one of my favorites: it is packed with flavor and offers a million (okay, eight) garnish options to appeal to just about everyone!

ingredients:

1 large onion, diced

1 red bell pepper, diced

1 green bell pepper, diced

3 cloves garlic, minced

2 boneless, skinless chicken breasts halves (about 1 pound)

1 (15-ounce) can crushed tomatoes

1 (4-ounce) can diced green chiles

3 cups chicken broth, homemade (page 354) or store-bought

2 teaspoons ground cumin

2 teaspoons chili powder

1 teaspoon fine sea salt

½ teaspoon paprika

Optional: ½ teaspoon cayenne pepper

¼ teaspoon freshly ground black pepper

¼ cup fresh cilantro leaves, finely chopped

2 teaspoons lime juice

OPTIONAL GARNISHES:

Crushed tortilla chips (see note)

Shredded cheese

Diced avocado

Diced onion

Chopped scallions

Jalapeño slices

Lime wedges

Chopped fresh cilantro

directions:

1. Combine all of the ingredients for the soup, minus the cilantro and lime juice, in a slow cooker. Stir the contents well.

2. Cover and cook on high for 3 to 4 hours or on low for 6 to 8 hours, until the chicken can easily be pulled apart with a fork.

3. Use two forks to shred the chicken right in the slow cooker. (If you have trouble, remove the chicken breasts to a cutting board and shred them there. Then simply return the chicken to the slow cooker and mix.)

4. Add the cilantro and lime juice and mix to combine. Serve hot with the desired garnishes.

5. You can refrigerate this soup for up to 5 days or freeze it for up to 3 months.

note: When buying tortilla chips, buy non-GMO and local if possible!

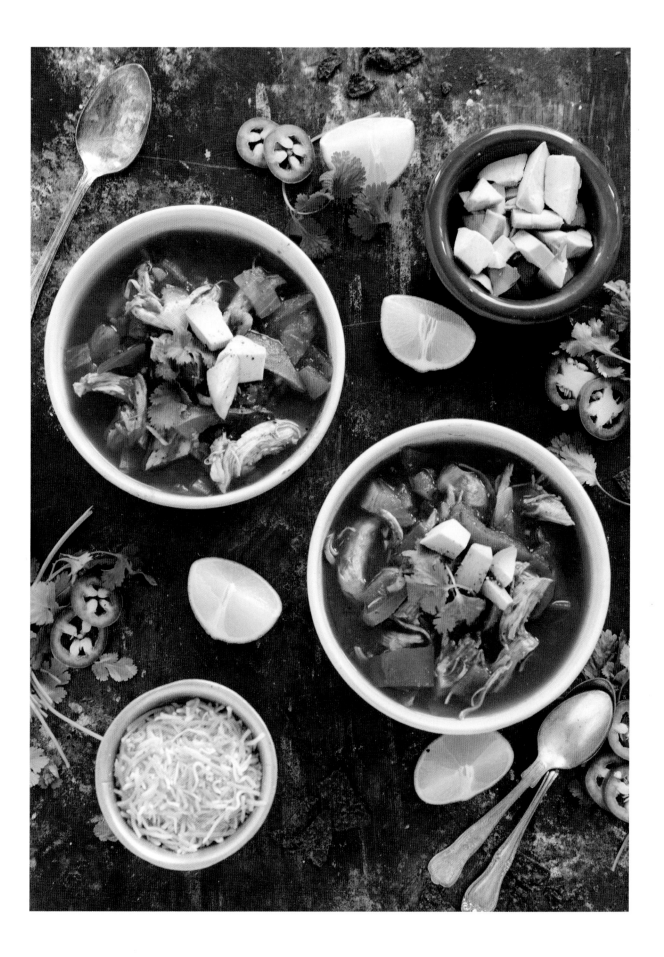

CIOPPINO STEW

serves 4 to 6   *prep time* 20 minutes   *cook time* 50 minutes

EGG-FREE / NUT-FREE / DAIRY-FREE OPTION: **use oil instead of butter** / PALEO-FRIENDLY

Fish stews are wonderfully hearty and light at the same time, making them great all year round. Serve this one up for a special weeknight meal—you will feel like you are dining in a fine restaurant!

ingredients:

2 tablespoons extra-virgin olive oil or unsalted butter

1 onion, finely diced or thinly sliced

1 shallot, finely diced

4 cloves garlic, minced

1 (28-ounce) can diced tomatoes with juice

1 (6-ounce) can tomato paste

4 cups chicken broth, homemade (page 354) or store-bought, or store-bought fish stock

½ cup dry white wine

Juice of ½ lemon

1 tablespoon Italian seasoning

1 teaspoon fine sea salt

½ teaspoon red pepper flakes

½ teaspoon freshly ground black pepper

Pinch of cayenne pepper

2 bay leaves

1 bunch fresh flat-leaf parsley, chopped, plus more for garnish

1 small bunch fresh basil, chopped, plus more for garnish

1½ pounds mussels, scrubbed and debearded

1½ pounds clams, scrubbed

Optional: 2 Mexican-style fresh (raw) chorizo links, casings removed and meat crumbled

1 pound cod fillet or firm white fish of choice, cubed

½ pound large shrimp, peeled and deveined

½ pound bay scallops

directions:

1. Heat the oil in a soup pot over medium heat, then add the onion, shallot, and garlic and sauté for 2 to 4 minutes, until soft.

2. To the pot, add the diced tomatoes, tomato paste, chicken broth, white wine, lemon juice, Italian seasoning, salt, red pepper flakes, black pepper, cayenne pepper, bay leaves, fresh parsley, and fresh basil. Bring to a boil, then lower the heat and simmer for 25 minutes to combine the flavors.

3. Add the mussels and clams, increase the heat to medium, and cook for about 5 minutes, until they begin to open. If adding chorizo, do so now. Lightly season the cod, shrimp, and scallops with salt and pepper and add to the soup. Reduce the heat to medium-low and simmer until the fish, shrimp, and scallops are cooked through, 5 to 10 minutes. Discard any clams and mussels that did not open.

4. Taste and add more red pepper flakes and/or salt, if desired. Serve hot, garnished with additional fresh basil and parsley.

notes: You can change the seafood in this recipe as desired. Don't want to use clams or mussels? Add more shrimp and white fish.

If you like, serve this stew with sliced and toasted All-Purpose Sandwich Bread (page 80), as pictured. Note that the bread contains both eggs and nuts.

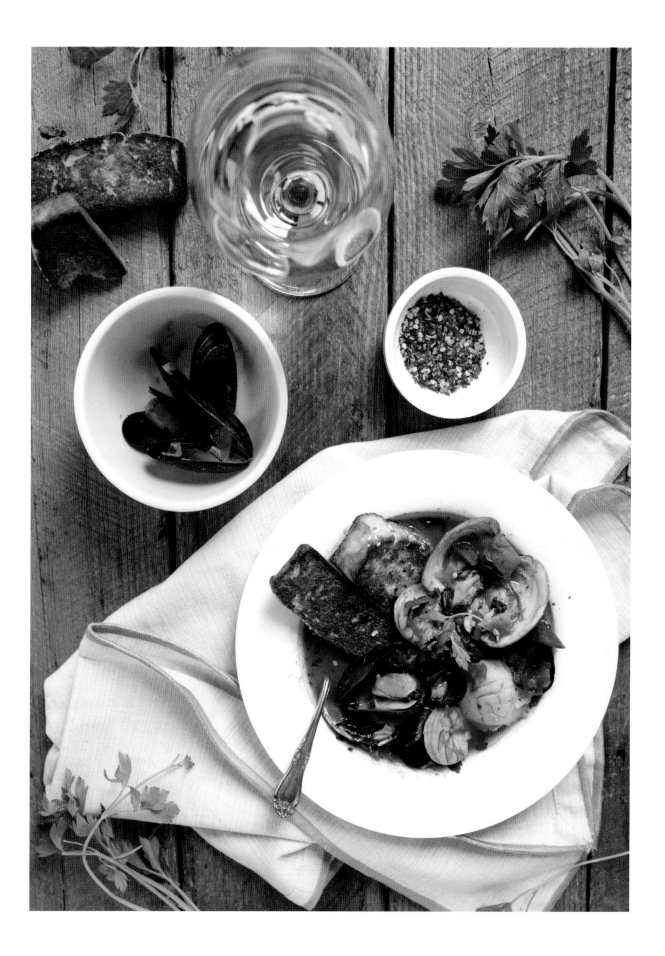

GREEK-INSPIRED LEMON CHICKEN SOUP

serves 3 to 4   *prep time* 10 minutes   *cook time* 45 minutes

NUT-FREE / DAIRY-FREE / PALEO-FRIENDLY

I absolutely love the flavors of Greek cuisine. We frequent a local Greek restaurant in our area, and I'm constantly trying new things on their menu. One day, I was in the mood for soup, and I devoured a comforting bowl of their lemony soup with egg mixed into it. It was a complete game-changer for me, and I knew I needed my own version. Think of this as traditional chicken soup with a totally unique and flavorful spin.

ingredients:

1 tablespoon extra-virgin olive oil

2 cloves garlic, minced

1 onion, diced

2 quarts (64 ounces) chicken broth, homemade (page 354) or store-bought

2 teaspoons grated lemon zest

Juice of 3 lemons

1 teaspoon fine sea salt

½ teaspoon freshly ground black pepper

2 cups shredded chicken (see page 152)

3 cups fresh spinach

4 large eggs

Optional: 1 cup Basic White Rice (page 247)

directions:

1. Heat the oil in a large pot over medium heat, then add the garlic. When the garlic is fragrant, after about 2 minutes, add the onion. Sauté for 5 minutes, until the onion is translucent.

2. Add the chicken broth, lemon zest, lemon juice, salt, and pepper and cook for 2 minutes.

3. Add the chicken and spinach. Reduce the heat and simmer for 15 minutes.

4. Crack the eggs into a bowl and lightly whisk them. Slowly pour the eggs into the soup while whisking the soup continuously and vigorously to separate the eggs into threadlike shapes as they cook. Once the eggs are cooked, remove the soup from the heat.

5. Add the rice, if using. Taste and add more salt and pepper, if desired. Simmer for an additional 2 to 4 minutes, then serve hot.

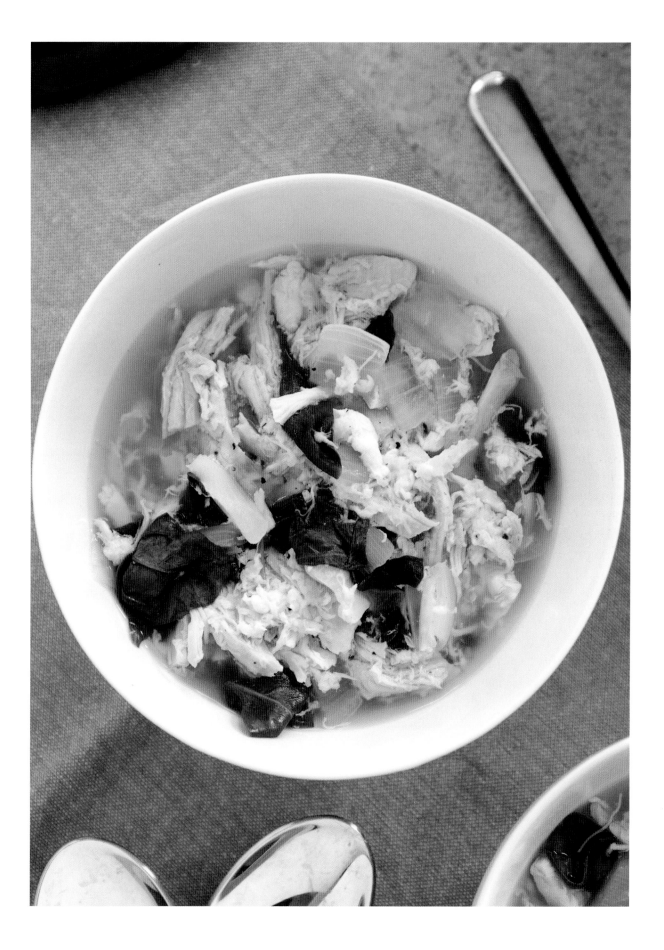

CREAMY PUMPKIN SOUP WITH ROASTED PUMPKIN SEEDS

serves 4 *prep time* 15 minutes *cook time* 1 hour

EGG-FREE / NUT-FREE / DAIRY-FREE OPTION: use oil instead of butter or ghee
PALEO-FRIENDLY OPTION: use ghee or oil instead of butter / VEGAN OPTION: use vegetable broth (page 356) instead of chicken broth and oil instead of butter or ghee

This soup is creamy and delicate, and pairs perfectly with any chicken, meat, or fish dish you are serving! It's best made with fresh pumpkin puree, but canned pumpkin works, too (see note below). Working with fresh pumpkin may seem daunting, but trust me, the hardest part is cutting it in half (use those muscles)!

ingredients:

1 small sugar pumpkin (3 to 4 pounds) (see note)

2 tablespoons unsalted butter, ghee (page 350), or oil of choice

½ onion, sliced

2 cloves garlic, minced

1 tablespoon pure maple syrup

1 teaspoon fine sea salt

½ teaspoon freshly ground black pepper

½ teaspoon ground cinnamon

¼ teaspoon ground nutmeg

Optional: ¼ teaspoon cayenne pepper

About 2 cups chicken broth, home-made (page 354) or store-bought

FOR THE ROASTED PUMPKIN SEEDS:

Pumpkin seeds (from above)

1 tablespoon extra-virgin olive oil or avocado oil

½ teaspoon fine sea salt

Optional: 1 teaspoon paprika

OPTIONAL GARNISHES:

1 to 2 tablespoons full-fat coconut milk

1 tablespoon chopped kale or other greens of choice

directions:

1. Have two oven racks in the oven, evenly spaced. Preheat the oven to 400°F.

2. Cut the stem off the pumpkin, then cut the pumpkin into 4 wedges. With a spoon or an ice cream scooper, scoop the pumpkin seeds into a small bowl and set aside. Place the pumpkin wedges cut side down on a rimmed baking sheet. Roast for 40 to 45 minutes, until fork-tender and golden brown. Peel off the skin and discard.

3. While the pumpkin wedges are roasting, make the roasted pumpkin seeds: Line a rimmed baking sheet with parchment paper. Rinse the pumpkin seeds to remove as much of the flesh and membrane as you can, then pat the seeds dry. Toss the seeds with the oil, salt, and paprika, if using. Spread the seeds in a single layer on the baking sheet. Roast for 25 minutes, until golden brown, stirring halfway through. Watch to avoid burning.

4. Melt the butter in a large Dutch oven over medium heat. Add the onion and garlic and sauté for about 4 minutes, until the onion is translucent.

5. Add the roasted pumpkin flesh, maple syrup, salt, and spices. Pour in just enough chicken broth to cover the pumpkin (this may take a little more or less than 2 cups). Bring to a boil, then reduce the heat and simmer, covered, for 10 minutes.

6. Transfer to a blender and blend until smooth (work in batches if needed). Taste and adjust the seasoning and spices as desired.

7. Serve the soup garnished with roasted pumpkin seeds and a drizzle of coconut milk and chopped kale, if desired. (*Note:* You will not need all of the roasted pumpkin seeds to garnish the soup. Store leftovers in a resealable plastic bag or container in the pantry for up to 1 week. They are great to snack on!)

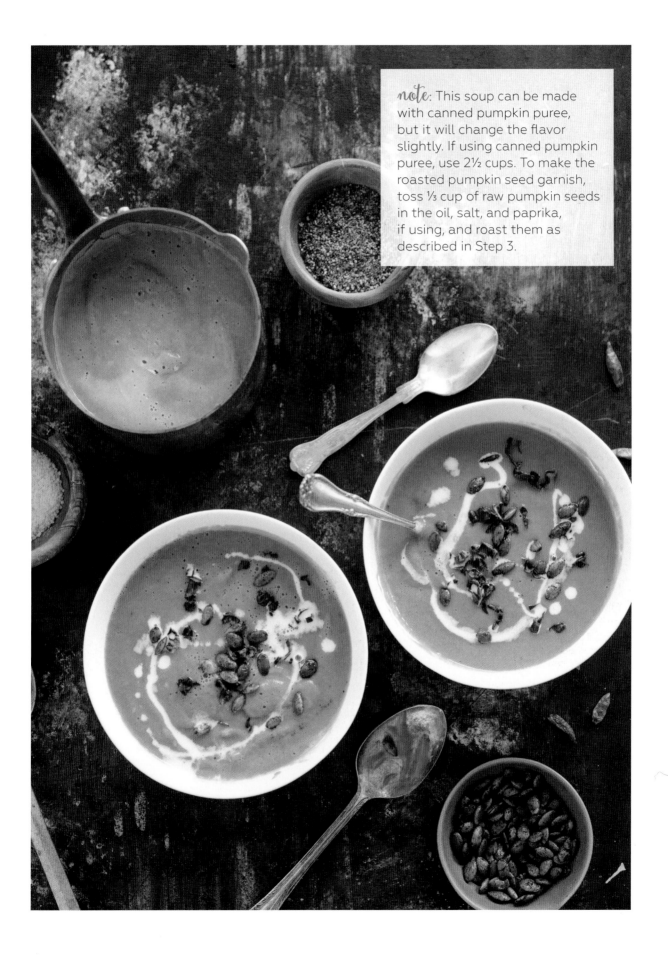

note: This soup can be made with canned pumpkin puree, but it will change the flavor slightly. If using canned pumpkin puree, use 2½ cups. To make the roasted pumpkin seed garnish, toss ⅓ cup of raw pumpkin seeds in the oil, salt, and paprika, if using, and roast them as described in Step 3.

EASY CHORIZO & KALE SOUP

serves 2 to 4 *prep time* 15 minutes *cook time* 45 minutes

EGG-FREE / NUT-FREE / DAIRY-FREE / PALEO-FRIENDLY

Veggies, spicy chorizo, and a little bit of heat come together to make a fabulous soup that's quick enough to whip up on a weeknight. And you may already have all of the ingredients sitting in your fridge and spice drawer!

ingredients:

- 1 tablespoon extra-virgin olive oil
- 2 large carrots, chopped
- 2 cloves garlic, minced
- 1 large onion, diced
- 2 links Mexican-style fresh (raw) chorizo, casings removed and meat crumbled
- 2½ cups chopped kale (about 1 bunch)
- 6 cups chicken broth, homemade (page 354) or store-bought
- ½ teaspoon ground cumin
- ½ teaspoon fine sea salt
- ½ teaspoon freshly ground black pepper

directions:

1. Heat the oil in a Dutch oven or medium-sized soup pot. Add the carrots, garlic, and onion and sauté for 5 minutes, until the mixture is fragrant and the carrots have begun to soften.

2. Add the chorizo and cook for 2 to 3 minutes, then add the kale and cook until wilted, 3 to 5 minutes.

3. Add the chicken broth, cumin, salt, and pepper. Bring to a boil, then reduce the heat and let summer for 30 minutes. Taste and adjust the seasonings as desired before serving.

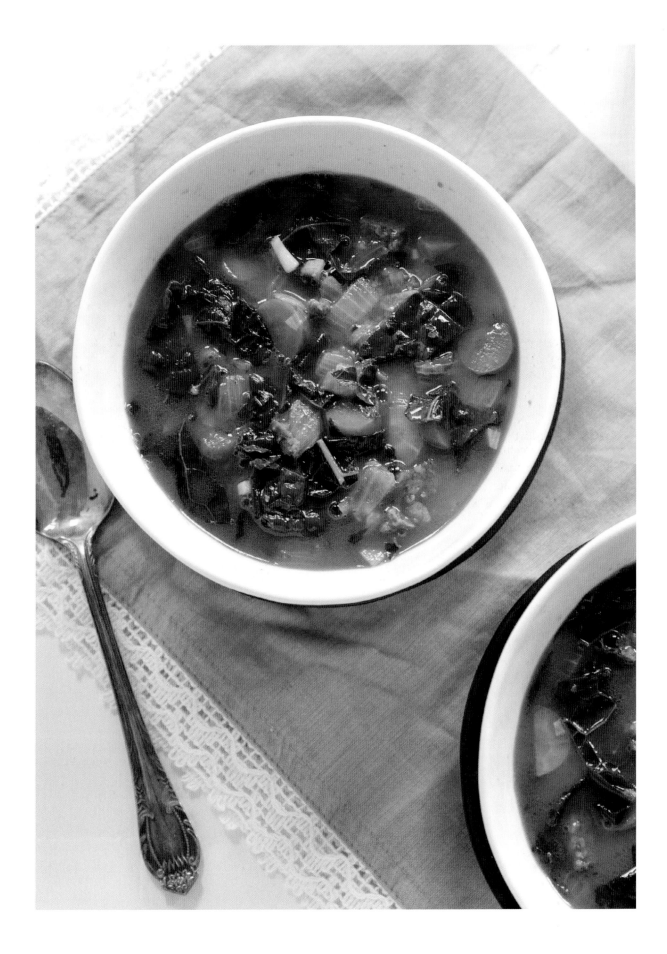

CURRY BUTTERNUT SQUASH SOUP

serves 4 to 6   *prep time* 10 minutes   *cook time* 40 minutes

EGG-FREE / NUT-FREE / DAIRY-FREE OPTION: use oil instead of ghee or butter
PALEO-FRIENDLY OPTION: use ghee or oil instead of butter / VEGAN OPTION: use vegetable broth
(page 356) instead of chicken broth and oil instead of ghee or butter

Curry and butternut squash together in soup form is divine. Simple as that. Packed with an enticing blend of flavors—a little sweetness and a punch of curry—this soup is bound to be a hit all fall and winter long (or spring and summer, if you enjoy soup year-round like I do)!

ingredients:

1 tablespoon ghee (page 350), unsalted butter, avocado oil, or extra-virgin olive oil

1 clove garlic, minced

1 large onion, diced

¼ cup coconut sugar

1½ tablespoons curry powder, plus more to taste

1 tablespoon ground cumin

½ teaspoon turmeric powder

½ teaspoon ground cinnamon

½ teaspoon freshly ground black pepper

2 teaspoons fine sea salt

1 butternut squash (about 3 pounds), peeled, seeded, and cubed

1 quart (32 ounces) chicken broth, homemade (page 354) or store-bought

½ cup full-fat coconut milk, plus more for garnish

Optional: 1 batch Croutons (page 82), for garnish

Chopped fresh cilantro, for garnish

directions:

1. In a large pot over medium heat, melt the ghee, then add the garlic. When the garlic is fragrant, after about 2 minutes, add the onion and sauté until translucent, about 5 minutes.

2. Add the coconut sugar, spices, and salt and cook until the spices are fragrant, about 2 minutes.

3. Add the cubed butternut squash and cook for 5 minutes, stirring often until the squash begins to soften. Add the chicken broth and coconut milk and bring to a boil. Once at a boil, turn down the heat and simmer until the squash is tender, about 20 minutes.

4. In a blender, puree the soup in batches until it is smooth and creamy.

5. Return the soup to the pot, bring to a boil, and let reduce for 10 minutes, until thickened slightly.

6. Taste the soup and add more curry powder, salt, and/or pepper, if desired.

7. Serve the soup garnished with croutons (if using), chopped cilantro, a drizzle of coconut milk, and a pinch of ground black pepper. Store any leftover soup in the refrigerator for up to 5 days.

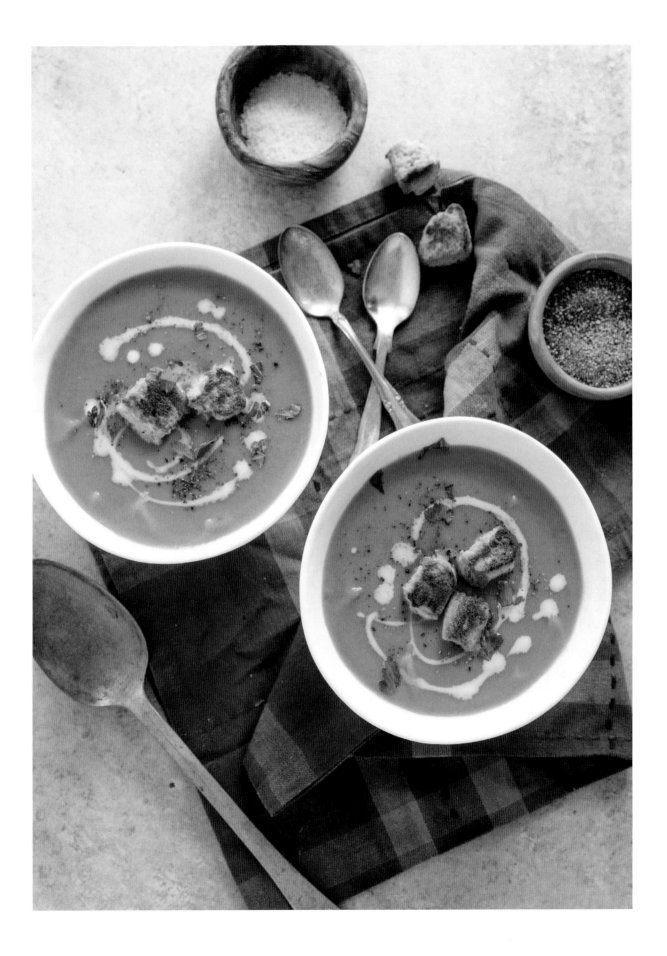

CHICKEN FAJITA SALADS

serves 4   *prep time* 15 minutes   *cook time* 20 minutes

EGG-FREE / NUT-FREE / DAIRY-FREE OPTION: omit cheese / PALEO-FRIENDLY OPTION: omit cheese

Chicken fajitas is my go-to order when I'm out at a Mexican restaurant, which is often! I love the spices and the flavors you get with *all* of the accompaniments. So why not throw it all together into an easy weeknight salad? I make this salad weekly, and we never tire of it. All of the flavors of your favorite fajitas at home in about thirty minutes! I also love using salsa as the dressing to switch things up.

ingredients:

FOR THE CHICKEN FAJITAS:

1 tablespoon extra-virgin olive oil

1 large onion, sliced

1 clove garlic, minced

1 large green bell pepper, sliced

2 red bell peppers, sliced

1 pound boneless, skinless chicken breasts, cubed or sliced

1 tablespoon paprika

1½ teaspoons garlic granules

1 teaspoon fine sea salt

½ teaspoon cayenne pepper

½ lime

FOR THE SALAD:

6 to 8 cups roughly chopped romaine lettuce

1 avocado, sliced

Optional: ¼ cup shredded cheddar cheese

1 cup salsa, homemade (page 336) or store-bought

directions:

1. In a large sauté pan or cast-iron skillet, heat the oil over medium heat. Add the onion and garlic and sauté for 3 minutes, until the onion starts to become soft and translucent. Add the sliced bell peppers and sauté for 5 minutes, until the peppers begin to soften.

2. While the vegetables are sautéing, combine the paprika, garlic granules, salt, and cayenne pepper in a small bowl. Season the chicken with the spice mixture.

3. Place the chicken in the skillet with the vegetables and cook for 4 minutes, then toss and cook until the chicken is golden brown and fully cooked, about 5 more minutes.

4. Squeeze the lime over the fajita mixture. Remove the skillet from the heat and set it aside.

5. To serve: Arrange the lettuce in four individual serving bowls or plates and top with the chicken fajitas, avocado slices, and shredded cheese, if using. Serve immediately, topped with salsa as the dressing.

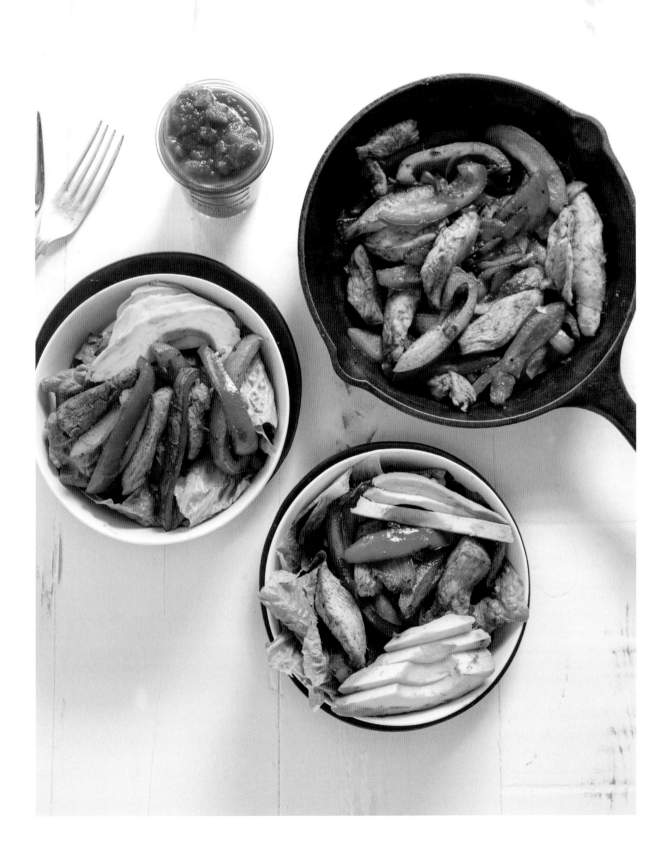

SRIRACHA LIME GRILLED CHICKEN SALAD

serves 2 *prep time* 15 minutes, plus 20 minutes to marinate chicken *cook time* 25 minutes

EGG-FREE / NUT-FREE / DAIRY-FREE / PALEO-FRIENDLY

A Lexi's Clean Kitchen reader favorite. This salad has taken over the Internet, and for good reason. It is the tastiest combination of flavors. Simple—yes. Light on flavor—nope! When it's time to get outside and grill, this is always one of the first recipes on my list.

ingredients:

FOR THE GRILLED CHICKEN:

¼ cup Sriracha sauce

Juice of 1 lime

2 boneless, skinless chicken breast halves

Pinch of fine sea salt

Pinch of freshly ground black pepper

Oil, for the grill

8 fresh pineapple rings, about ¼ inch thick, or 2 cups cubed pineapple (from ½ medium pineapple)

FOR THE LIME VINAIGRETTE:

⅓ cup extra-virgin olive oil or avocado oil

¼ cup apple cider vinegar

2 teaspoons honey

1 teaspoon grated lime zest

Juice of 2 limes

Pinch of fine sea salt

6 to 8 cups mixed greens or chopped romaine lettuce

1 avocado, sliced or cubed

1 cup grape tomatoes, halved

½ red onion, diced

directions:

1. Marinate the chicken: In a glass bowl or dish or a resealable plastic bag, combine the Sriracha and lime juice. Season the chicken with the salt and pepper, then add the chicken to the marinade bowl. Let the chicken marinate at room temperature for 20 minutes or in the refrigerator for up to 2 hours—the longer the better!

2. Preheat a grill to medium heat.

3. While the grill is heating, prepare the pineapple: Remove the top and peel the pineapple, then either slice it into rings using a pineapple corer or cut it into ½-inch cubes.

4. Grease the hot grill grate, then place the pineapple on the grill and cook for 4 minutes on each side, until the pineapple is warm and grill marks are visible. Set aside.

5. Place the chicken on the grill and cook for about 8 minutes on each side, depending on thickness, until no pink remains.

6. While the chicken is grilling, whisk together the ingredients for the vinaigrette.

7. Arrange the salad: Divide the greens between two bowls or plates. Slice or cube the chicken and place it on the salad. Top with the avocado, tomatoes, red onion, and grilled pineapple. Drizzle with the lime vinaigrette and serve immediately.

note: Try taking this salad to go in mason jars! Place 2 tablespoons of the lime vinaigrette in a quart-size jar. Add half of the salad ingredients in this order: tomatoes, onion, pineapple, chicken, avocado, and greens. Repeat with another quart-size jar. When ready to serve, pour into a bowl and enjoy! These mason jar salads will keep in the refrigerator for up to 5 days. The key is that the dressing and the greens are at opposite ends of the jar!

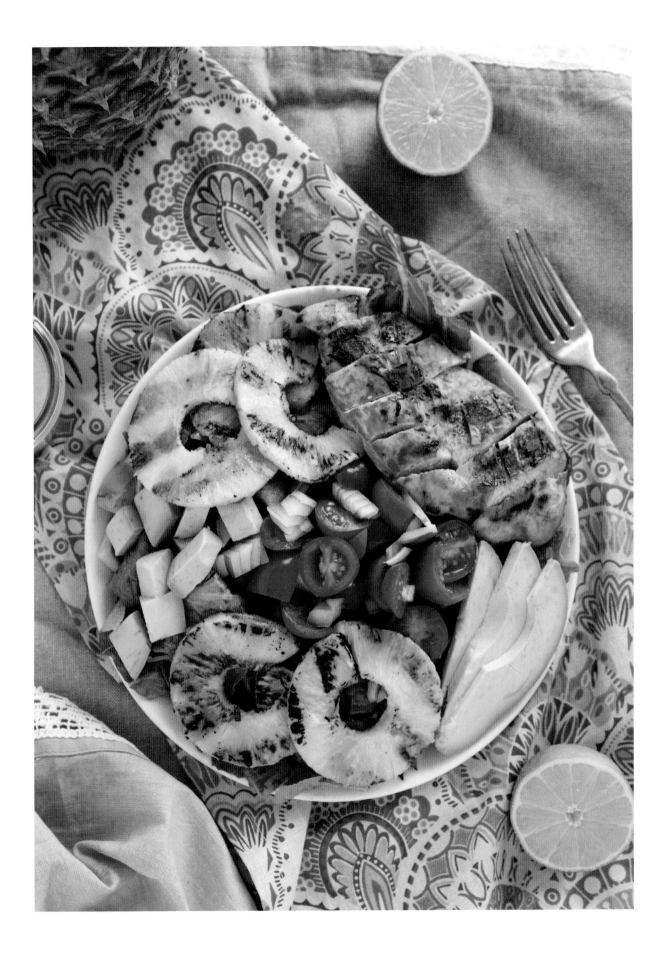

WINTER HARVEST SALAD

serves 2 to 4   *prep time* 10 minutes   *cook time* 40 minutes

EGG-FREE / DAIRY-FREE OPTION: use oil instead of butter
PALEO-FRIENDLY OPTION: use oil instead of butter / VEGAN OPTION: use oil instead of butter

FLAVOR TOWN! I adore this salad. Chopped kale, roasted squash, a hint of sweetness, and a bit of crunch, all topped with my favorite dressing, make this the ultimate salad all fall and winter long.

ingredients:

FOR THE ROASTED SQUASH:

1 medium kabocha squash

2 tablespoons extra-virgin olive oil, avocado oil, or unsalted butter

Pinch of fine sea salt

Pinch of ground cinnamon

6 to 8 cups destemmed and chopped kale

1 tablespoon extra-virgin olive oil or avocado oil

½ cup raw pecans

⅓ cup pomegranate seeds or dried cranberries

1 batch Maple Balsamic Dressing (page 322)

note: You can also use 2 acorn squash (since they're smaller) or 1 large butternut squash in this recipe! If using either of these two squashes, peel them and then roast as directed in Step 2.

directions:

1. Preheat the oven to 400°F. Line a rimmed baking sheet with parchment paper.

2. Slice the squash in half and scrape out the seeds. Cut the squash into ½-inch slices and toss with the 2 tablespoons of oil, salt, and cinnamon. Place the squash on the lined baking sheet and roast for 40 minutes, until fork-tender. Once done, let cool for 5 to 10 minutes. (There's no need to peel the skin of kabocha squash; it's edible!)

3. While the squash is roasting, massage the kale with the 1 tablespoon of oil for 1 to 2 minutes, until evenly coated. Set aside.

4. In a small sauté pan over medium-low heat, toast the pecans until lightly browned and fragrant, about 5 minutes, stirring often to ensure that they don't burn.

5. Assemble the salad: Divide the kale between two plates or place it in a large serving bowl. Top with the roasted kabocha squash, pomegranate seeds, and toasted pecans. Dress the salad with as much dressing as you'd like and serve immediately.

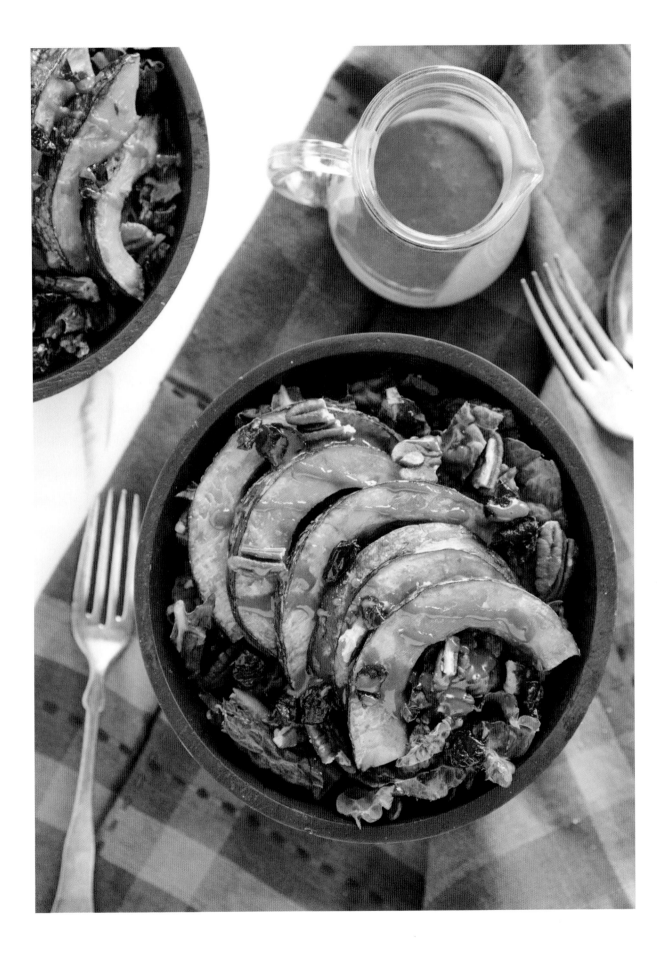

WATERMELON & MINT SALAD

serves 4 *prep time* 10 minutes *cook time* 10 minutes

EGG-FREE / NUT-FREE OPTION: omit almonds / DAIRY-FREE OPTION: omit cheese
PALEO-FRIENDLY OPTION: omit cheese

Can you say "summer"? That is exactly what this salad screams. Toss together some juicy and sweet watermelon, crunchy toasted almonds, spicy red onion, and fresh mint and you're all set—or throw in some feta and bacon for even more flavor. Plus, it's a perfect dish for a BBQ, since you can make a whole lot of it!

ingredients:

FOR THE BASIL GINGER DRESSING:

2 tablespoons fresh basil leaves

2 tablespoons water

1 teaspoon honey

1 teaspoon minced fresh ginger

⅓ cup raw sliced almonds

8 to 10 cups cubed watermelon (11 to 12 pounds watermelon with rind)

1 tablespoon extra-virgin olive oil

Pinch of fine sea salt

½ red onion, thinly sliced

1 small handful fresh mint leaves, chopped, plus additional leaves for garnish

Optional: ½ cup crumbled feta cheese (about 4 ounces)

Optional: 4 strips bacon, cooked until crispy and then crumbled

note: For a party, grab the biggest watermelon you can find and increase the rest of the ingredients proportionally!

directions:

1. Make the dressing: Place all of the dressing ingredients in a blender and blend on high for 30 seconds, until smooth. Taste and add additional honey, if desired.

2. In a medium-sized skillet over medium-low heat, toast the almonds until lightly browned and fragrant, about 4 minutes, stirring from time to time and watching carefully to avoid burning.

3. Assemble the salad: Place the cubed watermelon in a large serving bowl. Drizzle with the olive oil and sprinkle with the salt. Add the sliced onion, toasted almonds, chopped mint leaves, and optional feta cheese and bacon. Drizzle as much dressing as you'd like over the salad, top with a few whole mint leaves, and serve immediately.

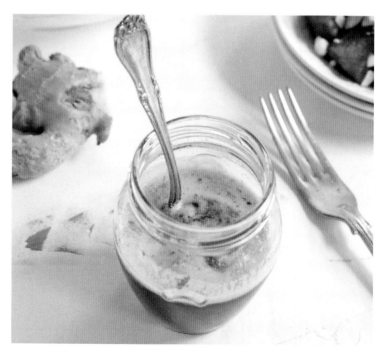

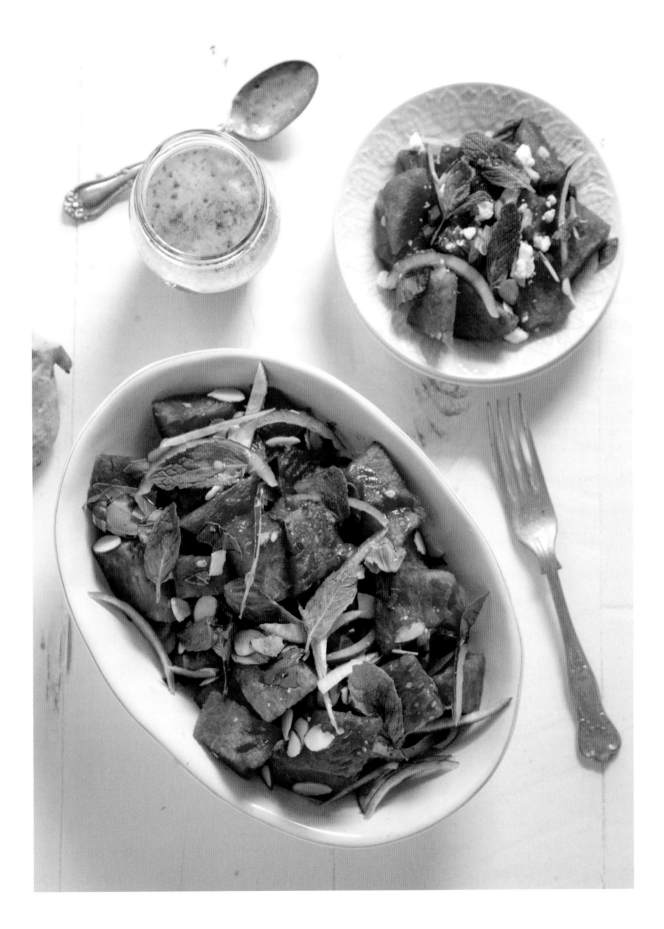

KALE CAESAR SALAD

serves 4 as a side *prep time* 10 minutes *cook time* 15 minutes

....

NUT-FREE / DAIRY-FREE OPTION: omit cheese / PALEO-FRIENDLY OPTION: omit cheese

....

Something about Caesar salad always seems a little naughty to me. Granted, it is usually junky. When I began my journey to eating clean, this was one of the first salads that I crossed off the menu when ordering at a restaurant. No more, though. I whip up a batch of my homemade croutons and my creamy Caesar dressing and chop up some kale, and we have ourselves a little make-your-own kale Caesar salad party!

ingredients:

6 to 8 cups destemmed and
   chopped kale

1 tablespoon extra-virgin olive oil

Juice of ½ lemon

Optional: ½ cup freshly grated
   Parmesan cheese

1 batch Creamy Caesar Dressing
   (page 320)

1 batch Croutons (page 82)

directions:

Place the kale, olive oil, and lemon juice in a large serving bowl and massage the kale for about 1 minute, until evenly coated. Toss the massaged kale with the Parmesan cheese, if using, and as much dressing as you'd like. Add the croutons and serve immediately.

variation:

Kale Chicken Caesar Salad. Prepare a batch of The Best Grilled Chicken (page 162), then slice it and place the grilled chicken atop the dressed Caesar salad. *Serves 2 as a meal.*

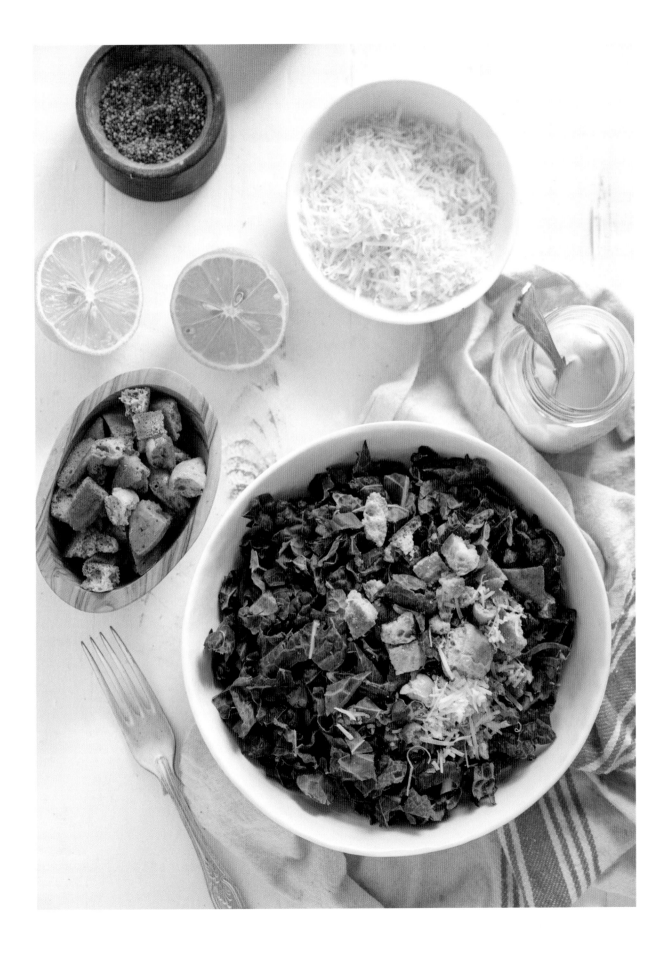

CHOPPED ANTIPASTO & GRILLED CHICKEN SALAD

serves 2   *prep time* 10 minutes (not including chicken)

EGG-FREE / NUT-FREE / DAIRY-FREE OPTION: **omit cheese**
PALEO-FRIENDLY OPTION: **omit cheese**

Oh, this salad! All of your favorite antipasto flavors in one hearty, crowd-pleasing dish. Once the chicken is marinated and grilled, this salad comes together very quickly.

ingredients:

4 to 6 cups roughly chopped lettuce

½ cup roasted red peppers, roughly chopped

1 cup roughly chopped tomatoes or quartered cherry tomatoes

1 cup sliced red onions

½ cup roughly chopped pepperoni of choice

½ cup roughly chopped salami

½ batch The Best Grilled Chicken (page 162), roughly chopped

Optional: 1 cup cubed fresh mozzarella cheese

1 teaspoon Italian seasoning

Fresh basil leaves, for garnish

FOR THE BASIL BALSAMIC DRESSING:

¼ cup extra-virgin olive oil

2 tablespoons balsamic vinegar

2 tablespoons finely chopped fresh basil

1 teaspoon Italian seasoning

directions:

1. Arrange the salad: Divide the chopped lettuce between two plates. Top with roasted red peppers, tomatoes, red onions, pepperoni, salami, grilled chicken, and fresh mozzarella, if using. Sprinkle the Italian seasoning on top. Garnish with fresh basil.

2. Whisk together the ingredients for the dressing. Pour over the salad and serve immediately.

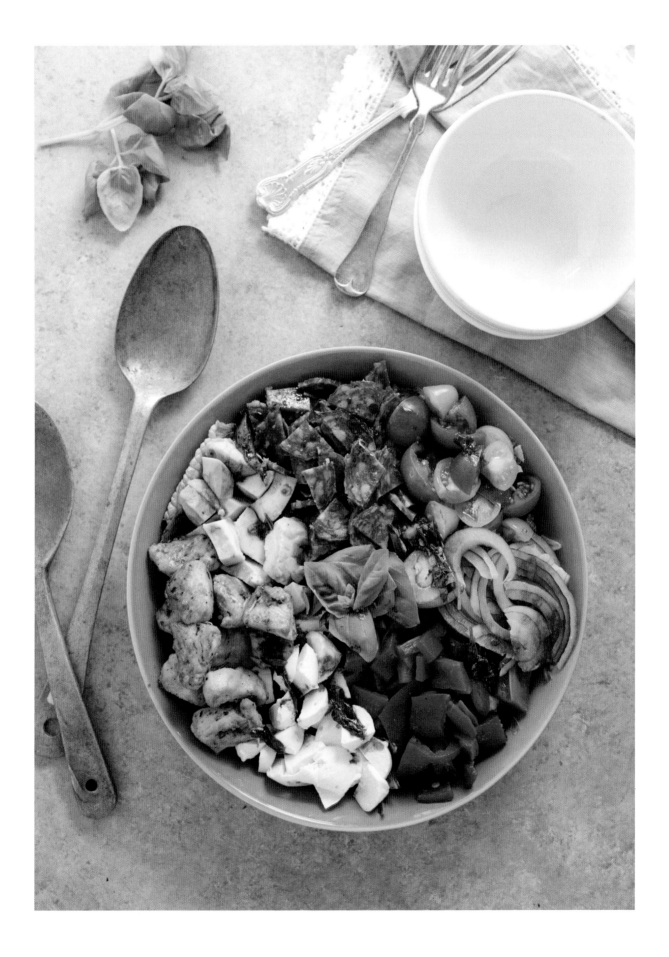

CHOPPED BBQ CHICKEN COBB SALAD

serves 2   *prep time* 10 minutes, plus 20 minutes to marinate chicken (not including caramelized onions)   *cook time* 8 minutes

---

NUT-FREE / DAIRY-FREE OPTION: **omit cheese** / PALEO-FRIENDLY OPTION: **omit cheese**

My husband, Mike, *loves* Cobb salad. He orders it wherever we go. I decided that a spin on the traditional Cobb was in order, and we can't seem to get enough of this version! There are a ton of fun flavors in this salad, like BBQ chicken and caramelized onions, because who doesn't love those two things together?

ingredients:

FOR THE BBQ CHICKEN:

1 pound boneless, skinless chicken breasts, cubed

1 cup Sweet & Smoky BBQ Sauce (page 328)

1 tablespoon extra-virgin olive oil

FOR THE CREAMY HONEY MUSTARD:

2 tablespoons mayo, homemade (page 312) or store-bought

2 tablespoons Dijon mustard

1 tablespoon whole-grain mustard

1 tablespoon honey

1 teaspoon apple cider vinegar

6 to 8 cups chopped lettuce

4 strips bacon, cooked until crispy and crumbled

4 hard-boiled eggs, diced (see page 66)

1 cup cherry tomatoes, halved or quartered

1 avocado, sliced or diced

1 cup Caramelized Onions (page 332)

Optional: ⅓ to ½ cup shredded cheddar cheese

directions:

1. In a glass dish or bowl or a resealable plastic bag, toss the chicken in the BBQ sauce. Let marinate at room temperature for 20 minutes or in the refrigerator for up to 6 hours.

2. Heat the olive oil in a large sauté pan over medium heat. When hot, place the chicken in the pan and cook for about 4 minutes on each side, depending on thickness, until the chicken is cooked through and no pink remains in the center. Let rest for 3 minutes to cool slightly.

3. In a bowl, whisk together the ingredients for the creamy honey mustard.

4. Arrange the salad: Divide the lettuce between two plates. Top with the BBQ chicken, bacon, hard-boiled eggs, cherry tomatoes, avocado, caramelized onions, and cheddar cheese, if using. Serve immediately, drizzled with the honey mustard.

note: This salad comes together very quickly when you have several of the ingredients precooked: the bacon, eggs, and caramelized onions can all be made a day ahead. What's more, the chicken can be placed in the marinade the day before you make the salad, and the BBQ sauce can be made up to a week in advance!

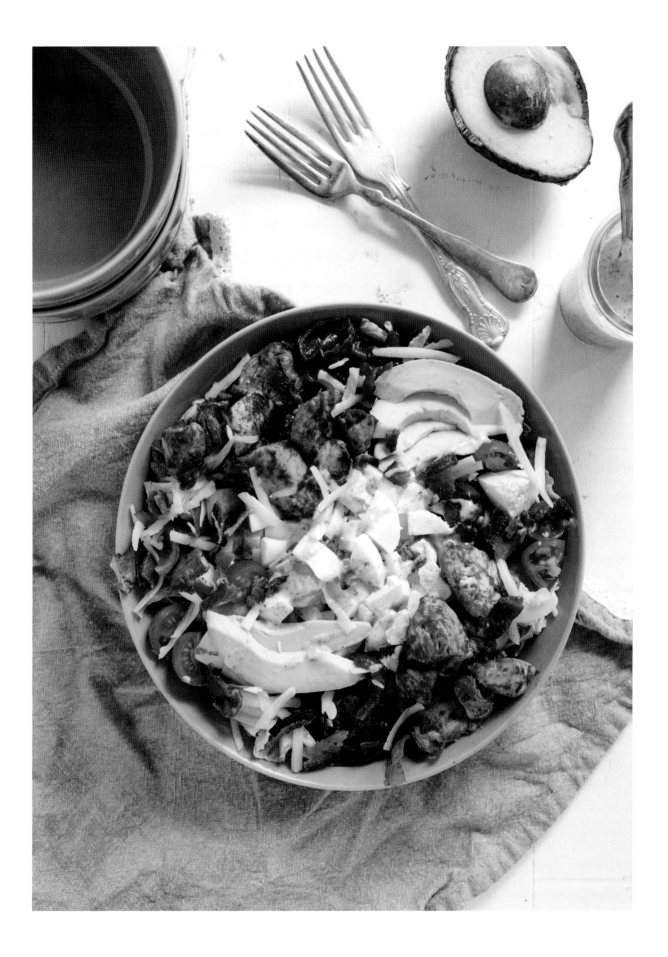

STRAWBERRY DATE SALAD WITH POPPY SEED DRESSING

serves 4 as a side   *prep time* 15 minutes   *cook time* 4 minutes

....

EGG-FREE / NUT-FREE OPTION: **omit almonds** / DAIRY-FREE / PALEO-FRIENDLY
VEGAN OPTION: **use maple syrup instead of honey**

....

When strawberries and spinach are in abundance at local farms in our area, I stock up and make a big, bold fresh salad. With a little added sweetness from the dates, a nice crunch from the sliced almonds, and a deliciously creamy poppy seed dressing, this recipe makes for the perfect summer salad.

ingredients:

½ cup sliced raw almonds

6 to 8 cups spinach leaves or mixed greens

6 dates, pitted and cut into ¼-inch pieces

2 cups sliced strawberries

FOR THE POPPY SEED DRESSING:

⅓ cup plus 2 tablespoons avocado oil or extra-virgin olive oil

¼ cup apple cider vinegar

2 tablespoons honey

1 tablespoon water, or more as needed

1 tablespoon poppy seeds

1 teaspoon Dijon mustard

½ teaspoon fine sea salt

directions:

1. In a medium-sized skillet over medium-low heat, toast the almonds until lightly browned and fragrant, about 4 minutes, stirring them from time to time and watching carefully to avoid burning.

2. Whisk together the dressing ingredients until smooth. Add more water as needed to reach your desired thickness.

3. Assemble the salad: Place the spinach leaves in a large bowl. Add the dates, strawberries, and toasted almonds. Top with the dressing and serve immediately.

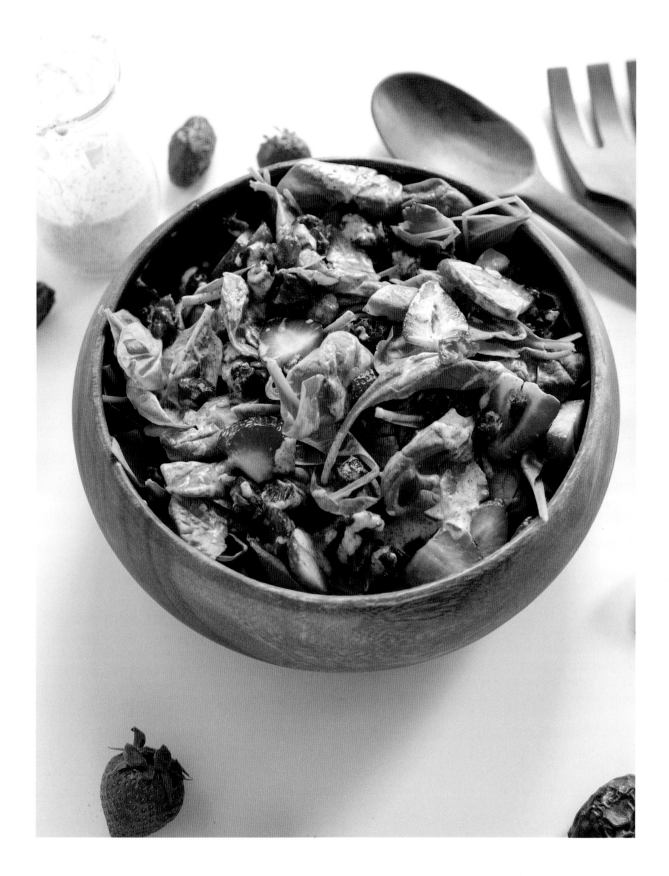

SESAME SEARED AHI TUNA SALAD WITH GINGER DRESSING

serves 2 *prep time* 15 minutes *cook time* 4 minutes

EGG-FREE / NUT-FREE / DAIRY-FREE / PALEO-FRIENDLY

Preparing seared ahi tuna at home might sound intimidating, but it actually comes together in a snap! This salad, topped with tuna encrusted with sesame seeds and seared to perfection and dressed with a delicious ginger dressing, will impress everyone who tries it!

ingredients:

FOR THE AHI TUNA:

2 tablespoons white sesame seeds

2 tablespoons black sesame seeds

1 pound sushi-grade ahi tuna steaks

1 tablespoon avocado oil

4 cups chopped romaine lettuce

½ cup shredded red cabbage

1 cup chopped cherry tomatoes

1 avocado, diced or sliced

¼ cup chopped red onions

1 mango, diced

1 batch Ginger Dressing (page 324)

Optional: 1 jalapeño pepper, sliced, for garnish

Optional: Lime wedges, for garnish

directions:

1. Place the sesame seeds in a shallow bowl. Press the tuna steaks into the seeds until the tuna is completely coated on all sides.

2. Heat the oil in a skillet over medium heat. When hot, add the tuna and cook for 2 minutes on each side, until the outside is seared and no longer pink. If you want your tuna cooked more than rare, cook it for a few minutes longer. Set aside to cool slightly, then cut into ½-inch slices.

3. Assemble the salad: Divide the lettuce, cabbage, cherry tomatoes, avocado, red onions, mango, and sliced tuna between two bowls. Top with the dressing and garnish with jalapeño slices and lime wedges, if desired. Serve immediately.

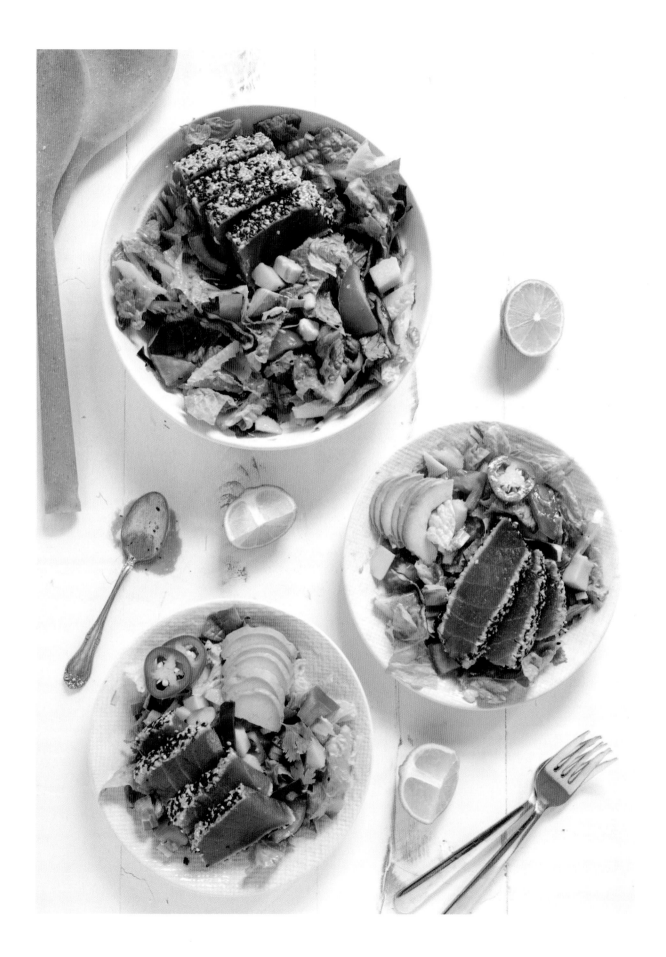

CHICKEN SALAD THREE WAYS

serves 2 (each)   *prep time* 15 minutes   *cook time* 4 minutes

EGG-FREE OPTION: make Pesto Chicken Salad / NUT-FREE OPTION: make Classic Chicken Salad, sub seeds for walnuts in Cranberry Walnut Chicken Salad, or make nut-free pesto for Pesto Chicken Salad / DAIRY-FREE OPTION: make Classic Chicken Salad or Cranberry Walnut Chicken Salad, or make dairy-free pesto for Pesto Chicken Salad / PALEO-FRIENDLY OPTION: make Classic Chicken Salad or Cranberry Walnut Chicken Salad, or make dairy-free pesto for Pesto Chicken Salad

Chicken salad can be made to satisfy everyone's taste buds—classic, savory, or sweet. These are my three favorite ways to prepare it, and each of them comes together for a fabulous meal! Pile it on top of a salad, wrap it in lettuce leaves, or enjoy it in a bowl for a snack or quick bite.

ingredients:

2 packed cups shredded chicken (see note)

FOR CLASSIC CHICKEN SALAD:

¾ cup finely chopped celery

¼ cup mayo, homemade (page 312) or store-bought

2 teaspoons Italian seasoning

Pinch of fine sea salt

FOR CRANBERRY WALNUT CHICKEN SALAD:

½ cup dried cranberries

½ cup raw walnuts, finely chopped

¼ cup mayo, homemade (page 312) or store-bought

1 tablespoon coconut sugar or granulated maple sugar

1 teaspoon ground cinnamon

Pinch of fine sea salt

FOR PESTO CHICKEN SALAD:

1 batch Lexi's Pesto (page 316)

Fine sea salt to taste

directions:

Place the shredded chicken in a large bowl. Add the ingredients for the salad of your choice and mix to combine. If it's a little dry, add more mayo or pesto. Taste and adjust the seasoning as desired.

How to Make Easy Shredded Chicken:

Place 2 whole boneless, skinless chicken breasts (1⅓ to 1½ pounds) in a slow cooker. Pour enough chicken broth over the chicken to cover, about 1 cup. Add 2 cloves of garlic, ½ cup of diced onions, 1 teaspoon of garlic powder, 1 teaspoon of fine sea salt, and ½ teaspoon of freshly ground black pepper. Cover and cook on high for 3 hours. Remove the chicken and shred with two forks. *Makes about 3 cups shredded chicken.*

note: Another great alternative for quick and easy meal prepping is to buy a whole rotisserie chicken!

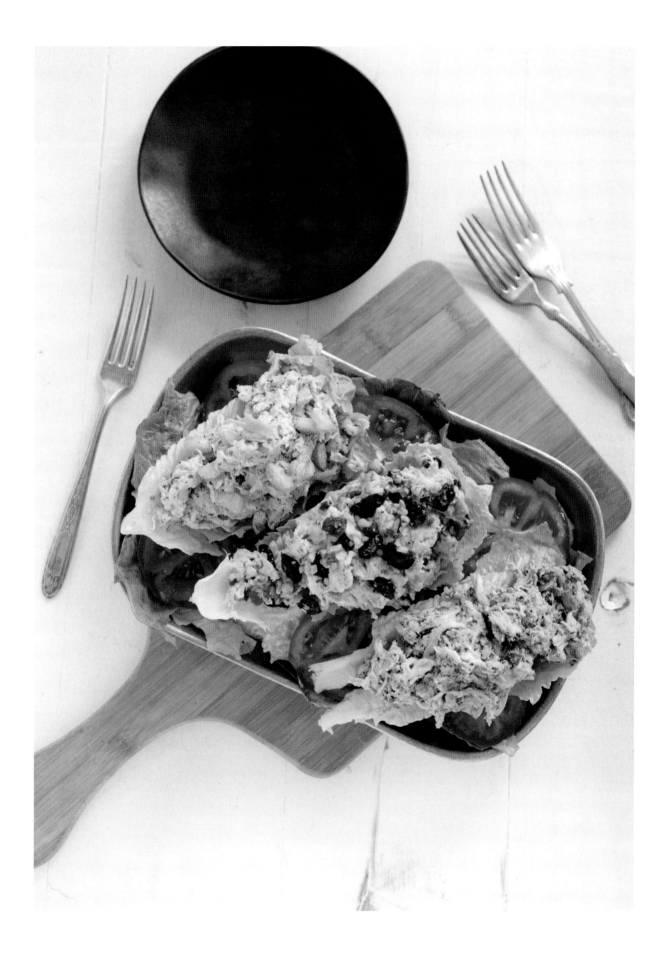

SHREDDED BRUSSELS SPROUTS SALAD

serves 4 as a side   *prep time* 15 minutes   *cook time* 5 minutes

EGG-FREE / PALEO-FRIENDLY OPTION: **omit cheese** / VEGAN OPTION: **omit cheese**

Shredded Brussels sprouts are a fantastic alternative to lettuce. If you haven't tried them, I highly recommend that you do! This salad is one of my favorites. I love the unique flavor of the hazelnuts and the crunch that they add. Topped with fresh Parmesan cheese and getting a hint of sweetness from the dried cranberries, the salad is finished with a light, classic red wine dressing for the perfect side.

ingredients:

1 cup raw hazelnuts, skins removed (see notes)

12 ounces Brussels sprouts

½ cup freshly grated Parmesan cheese, plus shaved Parmesan for garnish

⅓ cup dried cranberries

Optional: Cracked black pepper

FOR THE RED WINE DRESSING:

¼ cup extra-virgin olive oil

2 tablespoons red wine vinegar

1 teaspoon Dijon mustard

¼ teaspoon fine sea salt, or more to taste

Pinch of freshly ground black pepper

directions:

1. Heat a small skillet over medium heat. Add the hazelnuts and toast in the pan for 5 minutes, tossing often to avoid burning. Set aside to cool, then roughly chop.

2. To shred the Brussels sprouts, place them in a food processor and pulse until fine shreds form. (You should have about 5 cups.)

3. Put the Brussels sprouts, toasted hazelnuts, grated Parmesan cheese, and cranberries in a large serving bowl.

4. In a small bowl, whisk together the ingredients for the dressing.

5. Toss the salad with some cracked pepper, if adding, and your desired amount of dressing. Serve immediately, garnished with shaved Parmesan cheese.

notes: To remove the hazelnut skins, preheat the oven to 400°F. Spread the hazelnuts on a rimmed baking sheet and bake for 10 minutes, until the nuts have darkened and the skins have begun to flake off. Watch closely to avoid burning. Remove from the oven and let cool for 5 minutes. Then place the hazelnuts in the center of a large kitchen towel, gather the sides of the towel together to form a pouch, and rub and shake until the brown skins of the nuts start to peel off. Continue rubbing and shaking until most of the skins are removed—don't worry if a few stubborn ones remain.

Want to make this salad a meal? Top it with grilled chicken!

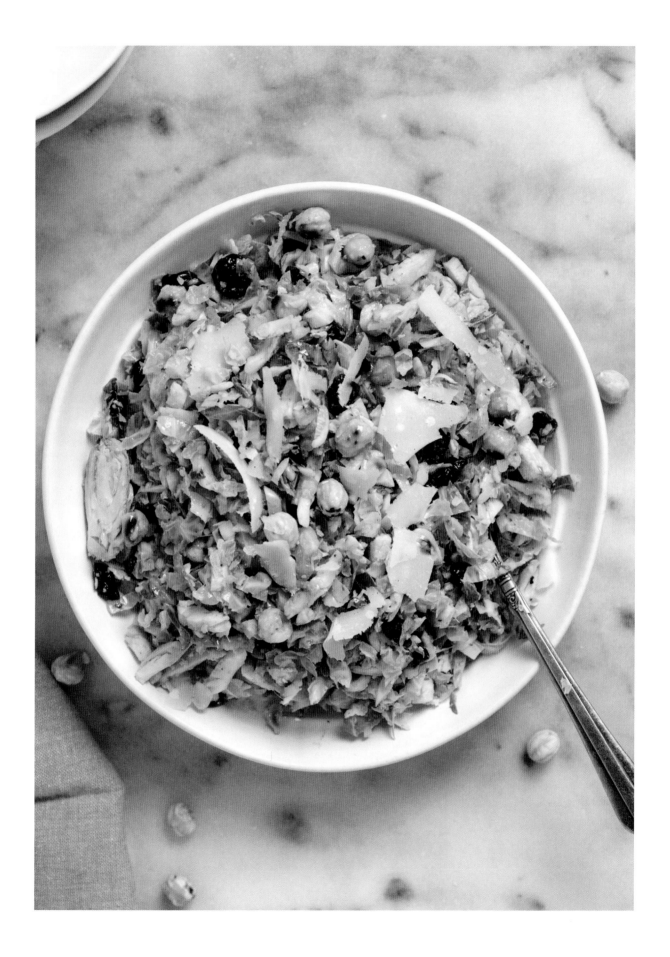

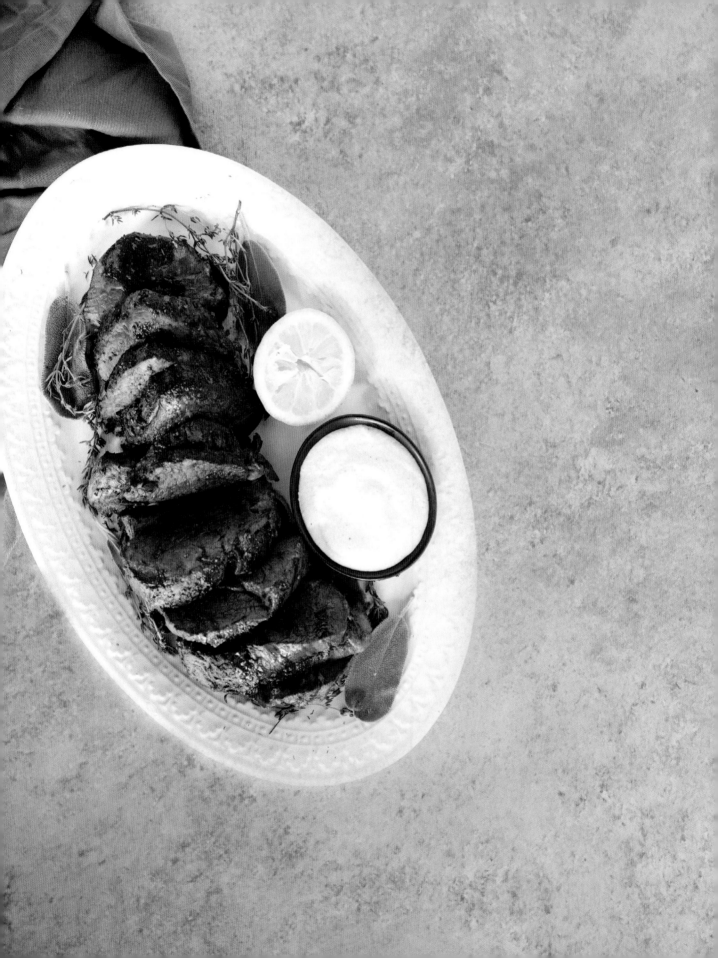

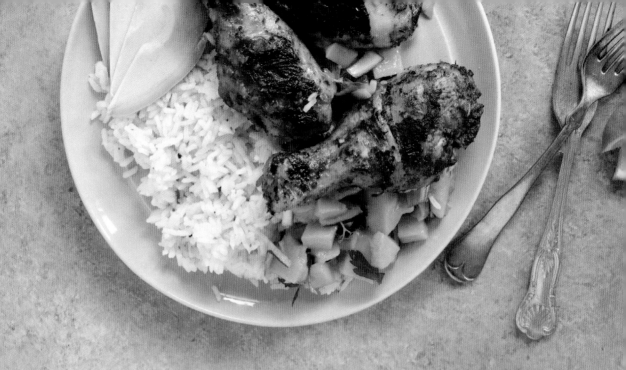

chapter 5

THE MAIN COURSE:

dinners for every night of the week

CLASSIC BAKED CHICKEN NUGGETS

serves 4   *prep time* 10 minutes   *cook time* 20 minutes

DAIRY-FREE / PALEO-FRIENDLY

As a kid, I really enjoyed fast-food chicken nuggets. Now, in my adult life, I can't believe how many Wendy's pit stops I made in my youth. Pretty disturbing. But guess what? Even in a clean-eating lifestyle, you can still have chicken nuggets that you'll rave about! These nuggets are seasoned just right, baked until golden and crispy, and served with a creamy honey mustard dipping sauce—all of the flavor with none of the junky ingredients.

ingredients:

1 cup blanched almond flour

1 tablespoon Italian seasoning

1 teaspoon garlic granules

1 teaspoon onion powder

½ teaspoon paprika

Pinch of freshly ground black pepper

½ teaspoon fine sea salt

1 large egg

1 teaspoon water

1 pound boneless, skinless chicken breasts, cubed

FOR THE CREAMY HONEY MUSTARD:

2 tablespoons mayo, homemade (page 312) or store-bought

2 tablespoons Dijon mustard

1 tablespoon whole-grain mustard

1 tablespoon honey

1 teaspoon apple cider vinegar

directions:

1. Preheat the oven to 375°F and line a rimmed baking sheet with parchment paper.

2. In a large bowl, mix together the almond flour, spices, and salt.

3. In a separate bowl, whisk together the egg and water until well combined.

4. Drop a few chicken cubes into the egg wash and turn them until coated. Transfer the coated chicken cubes to the spice bowl and dredge until evenly coated with the seasoning mixture. Place the coated chicken on the lined baking sheet.

5. Repeat until all of the chicken is coated, making sure to spread the cubes evenly on the baking sheet and leave some space between them.

6. Bake for 10 minutes, then flip and bake for an additional 8 minutes, until the chicken is golden and crispy and no pink remains in the center.

7. While the chicken is baking, whisk together the ingredients for the honey mustard or prepare another dipping sauce of choice (see suggestions below). Serve immediately with the nuggets.

serve with:

342
Ketchup

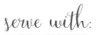
338
All-Purpose Marinara Sauce

328
Sweet & Smoky BBQ Sauce

312
Spicy Mayo

226
Sweet Potato Truffle Fries

variation: **Spicy Chicken Nuggets.** Make 'em spicy! Just add ¼ to ½ teaspoon of cayenne pepper and ½ teaspoon of chili powder to the spice mixture.

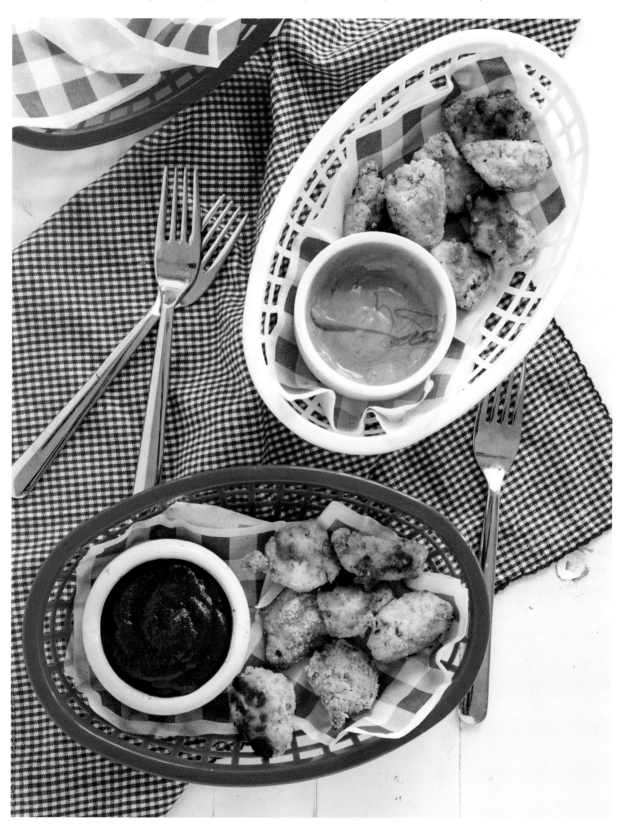

NANNY'S POTTED CHICKEN

serves 4   *prep time* 15 minutes   *cook time* 1 hour 40 minutes

EGG-FREE / NUT-FREE / DAIRY-FREE / PALEO-FRIENDLY

My nanny (grandma) has always been the cook in our family. Holidays are filled with her sweet and sour meatballs, brisket, stuffed cabbage rolls, and this potted chicken. Nanny lovingly gave me this recipe, and I am so glad to share it here, from my family's kitchen to yours! It's a special recipe that makes me think of the holidays, gathering around the dining room table with family, and of course, HER! Tender fall-off-the-bone chicken cooked slowly in a delicious sauce makes for the most fantastic meal.

ingredients:

1 tablespoon extra-virgin olive oil or avocado oil

2 onions, diced

6 cloves garlic, minced

4 carrots, diced

1 (28-ounce) can crushed tomatoes

¾ cup chicken broth, homemade (page 354) or store-bought

1 teaspoon dried basil

½ teaspoon dried oregano leaves

¼ teaspoon fine sea salt

¼ teaspoon black pepper

Pinch of red pepper flakes, or more to taste

1 whole chicken (about 4 pounds), cut into 8 pieces

1 teaspoon paprika

FOR SERVING:

1 batch Basic Cauliflower Rice (page 246), Basic White Rice (page 247), or Spaghetti Squash Noodles (page 248)

directions:

1. In a large braising pan or Dutch oven, heat the oil over medium heat. Add the onions and garlic and sauté for 2 minutes, until fragrant. Add the carrots and sauté for 2 to 3 minutes, until the carrots and onions begin to soften.

2. To the pot, add the crushed tomatoes, chicken broth, basil, oregano, salt, black pepper, and red pepper flakes. Mix to combine.

3. Season the chicken pieces generously with salt and pepper and add the chicken to the pot. Sprinkle the paprika over the chicken.

4. Lower the heat to medium-low and simmer, covered, for 90 to 100 minutes, until the chicken is tender. Taste the sauce and adjust the spices and seasoning as desired.

5. Serve hot over cauliflower rice, white rice, or spaghetti squash noodles.

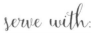

serve with:

Garlicky Blistered Green Beans

Burnt Broccoli

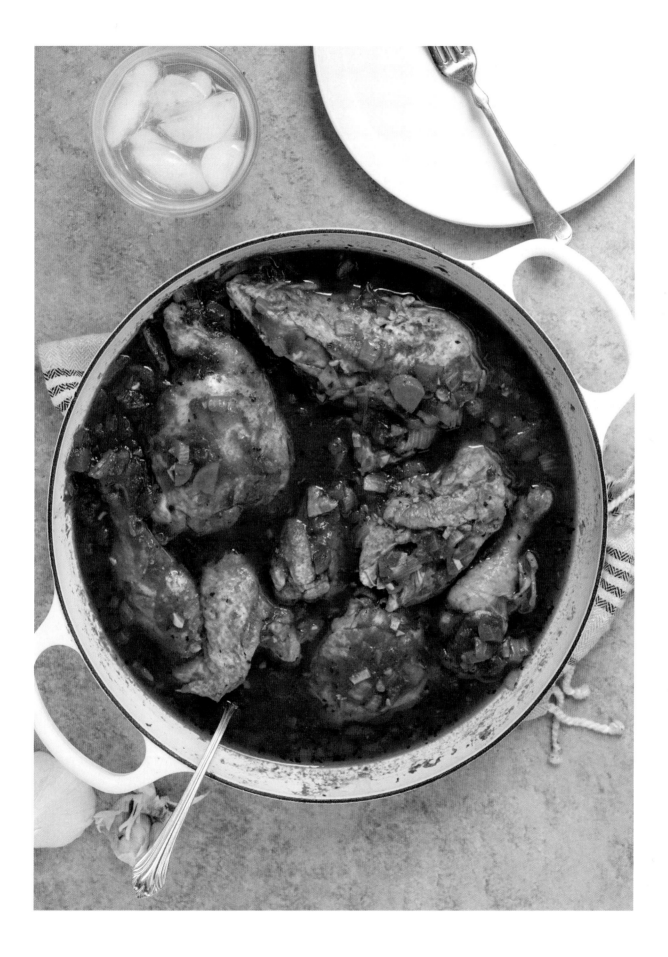

THE BEST GRILLED CHICKEN

serves 4   *prep time* 5 minutes, plus 30 minutes to marinate chicken   *cook time* 15 minutes

EGG-FREE / NUT-FREE / DAIRY-FREE / PALEO-FRIENDLY

When you take the time to marinate chicken with this seasoned wet rub before grilling it, you are rewarded with the best grilled chicken ever. I mean it!

ingredients:

FOR THE WET RUB
(MAKES ABOUT ¼ CUP):

2 tablespoons extra-virgin olive oil

2 cloves garlic, minced

1 tablespoon Italian seasoning

1 teaspoon fine sea salt

½ teaspoon freshly ground black pepper

½ teaspoon onion powder

½ teaspoon turmeric powder

Optional: ¼ to ½ teaspoon red pepper flakes, as desired

1½ pounds boneless, skinless chicken breasts or thighs, cubed

directions:

1. Make the wet rub: Place all of the ingredients for the rub in a small bowl and whisk to combine.

2. Put the cubed chicken in a glass or ceramic dish or resealable plastic bag, then add the wet rub. Turn the chicken in the rub, making sure that all the pieces are well coated. Place the chicken in the refrigerator for at least 30 minutes or up to 8 hours, until ready to cook.

3. Thirty minutes before you're ready to cook the chicken, preheat a grill or grill pan to medium heat.

4. Grease the hot grill grate. Place the chicken on the grill and cook for 5 to 7 minutes on each side, until no pink remains in the center. Remove from the heat and serve immediately.

note: If you don't have a jar of store-bought Italian seasoning, you can make your own by mixing together 1 tablespoon of dried basil leaves, 1 tablespoon of dried oregano leaves, 1 tablespoon of dried thyme leaves, 1 tablespoon of dried rosemary leaves, and 1 tablespoon of dried marjoram leaves. Store in a spice jar in a cabinet for up to a year (discard when it's no longer aromatic).

use in:

144
Chopped Antipasto & Grilled Chicken Salad

142
Kale Caesar Salad

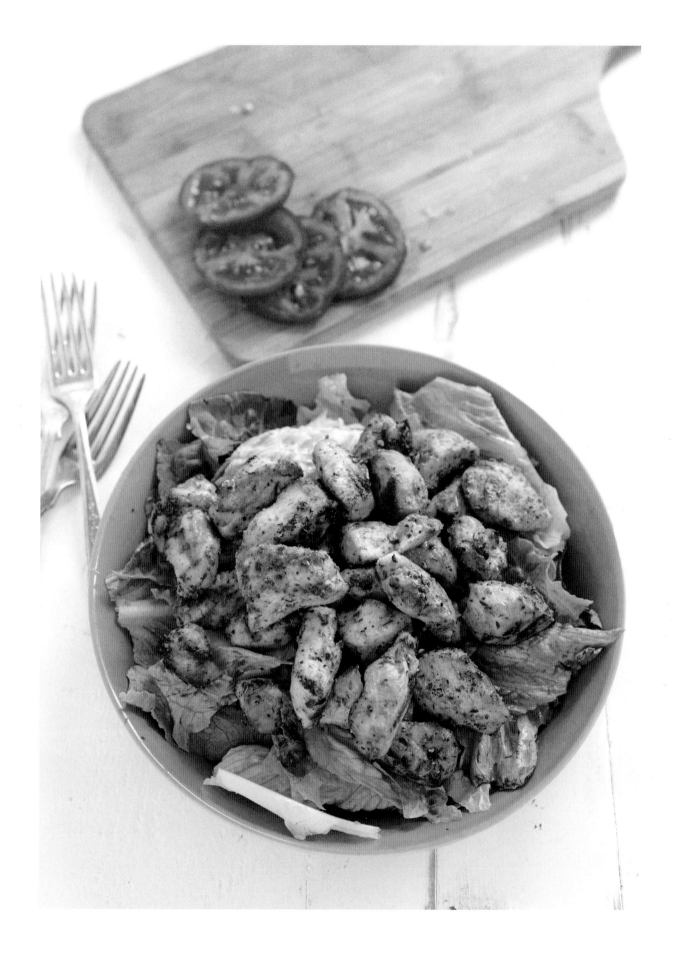

CHICKEN ENCHILADAS

serves 3   *prep time* 20 minutes (not including tortillas)   *cook time* 25 minutes

EGG-FREE / NUT-FREE / DAIRY-FREE OPTION: **omit cheese and use oil instead of ghee or butter**
PALEO-FRIENDLY OPTION: **omit cheese and use ghee or oil instead of butter**

Enchiladas are a heavenly combination of tortillas, veggies, chicken, and delicious sauce, plus cheese. Need I say more? This fun and hearty weeknight dinner makes for great leftovers the following day! Save yourself some time the day of by making the enchilada sauce ahead of time (it will keep for two weeks in the fridge). In addition to using the sauce in this recipe, try adding some to your morning eggs, to slow cooker shredded chicken (page 152), and so much more!

ingredients:

FOR THE ENCHILADA SAUCE (MAKES ABOUT 2 CUPS):

2 tablespoons avocado oil or extra-virgin olive oil

½ cup tomato sauce

1 tablespoon chili powder

½ teaspoon garlic powder

½ teaspoon onion powder

½ teaspoon ground cumin

½ teaspoon fine sea salt

1 cup chicken broth, homemade (page 354) or store-bought

2 teaspoons arrowroot flour

2 teaspoons water

1 batch Tortillas (page 72)

FOR THE CHICKEN ENCHILADAS:

1 tablespoon ghee (page 350), unsalted butter, or extra-virgin olive oil

1 onion, finely diced (omit if using caramelized onions; see below)

1 clove garlic, minced

1 pound boneless, skinless chicken breasts, cut into ½-inch cubes

1 (4-ounce) can diced green chiles

1 teaspoon paprika

½ teaspoon onion powder

¼ teaspoon ground cumin

¼ teaspoon freshly ground black pepper

½ teaspoon fine sea salt

1 cup baby spinach

Optional: ½ cup Caramelized Onions (page 332)

Optional: 1 cup shredded cheddar cheese, divided

Chopped fresh cilantro, for garnish

Diced avocado, for garnish

note: You can omit the cheese to make this dish dairy-free and Paleo-friendly, but if you tolerate it, I really do recommend it in this recipe.

directions:

1. Make the sauce: Heat the oil in a small saucepan over medium-high heat. Add the tomato sauce and stir in the spices and salt. Whisk in the chicken broth. Make a slurry with the arrowroot flour and water, then add the slurry to the sauce and whisk well.

2. Lower the heat and simmer for 10 minutes, or until the sauce is reduced by about one-quarter and coats the back of a spoon. Remove from the heat and let cool to room temperature.

3. While the sauce is reducing, prepare the chicken filling: In a large skillet over medium heat, melt the ghee. Add the onion and garlic and sauté for 2 minutes, until fragrant. (Omit the onion here if using caramelized onions.)

4. Add the chicken, diced green chiles, spices, and salt to the skillet and cook for 5 to 7 minutes, until no pink remains in the center of the chicken. Add the spinach and sauté for 1 minute, until wilted. Remove the pan from the heat and set aside. If adding caramelized onions, mix them in here.

5. Preheat the oven to 375°F. Spoon some of the sauce into the bottom of a 9 by 13-inch baking dish.

6. Assemble the enchiladas: Spread 1 tablespoon of the enchilada sauce on a tortilla, then place a spoonful or two of the chicken filling in the middle. Drizzle an additional teaspoon or two of the sauce over the chicken, then sprinkle with about a tablespoon of cheese, if using. Fold the sides of the tortilla up and over the filling and place the tortilla, seam side down, in the baking dish. Repeat with the rest of the tortillas, sauce, filling, and cheese, if using (reserving some cheese for the top).

7. When all the tortillas are stuffed and in the baking dish, top them with the rest of the enchilada sauce and the rest of the cheddar cheese, if using.

8. Bake for 15 minutes, or until the edges of the tortillas crisp up slightly and the cheese, if used, is melted.

9. Garnish with chopped cilantro and diced avocado and serve immediately.

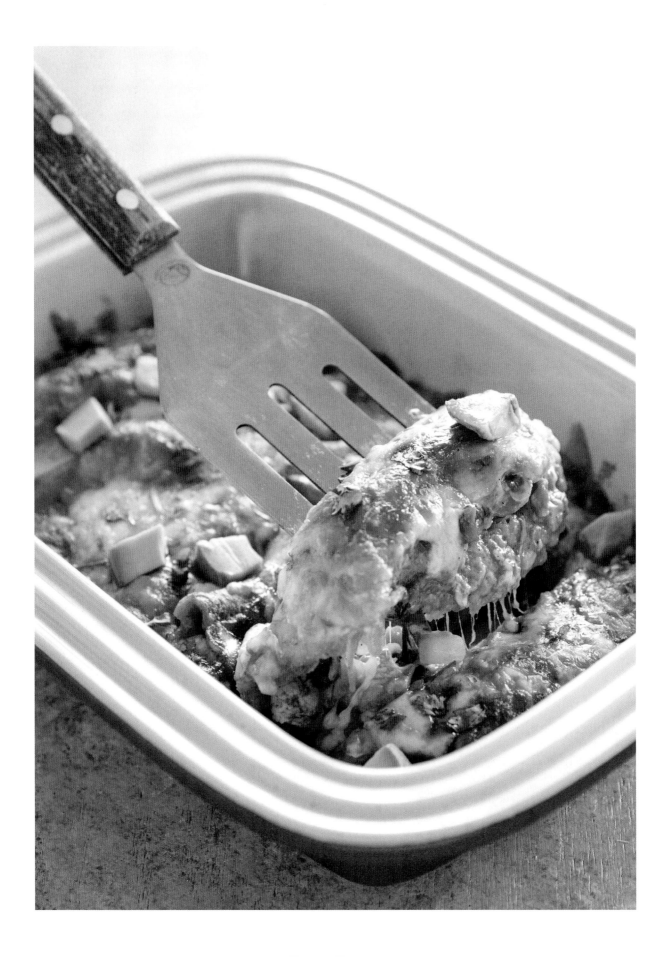

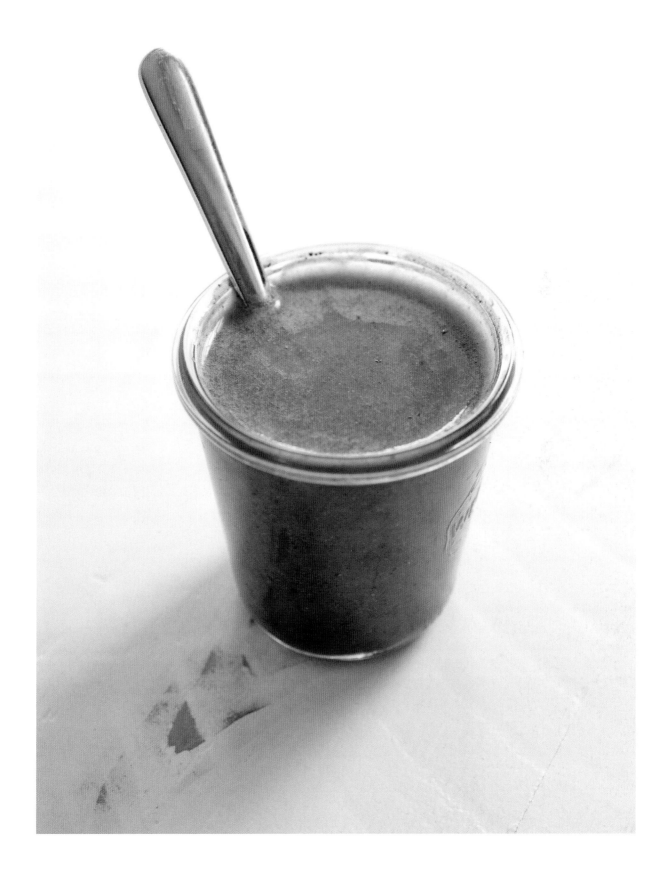

JERK CHICKEN WITH CARIBBEAN RICE & MANGO SALSA

serves 4   *prep time* 20 minutes, plus 4 hours to marinate chicken   *cook time* 25 minutes

EGG-FREE / NUT-FREE / DAIRY-FREE OPTION: use avocado oil instead of butter for rice
PALEO-FRIENDLY OPTION: use avocado oil instead of butter for rice

When we were in Jamaica, I fell in love with the jerk chicken made right on the beach. It packed a mean punch, and wow, was the spicy flavor and delicious charred skin incredible! A key ingredient in authentic jerk is the native Jamaican scotch bonnet pepper. If you can't find scotch bonnets (it can take a little digging here in the States), habañero is a good substitute. Warning: It gets SPICY!

ingredients:

FOR THE JERK SEASONING:

1 scotch bonnet or habañero chile, stemmed and roughly chopped

1 bunch scallions, chopped

2 cloves garlic, smashed with the side of a knife and peeled

1 tablespoon peeled and minced fresh ginger

2 tablespoons coconut aminos

1 tablespoon white vinegar

1 tablespoon lime juice

1 tablespoon coconut sugar

1 tablespoon ground allspice

1 teaspoon ground cinnamon

1 teaspoon dried thyme leaves

1 teaspoon fine sea salt

½ teaspoon freshly ground black pepper

2 tablespoons extra-virgin olive oil, plus more for the grill

2 pounds chicken drumsticks

FOR THE MANGO SALSA:

1 cup diced mangoes (about 2 mangoes)

¼ cup finely diced red onions

2 tablespoons chopped fresh cilantro

1 teaspoon lime juice

FOR THE CARIBBEAN RICE:

1 tablespoon unsalted butter

1 teaspoon peeled and grated fresh ginger

1 clove garlic, minced

1 cup jasmine rice

2 cups water

1 cup full-fat coconut milk

1 teaspoon fine sea salt

½ teaspoon freshly ground black pepper

½ teaspoon grated lime zest

1 avocado, sliced, for serving

directions:

1. Make the jerk seasoning: Place the ingredients for the seasoning in a food processor or blender. Pulse for 10 seconds, until the mixture is combined but not totally smooth. Set aside ¼ cup of the marinade, then transfer the rest to a large glass or ceramic dish or resealable plastic bag. Place the ¼ cup of marinade in the fridge.

2. Marinate the chicken: Pat the drumsticks dry, season them with a pinch of salt, and add them to the dish or plastic bag with the jerk seasoning. Mix to coat the chicken evenly, then marinate in the refrigerator for a minimum of 4 hours or up to 24 hours.

3. Thirty minutes before you're ready to cook the chicken, remove the chicken from the marinade and allow it to come to room temperature. Preheat a grill to medium heat. Meanwhile, prepare the rice and salsa.

4. Combine the ingredients for the salsa in a bowl and set aside.

5. Make the Caribbean rice: In a skillet that has a lid, melt the butter over medium heat. Add the ginger and garlic and sauté until fragrant, about 1 minute.

6. Add the rice and stir until all of the rice is coated in the butter, about 1 minute, then add the water, coconut milk, salt, pepper, and lime zest. Bring to a boil over medium heat, then reduce the heat to low and cover. Cook for 15 minutes, or until the rice is fluffy. Drain off any remaining liquid.

7. While the rice is cooking, grill the chicken: Brush the hot grill grate with oil. Place the chicken on the grill and cook for 8 minutes, then flip, brush with the reserved marinade, and grill for an additional 8 minutes. Turn the chicken over one last time, brush again with the remaining marinade, and cook for 5 more minutes, or until no pink remains in the center of the chicken and the skin is crispy.

8. To serve: Place the rice on plates, then add the chicken, mango salsa, and sliced avocado.

notes: This recipe works well with bone-in, skin-on chicken thighs. Having skin on the chicken is ideal here, as the skin allows the jerk flavor to really seep into the chicken.

Scotch bonnets are *very hot* chiles that are commonly used in Caribbean cooking and in authentic Jamaican jerk. On the heat scale, the scotch bonnet is one of the hottest peppers there is. Therefore, adjust accordingly for your desired taste. The best substitute is a habañero pepper, which has about the same level of spiciness and is more commonly found in supermarkets. If you don't love tons of heat, a bird's-eye or any other milder chile pepper is an adequate substitute. Simply do a taste test of the marinade to get the spiciness to your preference.

If using a scotch bonnet or habañero pepper, wear food-safe plastic gloves if you can, and wash your hands and the blender or food processor *thoroughly* after working with the pepper, especially before touching or rubbing your eyes!

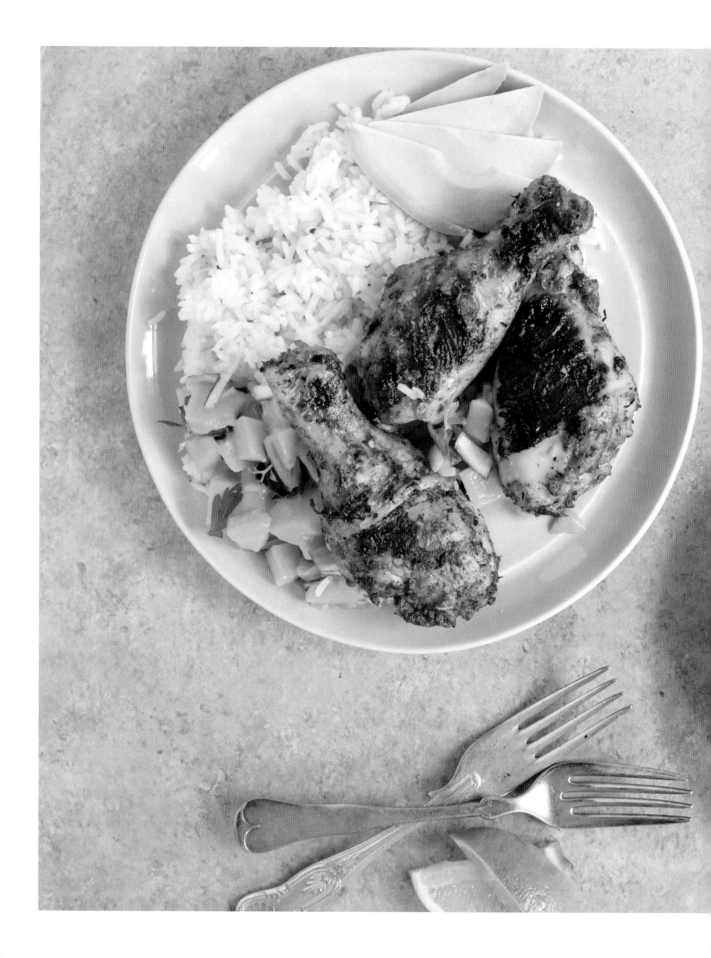

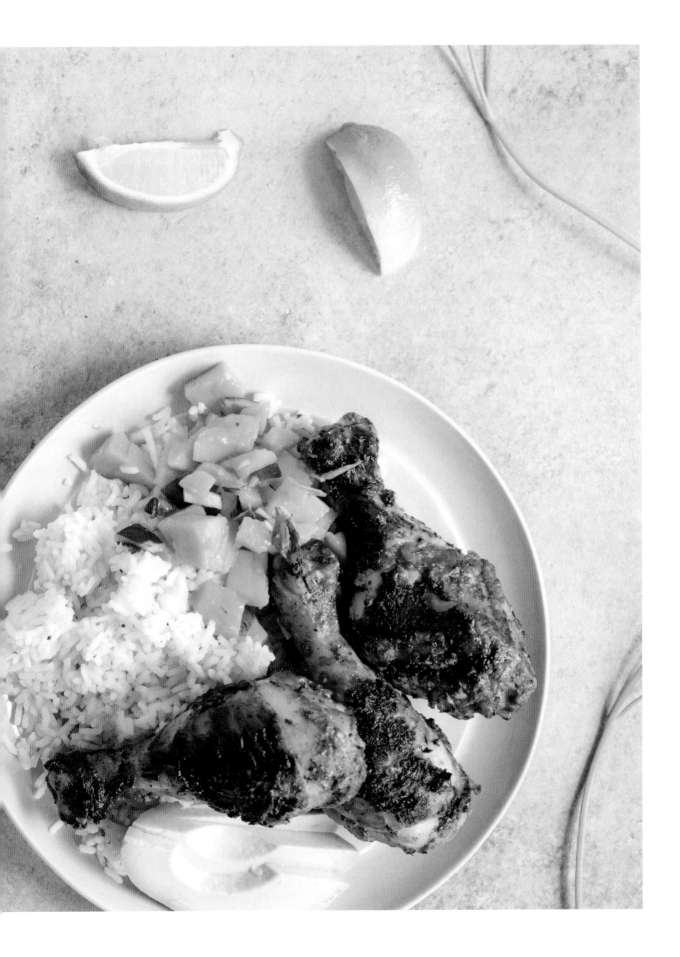

CHICKEN IN MUSHROOM SAUCE

serves 4   *prep time* 10 minutes   *cook time* 40 minutes

EGG-FREE / NUT-FREE / DAIRY-FREE OPTION: use extra-virgin olive oil or avocado oil instead of butter / PALEO-FRIENDLY OPTION: use extra-virgin olive oil or avocado oil instead of butter

This easy-to-prepare dinner is for all you mushroom fans out there! Pan-fried chicken is cooked to tender perfection in a delicious, buttery mushroom sauce that is so flavorful. Sop up the remaining sauce with some of my sandwich bread (page 80) or pair it with Garlic Mashed Parsnips (page 238) for the ultimate comfort meal.

ingredients:

FOR THE CHICKEN:

1½ pounds boneless, skinless chicken breasts

½ teaspoon fine sea salt

¼ teaspoon freshly ground black pepper

3 tablespoons arrowroot flour, plus more as needed to coat the chicken

1 tablespoon unsalted butter

FOR THE MUSHROOM SAUCE:

2 tablespoons unsalted butter

1 onion, diced

3 cloves garlic, minced

3 cups sliced cremini or baby portabella mushrooms (about 8 ounces)

1½ cups chicken broth, homemade (page 354) or store-bought

2 tablespoons red wine

Leaves from 4 sprigs fresh thyme or 1 teaspoon dried thyme leaves

1 bay leaf

½ teaspoon fine sea salt

½ teaspoon freshly ground black pepper

directions:

1. Pat the chicken breasts dry, then sprinkle them with the salt and pepper. Dredge the chicken breasts in the arrowroot flour.

2. Melt the 1 tablespoon of butter in a medium skillet over medium heat. Add the chicken and cook for about 3 minutes on each side, until golden brown but not fully cooked through. Remove from the pan and set aside.

3. Make the sauce: Melt the 2 tablespoons of butter in the same skillet over medium heat. Add the diced onion and minced garlic and sauté until fragrant, about 5 minutes.

4. Add the mushrooms and sauté for 2 minutes, until their color deepens.

5. Add the chicken broth, wine, thyme, bay leaf, salt, and pepper. Give the sauce a little stir and return the chicken to the pan.

6. Bring to a boil, then reduce the heat and simmer for 20 minutes, or until the sauce thickens slightly. Taste and adjust the seasoning as desired.

7. Serve immediately with extra mushroom and onion sauce spooned over the top of the chicken.

note: Feel free to use extra-virgin olive oil or avocado oil if you need to make this dish dairy-free or Paleo-friendly, but the butter does add significantly to the flavor.

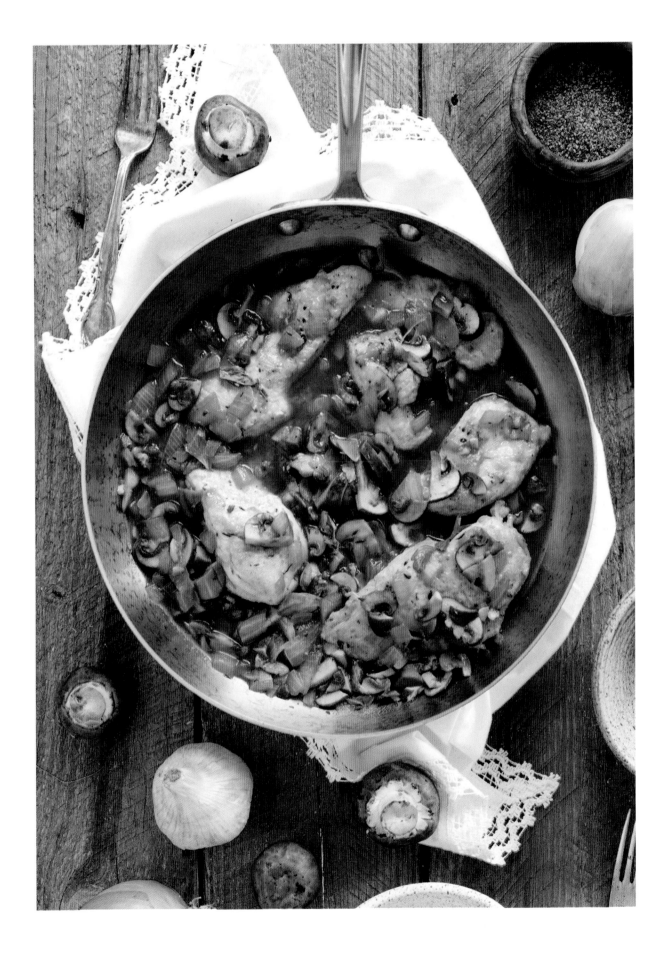

CREAMY CHICKEN BACON SPAGHETTI SQUASH BOATS

serves 4   *prep time* 10 minutes   *cook time* 50 minutes

NUT-FREE / DAIRY-FREE OPTION: omit cheese / PALEO-FRIENDLY OPTION: omit cheese

Move over, pasta! Spaghetti squash is a great alternative to traditional pasta, and serving it as a boat is a fun way to eat your "pasta" dinner, right out of the squash shell! You will love this garlic-infused creamy "pasta" dish made with chicken and bacon.

ingredients:

FOR THE "PASTA":

2 small or medium spaghetti squashes (about 8 pounds)

1 tablespoon extra-virgin olive oil

Fine sea salt and freshly ground black pepper

FOR THE SAUCE:

4 strips bacon

3 cloves garlic, minced

2 tablespoons extra-virgin olive oil

1 small onion, finely diced

1 pound boneless, skinless chicken breasts, cubed

1 teaspoon Italian seasoning

½ teaspoon garlic powder

½ teaspoon onion powder

½ teaspoon fine sea salt

Pinch of freshly ground black pepper

Pinch of red pepper flakes, or more if desired

⅓ cup mayo, homemade (page 312) or store-bought

Optional: ½ cup shredded mozzarella cheese

Roughly chopped fresh basil, for garnish

directions:

1. Preheat the oven to 400°F.

2. Make the "pasta": Cut the spaghetti squash in half lengthwise and scrape out the seeds. Drizzle the cut sides of the squash with the 1 tablespoon of oil and sprinkle with salt and pepper. Place the squash facedown on a rimmed baking sheet and add 2 tablespoons of water to the baking sheet. Bake for 35 to 40 minutes, until the squash is fork-tender and the skin gives when you press your finger into it. Remove from the oven and set aside to cool. Leave the oven on, but reduce the temperature to 350°F.

3. While the squash is baking, prepare the sauce: In a large sauté pan over medium heat, cook the bacon until crispy, about 10 minutes. Remove to a paper towel to cool, then crumble it.

4. In a medium skillet over medium heat, sauté the garlic in the 2 tablespoons of oil for 2 minutes, until fragrant. Add the onion and sauté for 2 minutes, until it beings to become translucent. Lightly salt and pepper the chicken, then add to the skillet and cook until golden and no pink remains. Add the Italian seasoning, garlic powder, onion powder, salt, black pepper, and red pepper flakes. Mix to combine.

5. Remove the skillet from the heat and mix in the mayo. Add the bacon and mix again.

6. Once the spaghetti squash has cooled, take two forks and fluff the threadlike spaghetti within the boats so it's no longer attached to the walls of the squash.

7. Add the chicken mixture to the center of each boat and mix to combine it with the "spaghetti."

8. Top with the cheese, if using, and bake for 10 minutes, until the cheese is bubbly. Garnish with basil and serve immediately.

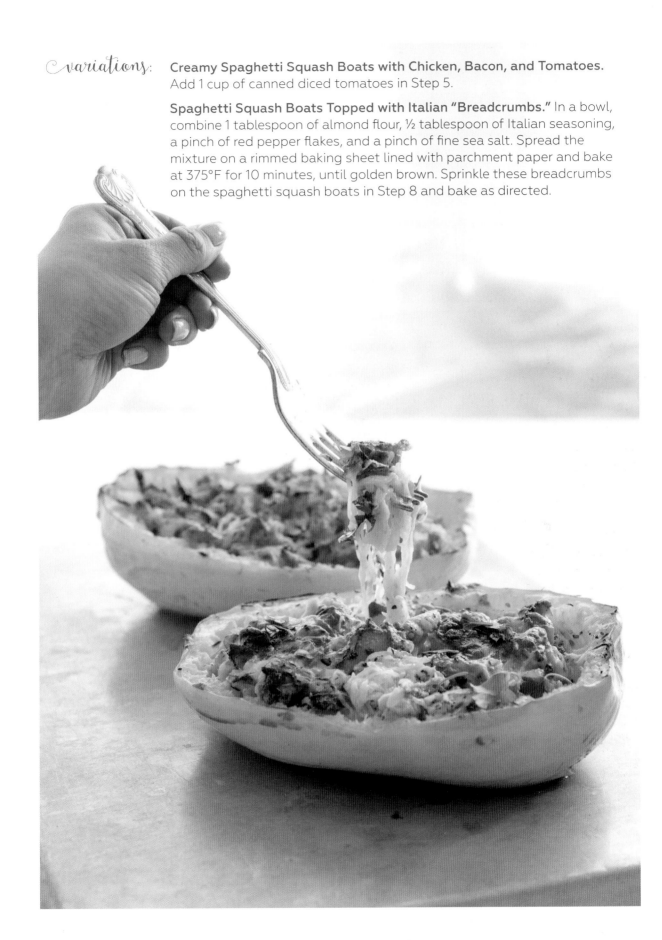

variations: **Creamy Spaghetti Squash Boats with Chicken, Bacon, and Tomatoes.** Add 1 cup of canned diced tomatoes in Step 5.

Spaghetti Squash Boats Topped with Italian "Breadcrumbs." In a bowl, combine 1 tablespoon of almond flour, ½ tablespoon of Italian seasoning, a pinch of red pepper flakes, and a pinch of fine sea salt. Spread the mixture on a rimmed baking sheet lined with parchment paper and bake at 375°F for 10 minutes, until golden brown. Sprinkle these breadcrumbs on the spaghetti squash boats in Step 8 and bake as directed.

BBQ CHICKEN PIZZA

serves 4 *prep time* 15 minutes (not including pizza crust or BBQ sauce) *cook time* 10 minutes

NUT-FREE / DAIRY-FREE OPTION: omit cheese / PALEO-FRIENDLY OPTION: omit cheese

My homemade BBQ sauce is both sweet and smoky, and it's perfect on top of pizza! Once the BBQ sauce and crust are made, this pizza comes together in no time flat.

ingredients:

1 tablespoon extra-virgin olive oil

1 pound boneless, skinless chicken breast, cut into ½-inch cubes

½ teaspoon fine sea salt

½ teaspoon freshly ground black pepper

1¼ cups Sweet & Smoky BBQ Sauce (page 328), divided, plus more if desired

1 par-baked Pizza Crust (page 76)

½ red onion, thinly sliced

Optional: ½ cup shredded cheddar cheese

Red pepper flakes, for serving

Optional: ⅓ cup Ranch Dressing (page 318), for serving

directions:

1. Preheat the oven to 350°F.

2. Heat the olive oil in a medium sauté pan over medium heat. Season the chicken with the salt and pepper and add to the pan.

3. Sauté the chicken for 5 minutes on each side, until golden and mostly cooked through. Add ¾ cup of the BBQ sauce and mix to coat the chicken.

4. Spread ½ cup of the BBQ sauce (or more, if desired) onto the par-baked pizza crust. Top with the chicken, red onion slices, and shredded cheese, if using.

5. Bake for 10 minutes, until the edges of the pizza are golden.

6. Serve immediately with red pepper flakes and ranch dressing, if using.

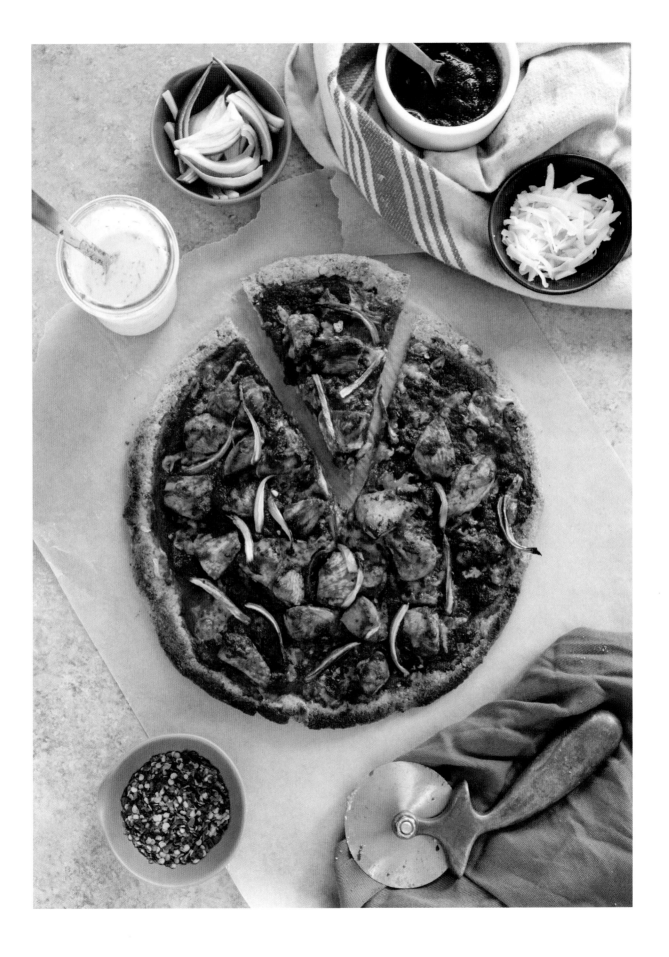

CREAMY CAJUN CHICKEN PASTA

serves 4 *prep time* 20 minutes (not including pasta) *cook time* 1 hour if making spaghetti squash noodles, or about 20 minutes if making zucchini noodles

....

NUT-FREE / DAIRY-FREE OPTION: **use oil instead of butter**
PALEO-FRIENDLY OPTION: **use oil instead of butter**

....

Cajun-spiced chicken is one of my favorites. Pair it with creamy "pasta" and I am a happy camper. This dish can be made two ways—with spaghetti squash or with zucchini noodles! Pick whichever one suits your fancy and devour.

ingredients:

FOR THE CAJUN SEASONING:

2 tablespoons paprika

1 teaspoon garlic powder

1 teaspoon onion powder

½ teaspoon cayenne pepper

½ teaspoon fine sea salt

½ teaspoon freshly ground black pepper

½ teaspoon ground white pepper

1½ pounds boneless, skinless chicken breasts

1 clove garlic, minced

1 tablespoon unsalted butter, extra-virgin olive oil, or avocado oil

1 onion, sliced

1 red bell pepper, sliced

½ teaspoon fine sea salt

¼ teaspoon freshly ground black pepper

4 cups cooked spaghetti squash noodles or 4 to 5 cups raw zucchini noodles (page 248)

⅓ cup mayo, homemade (page 312) or store-bought

directions:

1. Preheat the oven to 350°F and line a rimmed baking sheet with parchment paper.

2. In a small bowl, combine the Cajun seasoning ingredients.

3. Pat the chicken dry, then rub with three-quarters of the Cajun seasoning mix until fully coated.

4. Place the chicken on the lined baking sheet and bake for 10 minutes, then flip the breasts over and bake for an additional 10 minutes, or until no pink remains in the center of the chicken.

5. While the chicken is baking, make the sauce: In a large skillet over medium heat, sauté the garlic in the butter for 2 minutes, until fragrant.

6. Add the sliced onion and bell pepper and sauté for 5 minutes, until they are soft. Season with the salt and pepper and mix to combine.

7. Lower the heat to medium-low, then add the noodles to the skillet and mix to combine. If using spaghetti squash, leave on the heat just long enough to heat through; if using zucchini, cook for about 2 minutes, until the zucchini noodles have softened but are still firm.

8. In a small bowl, whisk together the mayo and the remaining Cajun seasoning mix. Add to the skillet and toss to coat the noodles.

9. Divide the creamy pasta among four serving bowls. Slice the chicken breasts and place on top of the pasta. Serve immediately.

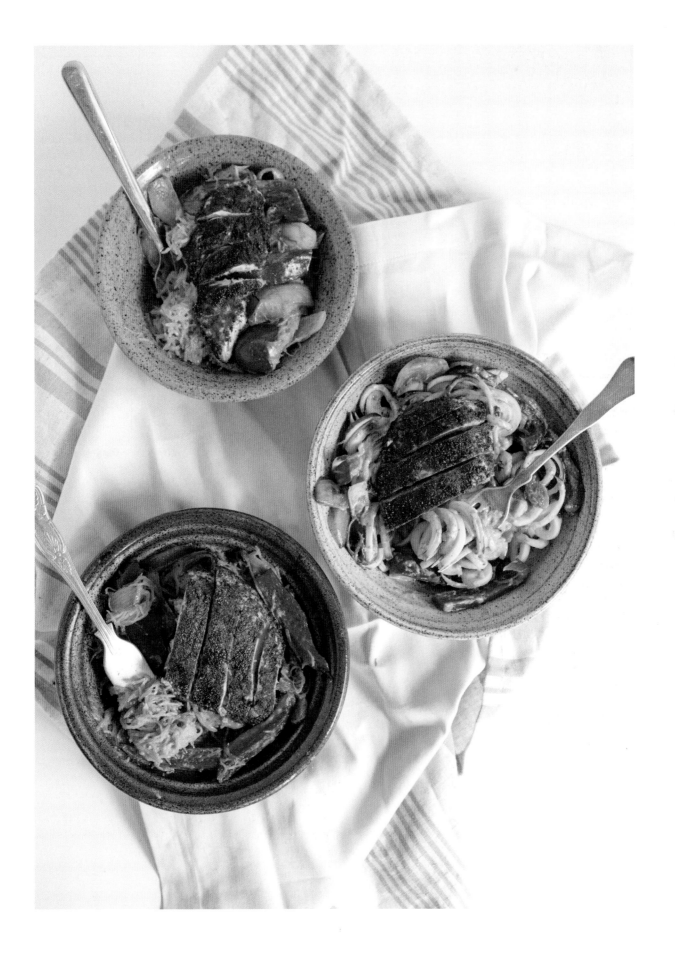

EASY ONE-PAN ARROZ CON POLLO

serves 4   *prep time* 10 minutes   *cook time* 45 minutes

EGG-FREE / NUT-FREE / DAIRY-FREE / PALEO-FRIENDLY

Arroz con pollo is a traditional Spanish and Latin American dish similar to paella. Authentic arroz con pollo is made with saffron, and we are keeping it traditional with this one-pan dish. It is one of my favorite one-pan picks!

ingredients:

3 cloves garlic, minced

1 tablespoon extra-virgin olive oil

1 onion, chopped

2 red bell peppers, chopped

1 cup frozen peas

1 pound boneless, skinless chicken breasts, cubed

1 cup white rice

2 cups chicken broth, homemade (page 354) or store-bought

½ cup diced canned tomatoes

1 teaspoon saffron

½ teaspoon ground cumin

¼ teaspoon turmeric powder

½ teaspoon fine sea salt

¼ teaspoon freshly ground black pepper

Optional: ¼ to ½ teaspoon red pepper flakes, as desired

directions:

1. In a large braising pan or Dutch oven over medium heat, sauté the garlic in the olive oil for 2 minutes, until fragrant.

2. Add the onion, peppers, and peas and sauté for 5 minutes, until the onion and peppers begin to soften.

3. Add the chicken and sear on all sides for 2 minutes (it does not need to fully cook here).

4. Add the rice and stir until the chicken, vegetables, and rice are thoroughly mixed together, about 1 minute.

5. Add the chicken broth, tomatoes, saffron, cumin, turmeric, salt, black pepper, and red pepper flakes, if using. Mix to combine.

6. Bring to a boil over medium heat, then reduce the heat to low, cover, and simmer for 30 minutes, until the rice is fluffy and no broth remains.

7. Serve hot with additional black pepper and red pepper flakes.

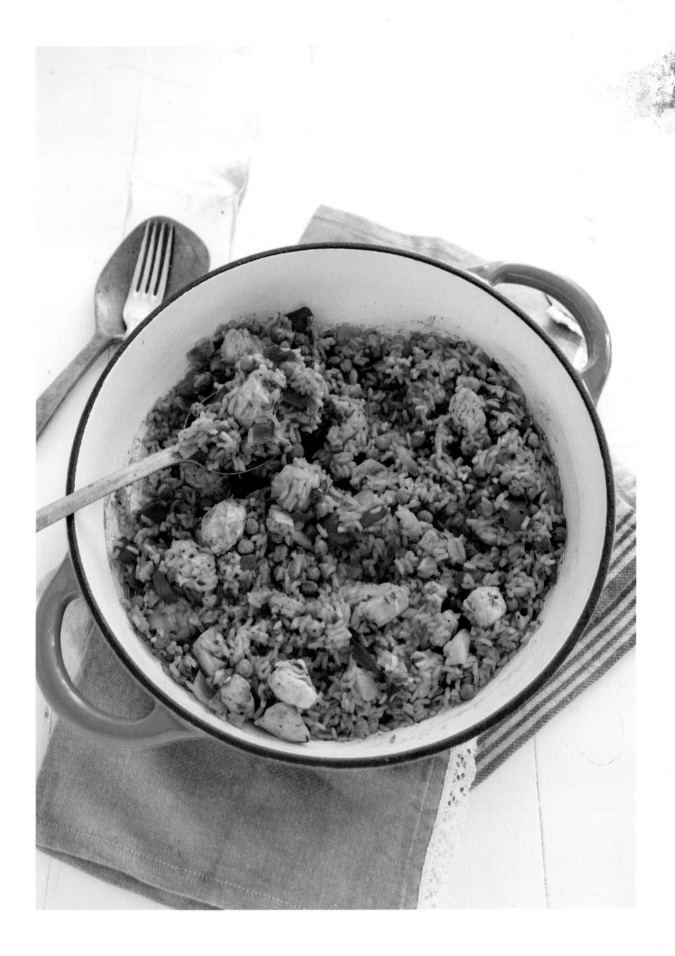

LOADED ITALIAN MEATBALLS

serves 4   *prep time* 10 minutes (not including zucchini noodles)   *cook time* 15 minutes

NUT-FREE / DAIRY-FREE / PALEO-FRIENDLY

You simply can't go wrong with these turkey meatballs for dinner—they are loaded with veggies *and* flavor.

ingredients:

FOR THE MEATBALLS:

1 pound ground turkey

10 ounces frozen spinach, thawed, drained, and excess water squeezed out

¼ cup finely chopped onions

1 large egg, whisked

1 teaspoon garlic powder

1 teaspoon onion powder

½ teaspoon dried basil

½ teaspoon dried oregano leaves

½ teaspoon Italian seasoning

½ teaspoon fine sea salt

¼ teaspoon freshly ground black pepper

FOR SERVING (OPTIONAL):

1 batch cooked zucchini noodles (page 248)

Marinara sauce, homemade (page 338) or store-bought, warmed

directions:

1. Preheat the oven to 350°F and line a rimmed baking sheet with parchment paper.

2. In a large mixing bowl, use your hands to mix together the ingredients for the meatballs until they're evenly combined.

3. Roll the mixture into 1-inch balls and place on the lined baking sheet. Bake for 15 minutes, or until no pink remains in their centers.

4. Serve immediately with cooked zucchini noodles and warmed marinara sauce, if desired.

note: This recipe works well with ground chicken, too.

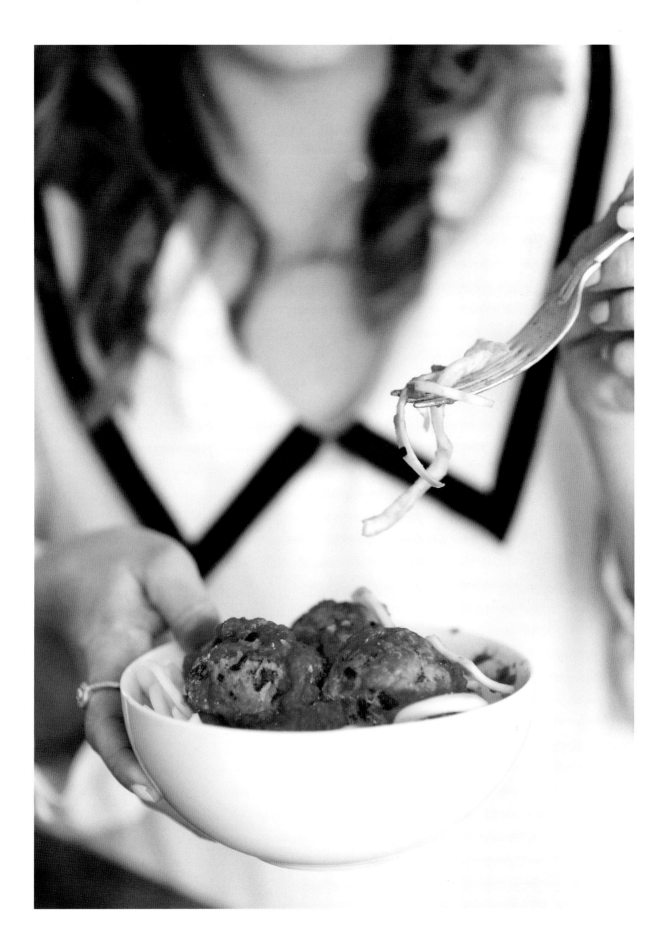

THAI MEATBALLS

serves 4 *prep time* 10 minutes *cook time* 15 minutes

EGG-FREE / NUT-FREE / DAIRY-FREE / PALEO-FRIENDLY

I love meatballs! I guess that's why this book contains multiple meatball recipes with a range of flavors. These Thai meatballs are wonderful and are an easy way to infuse Thai flavors into your dinner!

ingredients:

FOR THE MEATBALLS:

1 pound ground turkey

½ cup shredded carrots

¼ cup chopped scallions

2 cloves garlic, minced

1 tablespoon peeled and grated fresh ginger

2 tablespoons coconut aminos

1 teaspoon chili paste or Sriracha sauce

¼ teaspoon fine sea salt

¼ teaspoon freshly ground black pepper

FOR THE SAUCE:

¼ cup coconut aminos

2 tablespoons extra-virgin olive oil

1 teaspoon fish sauce

1 clove garlic, crushed to a paste

2 teaspoons peeled and grated fresh ginger

1 teaspoon chili paste or Sriracha sauce

2 tablespoons chopped scallions

directions:

1. Preheat the oven to 350°F and line a rimmed baking sheet with parchment paper.

2. In a large bowl, use your hands to mix together the ingredients for the meatballs until they're evenly combined.

3. Roll the mixture into 12 large or 15 medium-sized balls and place on the lined baking sheet. Bake for 15 minutes, or until no pink remains in their centers.

4. While the meatballs are baking, make the sauce: In a small saucepan, whisk together the sauce ingredients. Bring the mixture to a boil over medium heat, then reduce the heat and simmer for 5 minutes, until the sauce thickens slightly.

5. Pour the sauce over the meatballs and serve immediately.

serve with:

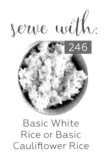
246

Basic White Rice or Basic Cauliflower Rice

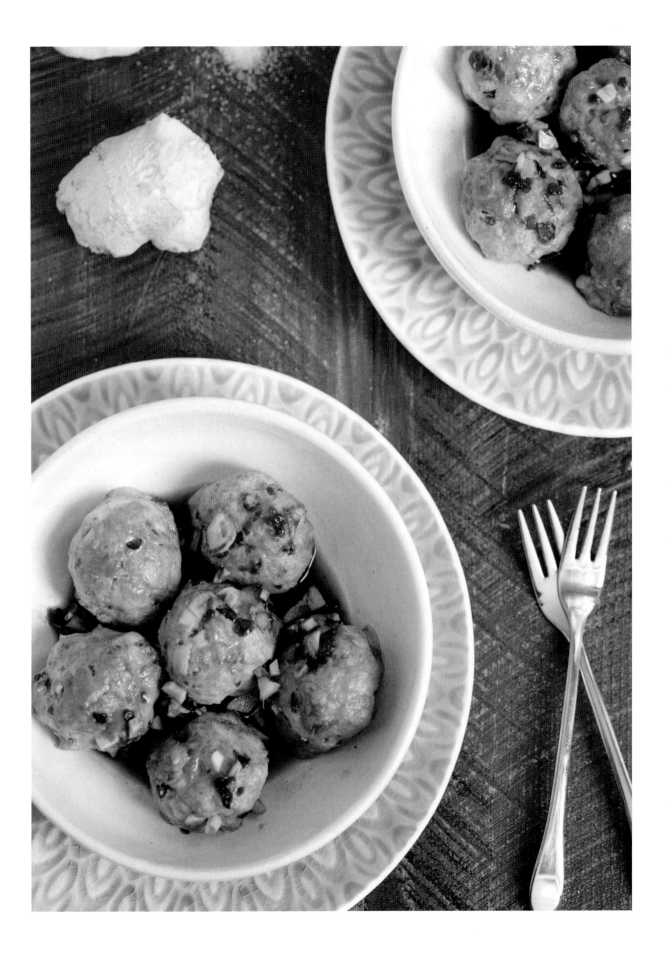

MAPLE-CRUSTED SALMON

serves 4 *prep time* 5 minutes *cook time* about 10 minutes

EGG-FREE / NUT-FREE / DAIRY-FREE / PALEO-FRIENDLY

This salmon is a reader favorite. It is simple to prepare, and the combination of the sweet and spicy rub and the moist, flaky salmon is so tasty. And topping it all off is a to-die-for maple crust!

ingredients:

- 1 tablespoon chili powder
- 1 tablespoon paprika
- 2 teaspoons coconut sugar or granulated maple sugar
- ½ teaspoon fine sea salt
- 1½ pounds salmon fillets, cut into 4 portions
- 3 tablespoons pure maple syrup

directions:

1. Place an oven rack in the top position and set the oven temperature to broil. Line a rimmed baking sheet with parchment paper, then grease the paper.

2. In a bowl, mix together the chili powder, paprika, sugar, and salt.

3. Evenly coat the tops of the salmon fillets with the spice rub.

4. Place the salmon on the prepared baking sheet and broil for 7 to 9 minutes, depending on how thin or thick your fillets are (about 7 minutes for a ½-inch piece or 9 minutes for a 1-inch piece).

5. Remove the salmon from the oven and brush the maple syrup over the tops to coat the spice rub. Return to the oven and broil for an additional 1 to 2 minutes, until the maple syrup is bubbling and has formed a crust. Serve immediately.

serve with:

Burnt Broccoli
230

Maple Bacon Brussels Sprouts
224

Garlicky Blistered Green Beans
234

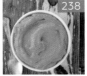
Creamy Mashed Roots
238

Asian Summer Slaw
232

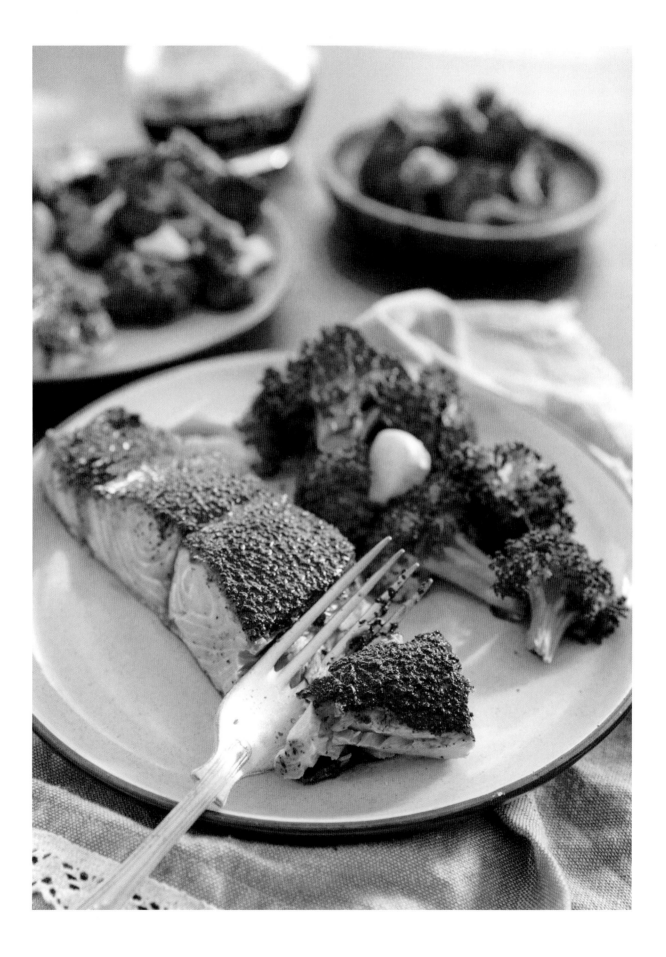

THAI BBQ SALMON

serves 4   *prep time* 8 minutes   *cook time* about 10 minutes

EGG-FREE / NUT-FREE / DAIRY-FREE / PALEO-FRIENDLY

One of my absolute favorite ways to prepare salmon is with this Thai BBQ Sauce.

ingredients:

FOR THE BBQ SAUCE:

2 tablespoons ketchup, homemade (page 342) or store-bought

2 tablespoons coconut aminos

1 tablespoon unseasoned rice vinegar

1 tablespoon coconut sugar

2 teaspoons chili paste

1 teaspoon toasted sesame oil

1 (1-inch) chunk fresh ginger, peeled and grated, or ¼ teaspoon ginger powder

½ teaspoon garlic powder

1½ pounds salmon fillets, cut into 4 portions

FOR GARNISH:

Sesame seeds

Sliced scallions

Mung bean sprouts

Red pepper flakes

directions:

1. Place an oven rack in the top position and set the oven temperature to broil. Line a rimmed baking sheet with parchment paper, then grease the paper.

2. In a bowl, whisk together the BBQ sauce ingredients.

3. Brush some of the sauce over the tops and sides of the salmon fillets, saving the remaining sauce for later.

4. Place the salmon on the prepared baking sheet and broil for 9 to 10 minutes, depending on how thin or thick your fillets are, until the salmon is cooked to your desired pinkness (about 7 minutes for a ½-inch piece or 9 minutes for a 1-inch piece).

5. While the salmon is broiling, heat the remaining sauce in a small saucepan over medium heat for 3 minutes, until bubbling.

6. Remove the salmon from the oven and brush the remaining sauce over the salmon.

7. Garnish with sesame seeds, scallions, bean sprouts, and red pepper flakes and serve immediately.

serve with:

246
Basic White Rice or Basic Cauliflower Rice

230
Burnt Broccoli

234
Garlicky Blistered Green Beans

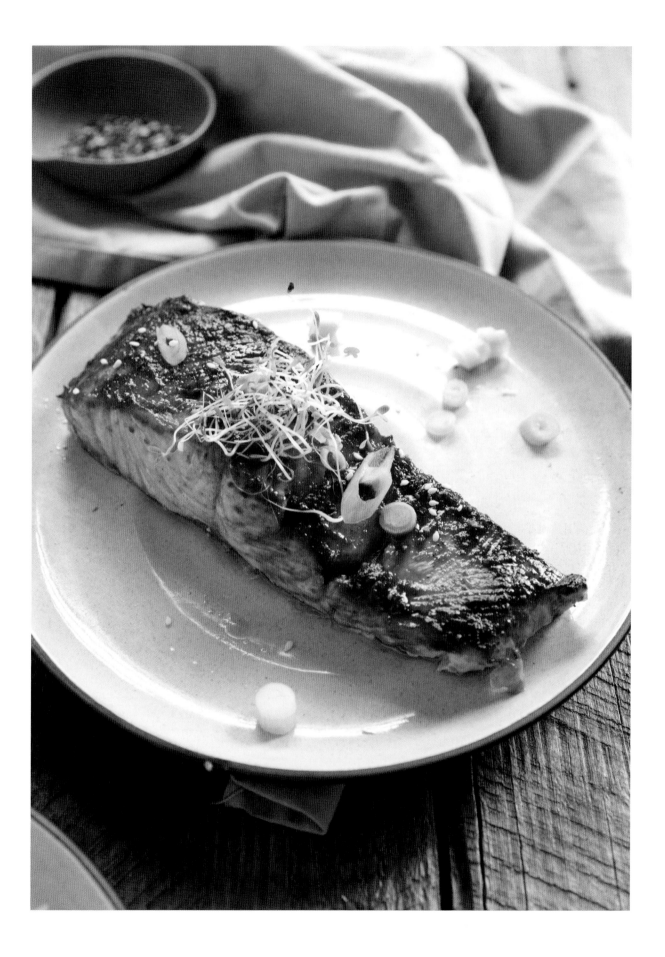

FISH TACOS WITH TROPICAL SALSA, SPICY SLAW & QUICK PICKLED CABBAGE

makes 6 tacos (2 to 3 per serving) *prep time* 20 minutes (not including tortillas, avocado crema, or spicy mayo) *cook time* 10 minutes

NUT-FREE / PALEO-FRIENDLY

These fish tacos are light, refreshing, and packed with flavor! They are sure to turn taco night into a family favorite.

ingredients:

FOR THE QUICK PICKLED CABBAGE:

2 cups shredded red cabbage

3 tablespoons apple cider vinegar

1 teaspoon honey

½ teaspoon fine sea salt

FOR THE TROPICAL SALSA:

1 mango, diced

1 orange, diced

1 avocado, diced

1 cup cherry tomatoes, chopped

¼ cup finely chopped red onions

1 tablespoon lime juice (½ to 1 lime)

1 tablespoon chopped fresh cilantro

¼ teaspoon garlic powder

FOR THE SPICY SLAW:

2 cups coleslaw mix

2 to 4 tablespoons Spicy Mayo (page 312)

FOR THE FISH:

1½ teaspoons chili powder

1 teaspoon ground cumin

1 teaspoon garlic powder

1 teaspoon onion powder

½ teaspoon fine sea salt

¼ teaspoon freshly ground black pepper

1 pound mahi mahi steaks or white fish steaks or fillets of choice, cubed

1 tablespoon plus 2 teaspoons extra-virgin olive oil or avocado oil

Juice of ½ lime

FOR SERVING:

1 batch Tortillas (page 72)

Avocado Crema (page 344)

Spicy Mayo (page 312)

Lime wedges

Fresh cilantro leaves

directions:

1. Place the pickled cabbage ingredients in a bowl and massage together with your hands for about 30 seconds, until the liquid begins to turn pink. Set aside for 20 minutes or up to overnight.

2. In a large bowl, mix together the salsa ingredients and set aside.

3. In a medium-sized bowl, mix together the spicy slaw ingredients.

4. In another bowl, mix together the spices and salt for the fish, then gently toss the fish cubes in the seasoning blend, 2 teaspoons of the oil, and the lime juice to coat. In a sauté pan, heat the remaining tablespoon of oil over medium heat and cook the fish until opaque.

5. Assemble the tacos: Place some fish on each tortilla, then top with the pickled cabbage, slaw, and salsa. Drizzle each taco with avocado crema and spicy mayo and serve immediately with lime wedges and cilantro.

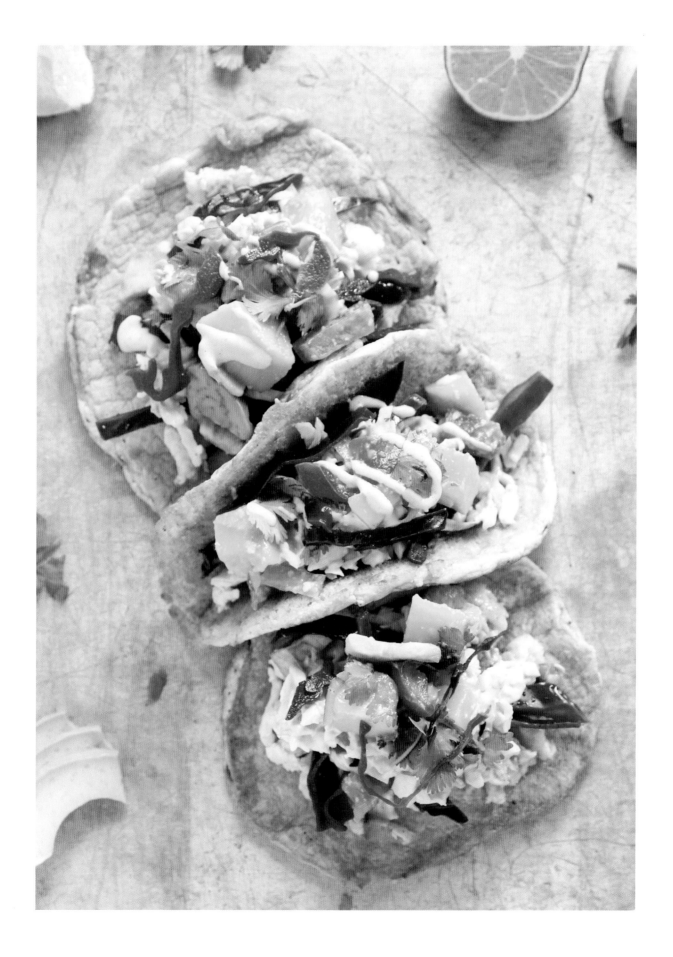

SCALLOPS PROVENÇAL

serves 4 *prep time* 10 minutes *cook time* 18 minutes

EGG-FREE / NUT-FREE

There are some tricks to getting perfectly crusted and seared scallops, and I'm going to share them with you right here. I love scallops, and if I had to pick just one preparation, it would be with this fabulous Provençal sauce. This recipe also works well for two people; simply reduce the number of scallops to eight or ten.

ingredients:

1 teaspoon extra-virgin olive oil or avocado oil

2 tablespoons unsalted butter

16 to 20 large sea scallops (4 or 5 per person)

Fine sea salt and freshly ground black pepper

FOR THE PROVENÇAL SAUCE:

½ cup chopped onion

2 cloves garlic, minced

½ cup dry white wine

3 tablespoons chopped fresh flat-leaf parsley, plus more for garnish

2 teaspoons arrowroot flour

1 teaspoon lemon juice

¼ teaspoon fine sea salt

¼ teaspoon freshly ground black pepper

1 lemon, cut into wedges, for serving

directions:

1. Preheat a large skillet over medium heat for about 2 minutes, until hot.

2. Put the oil and butter in the skillet (the oil keeps the butter from burning) and give the two a stir to combine.

3. Pat the scallops dry with a paper towel and season generously with salt and pepper. When the butter mixture is hot, add the scallops to the skillet and sear for 2 minutes without touching them (this is important to get a nice crust to form). Once the underside has a nice sear, flip the scallops over and sear the other side for 2 minutes without touching them. When both sides have a nice sear, transfer the scallops to a plate.

4. Make the sauce: Place the onion and garlic in the same skillet (add more butter if the skillet is too dry) and sauté for 3 to 4 minutes, until fragrant.

5. Whisk together the white wine, parsley, arrowroot flour, lemon juice, salt, and pepper. Pour the sauce into the skillet, then stir to combine with a wooden spatula, scraping the bottom of the pan. Reduce the heat and simmer for 5 to 7 minutes, until the sauce thickens slightly.

6. Pour the sauce over the scallops and serve with lemon wedges.

serve with:

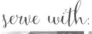

Garlicky Blistered Green Beans

Lemon Herb Spring Vegetable Risotto

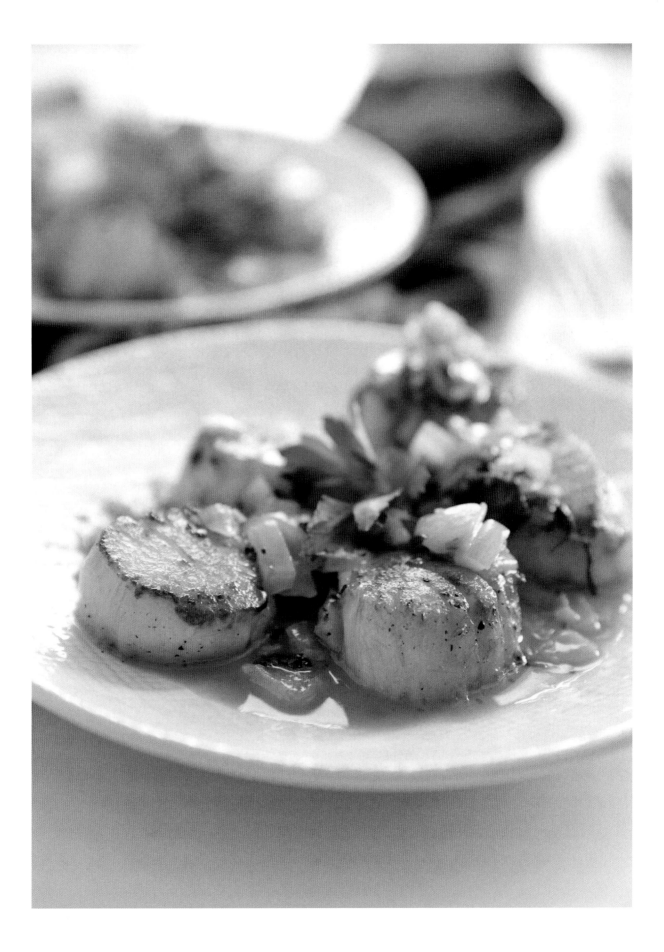

CHIMICHURRI SHRIMP

serves 4   *prep time* 10 minutes (not including chimichurri)   *cook time* 6 minutes

EGG-FREE / NUT-FREE / DAIRY-FREE / PALEO-FRIENDLY

This light, refreshing, and flavorful shrimp dish pairs well with any side!

ingredients:

1½ pounds large shrimp, peeled and deveined

Pinch of fine sea salt and freshly ground black pepper

1 batch Chimichurri (page 352), divided

1 tablespoon extra-virgin olive oil

directions:

1. Pat the shrimp dry with a paper towel and season with salt and pepper.

2. Toss the shrimp with half of the chimichurri and set aside for 10 minutes.

3. In a large skillet, heat the olive oil over medium heat, then add the shrimp and cook for 3 minutes on each side, until they begin to look opaque. Add the remaining chimichurri and mix to combine.

4. Serve immediately.

serve with:

247
Basic White Rice

Over a salad

use in:

144
Chopped Antipasto Salad: sub shrimp for the chicken

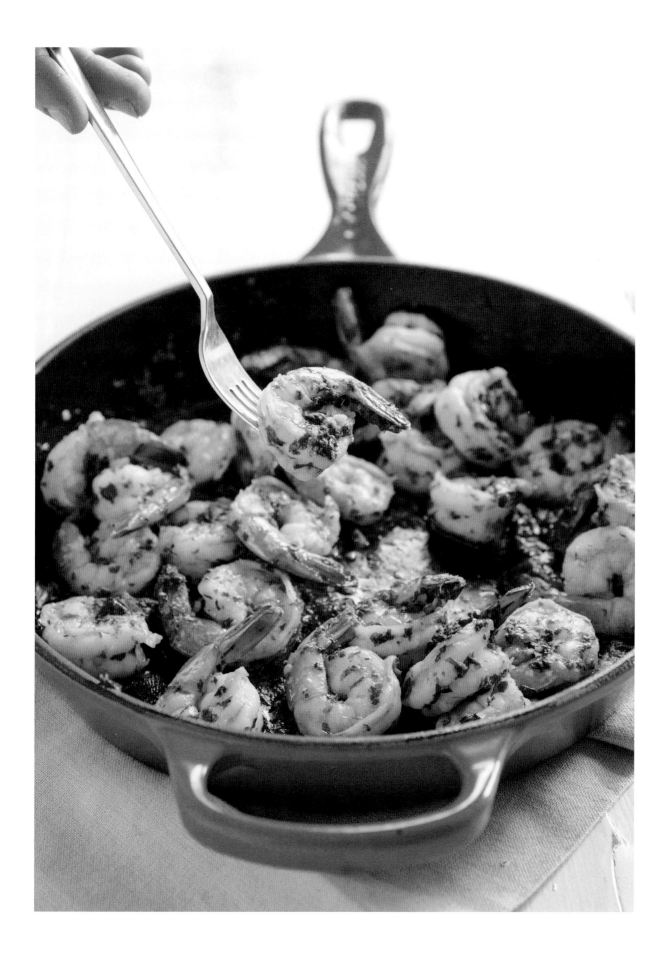

NEW ENGLAND LOBSTER ROLLS

serves 4   *prep time* 15 minutes (not including bread or time to cook lobsters)

DAIRY-FREE OPTION: use oil instead of butter / PALEO-FRIENDLY OPTION: use oil instead of butter

Summertime in New England means fresh seafood and lobster rolls. It's totally New Englanders' thing. Here's my beef with lobster rolls, though: I want delicious lobster, but I don't want a standard hot dog roll. Not only because I stay away from gluten, but because I feel like we can do better than that. Know what I mean? My lobster salad is fresh, fresh, fresh—and it's piled high on buttery toasted homemade bread for the ultimate lobster roll experience.

ingredients:

1½ pounds precooked and chilled lobster meat (see notes)

⅓ to ½ cup mayo, homemade (page 312) or store-bought

2 celery stalks, finely chopped

¼ cup chopped scallions

2 tablespoons lemon juice (about 1 lemon)

1 tablespoon chopped fresh flat-leaf parsley

Fine sea salt and freshly ground black pepper

2 tablespoons unsalted butter or avocado oil, or more if needed

1 loaf All-Purpose Sandwich Bread (page 80), cut into 8 slices

Lemon wedges, for serving

directions:

1. In a large bowl, combine the lobster meat, mayo (starting with ⅓ cup and adding more as desired), celery, scallions, lemon juice, parsley, and salt and pepper to taste.

2. When ready to serve, heat 1 tablespoon of butter in a large heavy-bottomed skillet over medium heat. Swirl to coat the pan. Place as many slices of bread as will comfortably fit in the skillet, cut side down, in the hot butter. Press down and move them around slightly until toasted and golden brown on one side. Add more butter and repeat on the other side and with the remaining bread.

3. Add the lobster salad to the toasted bread and serve immediately with lemon wedges.

notes: Precooked lobster meat is often available at local fish markets and comes without the shell on. I don't recommend purchasing frozen lobster meat. Fresh is always best!

To cook fresh lobsters at home rather than buy precooked, shelled meat, you will need four 1½-pound lobsters. Cook them using your desired method. I like to steam them. To do so, add about 2 inches of water to a large pot, then add 1 tablespoon of fine sea salt for each quart of water. When the water is boiling, quickly add the lobsters (headfirst) to the pot and cover. Steam the lobsters, shaking the pot occasionally, until cooked through, about 13 minutes for 1½- to 2-pound lobsters, about 12 minutes for 1- to 1¼-pound lobsters, and about 10 minutes for ¾- to 1-pound lobsters.

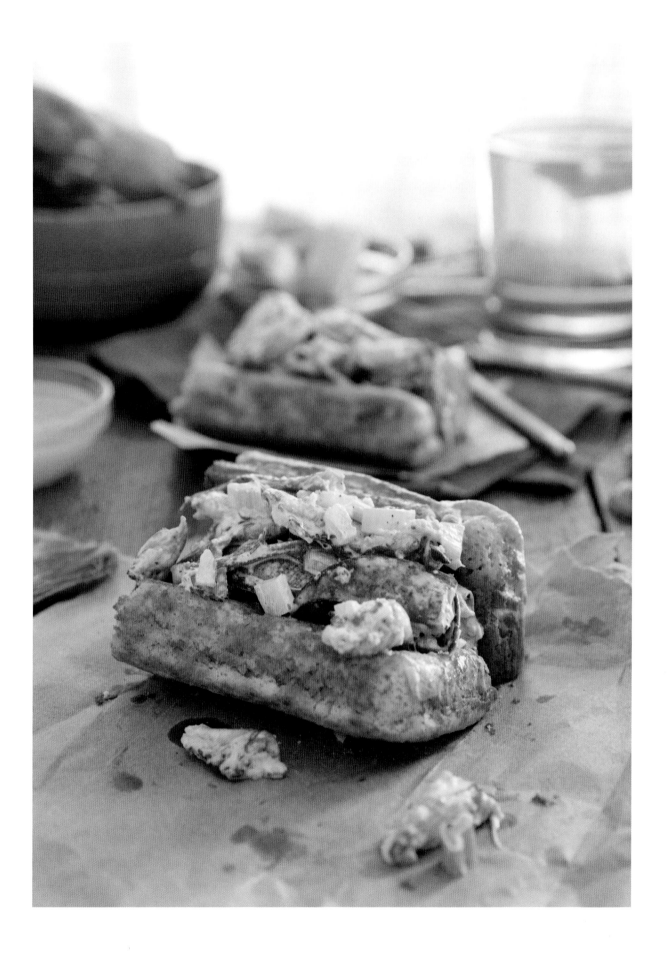

ALL-AMERICAN BURGERS

serves 4 *prep time* 10 minutes (not including buns or homemade toppings)
cook time about 8 minutes

EGG-FREE OPTION: omit buns and use large lettuce leaves to wrap burgers / NUT-FREE OPTION:
omit buns and use large lettuce leaves to wrap burgers / DAIRY-FREE OPTION: omit cheese
PALEO-FRIENDLY OPTION: omit cheese

I love burgers year-round, but especially during the spring and summer months and even into the early fall. There's nothing like a perfectly cooked burger with ALL THE FIXIN'S—and truffle sweet potato fries on the side, of course.

ingredients:

1 pound ground beef

¼ cup finely diced or grated onions

1 clove garlic, minced

1½ teaspoons Sriracha sauce or Dijon mustard

½ teaspoon fine sea salt

½ teaspoon freshly ground black pepper

½ teaspoon onion powder

Avocado oil, for the grill

4 All-Purpose Sandwich Buns, plain or "Everything" (page 80), split and toasted

TOPPING IDEAS:

Caramelized Onions (page 332)

Red onion slices

Cheddar cheese slices

Lettuce leaves

Tomato slices

Avocado slices

Cooked bacon slices

Pickles

Ketchup, homemade (page 342) or store-bought

Mayo, spicy or regular, homemade (page 312) or store-bought

directions:

1. Preheat a grill to medium.

2. Put the beef, onions, garlic, Sriracha or mustard, salt, and spices in a large mixing bowl. Using your hands or a fork, mix everything together until evenly combined.

3. Gently shape the meat mixture into four ¾- to 1-inch-thick burger patties. Using your thumb, make a shallow depression in the center of each burger.

4. Oil the hot grill grate and place the burgers on the grill. Close the lid and grill for 3 to 4 minutes, then turn and move the burgers so they aren't directly over the flame and grill for another 3 to 4 minutes, until no pink remains. The insides of the burgers should read 160°F on an instant-read thermometer. (This will give you medium-done burgers.)

5. Serve immediately on toasted buns, with your favorite toppings.

note: Don't press the burgers with a spatula, flip more than once, or prick with a fork. This will release juices that you want to keep inside your burgers!

serve with:

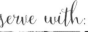

Sweet Potato Truffle Fries

Summer's Best Grainy Mustard Potato Salad

Asian Summer Slaw

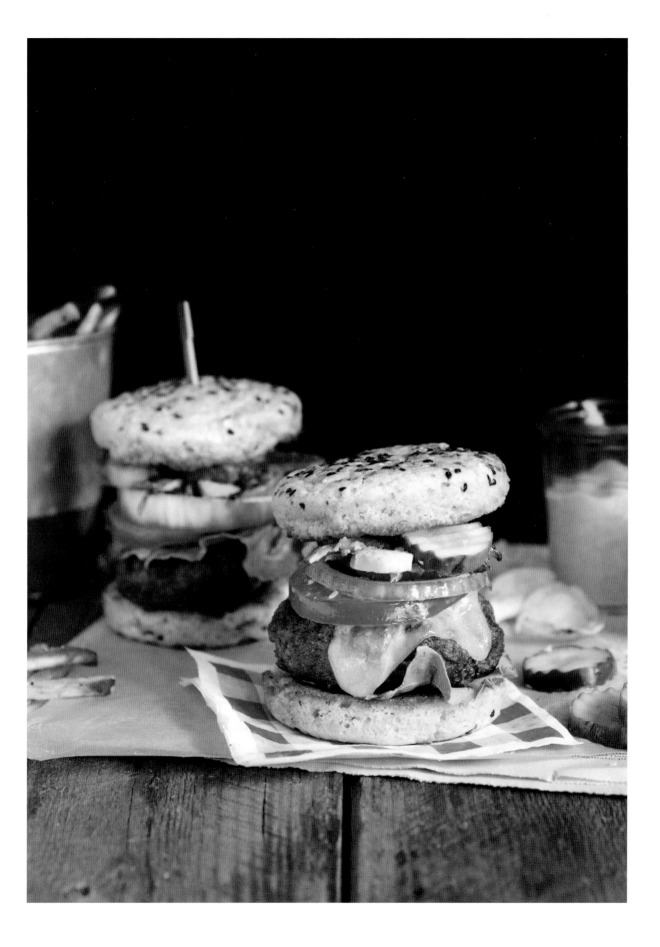

MEDITERRANEAN GRILLED LAMB KEBABS

serves 6   *prep time* 15 minutes, plus 2 hours to marinate lamb   *cook time* 20 minutes

EGG-FREE / NUT-FREE / DAIRY-FREE / PALEO-FRIENDLY

In addition to Mexican fare, you'll find Mediterranean dishes throughout this book. I love the fresh flavors and light nature of that cuisine! These marinated, grilled lamb skewers are loaded with Mediterranean flavor in an easy meal-in-one preparation. They are wonderful alone or over a simple Mediterranean salad!

ingredients:

FOR THE MARINADE:

3 tablespoons fresh flat-leaf parsley leaves

2 tablespoons fresh marjoram leaves

2 tablespoons extra-virgin olive oil

2 teaspoons lemon juice

2 cloves garlic, roughly chopped

1 teaspoon fine sea salt

½ teaspoon freshly ground black pepper

FOR THE SKEWERS:

2 pounds top round lamb, cut into 1½-inch cubes

Fine sea salt and freshly ground black pepper

1 red bell pepper, cut into 1-inch pieces

1 green bell pepper, cut into 1-inch pieces

1 large red onion, cut into 1-inch chunks

Lemon wedges, for garnish

SPECIAL EQUIPMENT:

Metal or soaked wooden skewers

serve with:

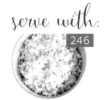

Basic
Cauliflower Rice

directions:

1. Combine the marinade ingredients in a food processor or blender and pulse until smooth.

2. Pat the lamb cubes dry and sprinkle generously with salt and pepper. Put the lamb and marinade in a glass dish or resealable plastic bag. Toss to evenly coat the meat and refrigerate for at least 2 hours or up to 24 hours.

3. Preheat a grill or grill pan to medium heat.

4. Place cubes of lamb on skewers, followed by peppers and onions. Repeat until the skewers are filled.

5. Oil the hot grill grate, then place the skewers on the grill. Cook the lamb to the desired doneness, turning the skewers every 1 to 2 minutes (7 to 8 minutes total for medium doneness).

variation:

Mediterranean Grilled Lamb and Veggie Salad. Make the lamb kebabs as directed above, then remove the grilled lamb and vegetables from the skewers and set aside. Place 4 cups of romaine lettuce in a large serving bowl. Add 2 cups of sliced tomatoes; 1 cucumber, sliced; ½ red onion, sliced; and ½ cup of feta cheese, if you tolerate dairy. Top with the grilled lamb and veggies and serve with lemon wedges. In a mason jar, combine ¼ cup of extra-virgin olive oil, 2 tablespoons of red wine vinegar, 1 clove of garlic, crushed to a paste, the juice of ½ lemon, ½ teaspoon of dried oregano leaves, and a pinch of salt and pepper. Shake vigorously, then pour the desired amount of dressing over the salad.

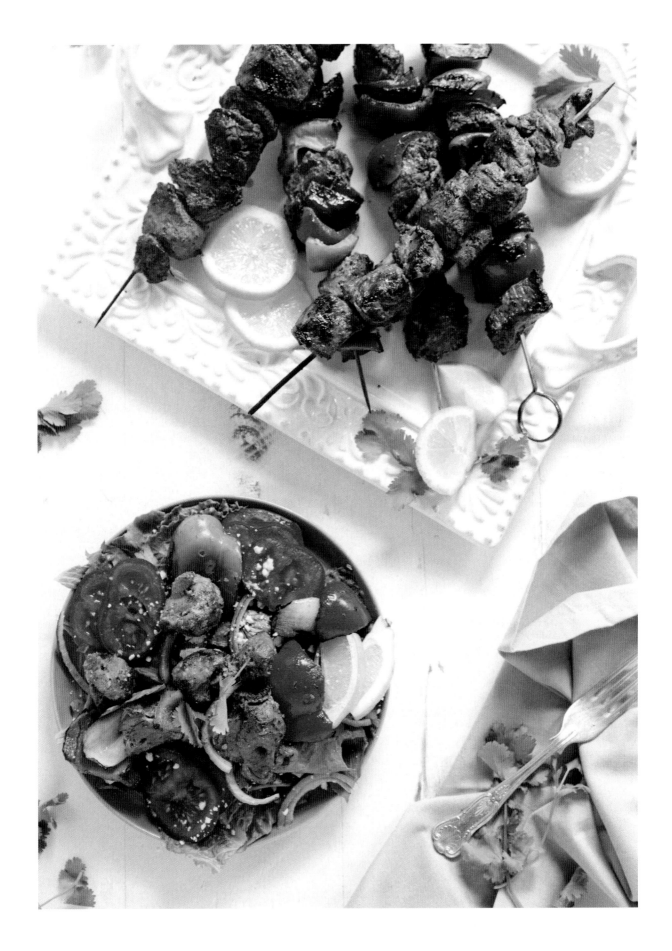

SLOW COOKER BEEF BARBACOA

serves 3 (2 tacos per person)   *prep time* 10 minutes   *cook time* 8 hours

....

EGG-FREE OPTION: use lettuce leaves instead of tortillas
NUT-FREE OPTION: use lettuce leaves instead of tortillas / DAIRY-FREE OPTION: omit cheese
PALEO-FRIENDLY OPTION: omit cheese

....

Slow cooker goodness! This beef barbacoa pairs remarkably well with just about anything. Set it and forget it for the perfect lunch and dinner. The barbacoa makes a good deal of meat, so you'll have plenty for tacos or lettuce wraps, to serve on top of a salad, or to serve with eggs for breakfast.

ingredients:

FOR THE RUB:
1 tablespoon chili powder
1 tablespoon paprika
1 teaspoon fine sea salt
1 teaspoon garlic granules
1 teaspoon onion powder
1 teaspoon dried ground oregano
½ teaspoon ground cumin
½ teaspoon freshly ground black pepper
¼ teaspoon cayenne pepper

2½ pounds boneless beef shoulder roast

FOR THE SAUCE:
1 (14½-ounce) can diced tomatoes
1 (4-ounce) can diced green chiles
1 onion, sliced
3 cloves garlic, minced
1 tablespoon apple cider vinegar
1 tablespoon pure maple syrup or honey
2 teaspoons paprika
1 teaspoon ground cumin
1 teaspoon fine sea salt

TOPPING IDEAS:
Sliced scallions
Chopped fresh cilantro
Shredded lettuce
Diced tomato
Diced mango
Diced avocado
Shredded cabbage
Shredded cheddar cheese
Fried sweet plantains

directions:

1. Place an oven rack in the center of the oven and set the broiler to high.

2. In a small bowl, mix together the ingredients for the rub. Press the rub onto the beef shoulder, coating it on all sides.

3. Place the beef on a rimmed baking sheet and broil for 4 minutes on each side.

4. While the meat is in the oven, combine the sauce ingredients in a slow cooker.

5. Place the beef in the slow cooker and turn to coat in the sauce. Cover and cook on low for 8 hours.

6. Shred the meat and mix in the sauce. Serve with the desired toppings.

serve with:

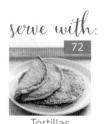

72

Tortillas

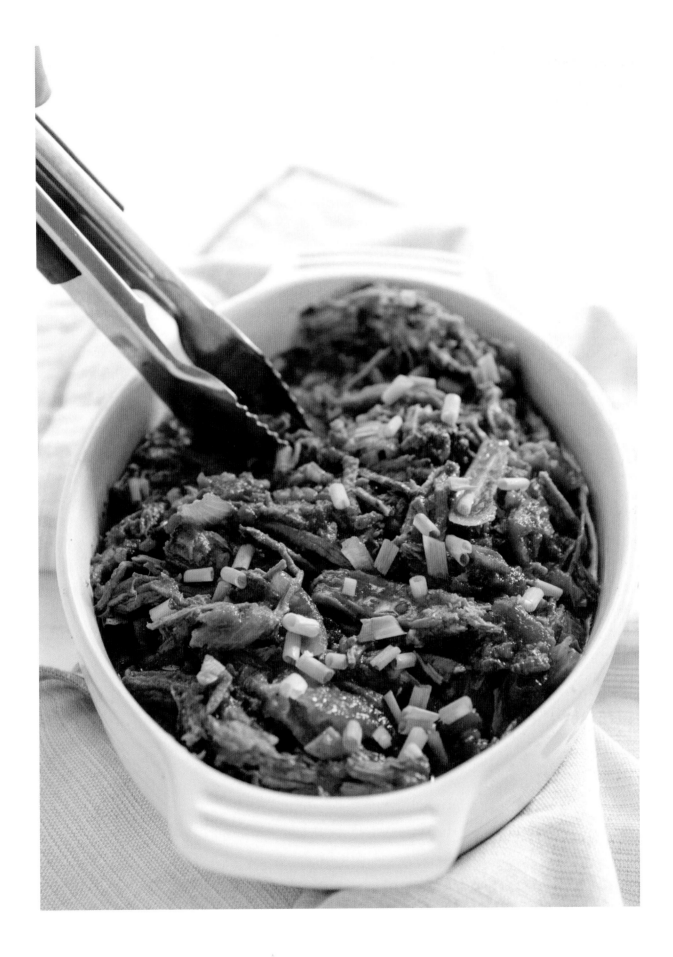

BALSAMIC BRAISED SHORT RIBS

serves 4   *prep time* 20 minutes (not including mashed parsnips)   *cook time* 2 hours

....

EGG-FREE / NUT-FREE / DAIRY-FREE / PALEO-FRIENDLY

....

Don't tell the others, but this melt-in-your-mouth short ribs dish might be my favorite recipe in this cookbook!

ingredients:

2 tablespoons extra-virgin olive oil, divided

3 pounds bone-in short ribs

Fine sea salt and freshly ground black pepper

1 onion, chopped

2 cloves garlic, minced

3 carrots, chopped

1 cup canned diced tomatoes

1 (6-ounce) can tomato paste

2 cups beef broth, homemade (page 354) or store-bought

5 tablespoons good-quality balsamic vinegar

1 tablespoon coconut sugar or granulated maple sugar

2 sprigs fresh thyme, plus additional sprigs for garnish

1 bay leaf

Optional: 1 batch Garlic Mashed Parsnips (page 238), for serving

note: These short ribs are good on their own, but are particularly good served on a bed of Garlic Mashed Parsnips to sop up all of the braising liquid. To bring this meal together seamlessly, start the mashed parsnips a half hour before the ribs are finished.

directions:

1. Preheat the oven to 375°F.

2. To sear the meat, heat 1 tablespoon of the olive oil in a Dutch oven over medium heat. Season the short ribs generously with salt and pepper. Working in batches if needed to avoid overcrowding, sear the short ribs for 1 minute on all sides until slightly browned. Remove and set aside.

3. Heat the remaining tablespoon of olive oil in the Dutch oven over medium heat. Add the onion and garlic and sauté for 3 minutes, until the mixture is fragrant and the onion starts to become translucent.

4. Add the carrots and sauté for 5 minutes, until they begin to soften.

5. Add the diced tomatoes, tomato paste, beef broth, balsamic vinegar, and sugar. Stir to combine.

6. Return the short ribs to the pot and add the thyme sprigs and bay leaf.

7. Cover and place in the oven. Bake for 2 hours, until the short ribs are tender and the sauce begins to brown on the sides of the pot. Using a wooden spoon or a spatula, scrape down the sides. Remove the bay leaf and serve hot with the mashed parsnips, if desired.

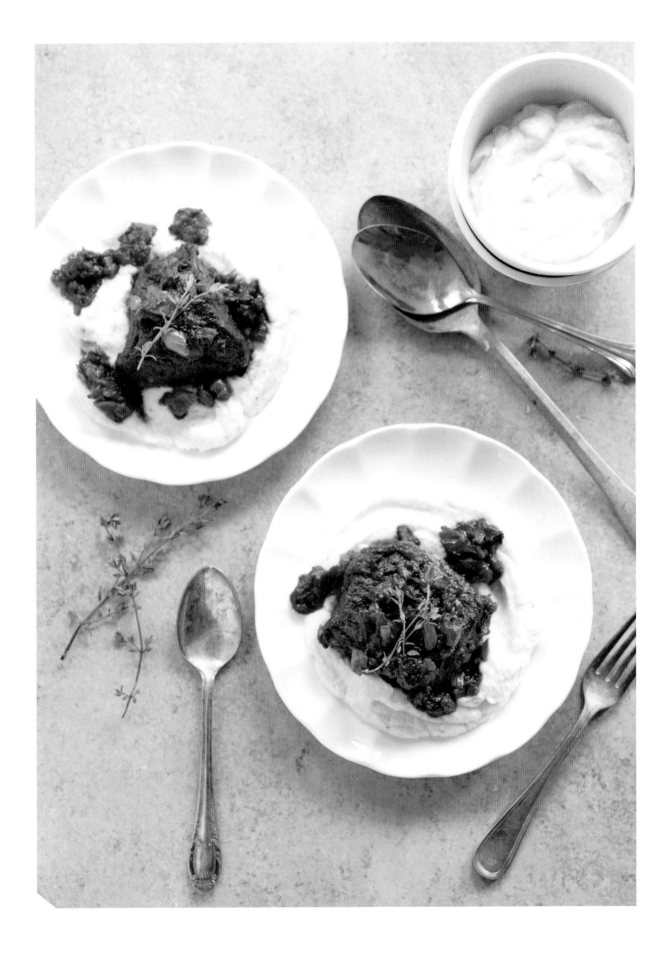

BEEF TENDERLOIN WITH CREAMY HORSERADISH SAUCE

serves 4 to 6   *prep time* 8 minutes   *cook time* 40 minutes

....

NUT-FREE / DAIRY-FREE / PALEO-FRIENDLY

....

Tender beef cooked to perfection and served with the absolute best creamy horseradish sauce—I can't think of anything better, especially for the holidays!

ingredients:

1 (2-pound) beef tenderloin

1 teaspoon fine sea salt

1 teaspoon freshly ground black pepper

1 tablespoon extra-virgin olive oil

FOR THE CREAMY HORSERADISH SAUCE:

½ cup prepared horseradish, homemade (page 346) or store-bought

¼ cup mayo, homemade (page 312) or store-bought

1 tablespoon Dijon mustard

1 teaspoon lemon juice

½ teaspoon white vinegar

⅓ cup water

Juice of ½ lemon

SPECIAL EQUIPMENT:

Kitchen twine

note: I prefer to use freshly prepared horseradish because I love the strong, fresh flavor it provides, but store-bought will work, too.

directions:

1. Preheat the oven to 350°F.

2. Secure the beef at 2-inch intervals with kitchen twine, then season generously with the salt and pepper. Heat the oil in a large oven-safe skillet over medium-high heat. Add the beef to the pan and sear for 5 minutes on each side, until browned. Transfer the pan to the oven and cook the tenderloin for 30 minutes for medium-rare or 40 minutes for medium.

3. While the beef is cooking, whisk together the ingredients for the horseradish sauce. Set aside, covered, in the refrigerator.

4. When the beef is cooked to your liking, remove it from the oven and transfer it to a cutting board; tent with foil and let it rest for 15 minutes.

5. While the meat is resting, make a pan sauce: Place the skillet over medium heat and pour in the water. Scrape the bottom of the skillet to release any browned bits. Bring to a boil, then lower the heat and simmer for 8 to 10 minutes, until slightly reduced.

6. After the tenderloin has rested, remove the twine and cut the meat into ½-inch to ¾-inch slices. Sprinkle with the lemon juice and season with additional salt and pepper.

7. Pour the pan sauce over the meat and serve immediately with the horseradish sauce.

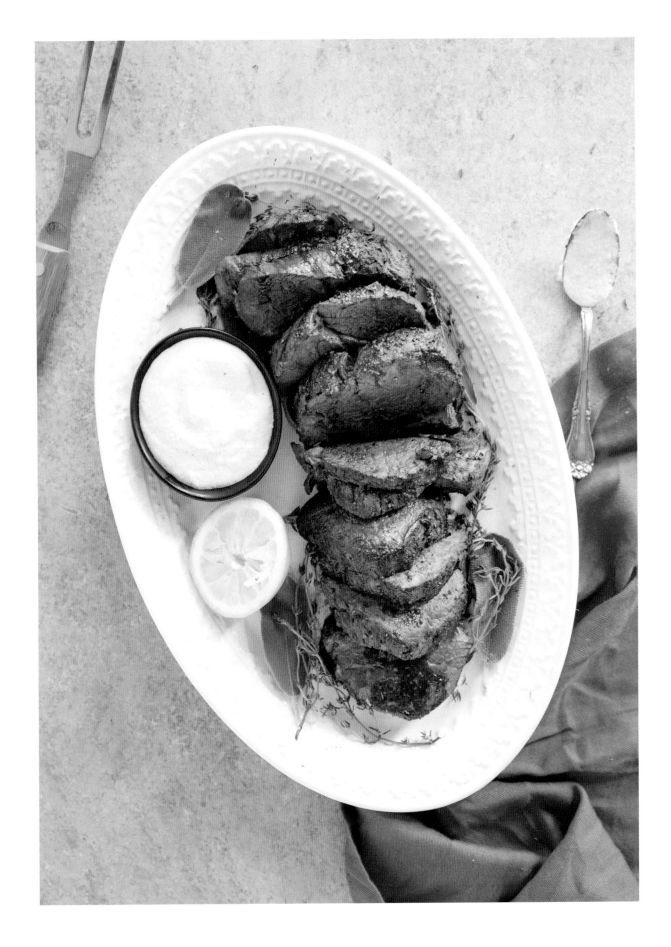

BEEF & BROCCOLI STIR-FRY

serves 4 *prep time* 8 minutes *cook time* 18 minutes

....

EGG-FREE / NUT-FREE / DAIRY-FREE / PALEO-FRIENDLY

....

Who needs takeout when you can make saucy, tender beef and broccoli at home? This dish is everything you want in a beef and broccoli stir-fry—just like the one you recall from your takeout days—but it won't make you feel junky after you eat it!

ingredients:

3 tablespoons extra-virgin olive oil or avocado oil, divided

3 cups broccoli florets

Fine sea salt and freshly ground black pepper

1 tablespoon water

1 pound flank steak or boneless steak of choice, cut into ¼-inch strips

FOR THE SAUCE:

¼ cup coconut aminos

1 teaspoon toasted sesame oil

1 clove garlic, minced

1 (1-inch) chunk fresh ginger, peeled and minced

1 teaspoon coconut sugar or granulated maple sugar

1 tablespoon arrowroot flour

1 tablespoon water

2 cups Basic White Rice (page 247), for serving

¼ cup sliced scallions, for garnish

Sesame seeds, for garnish

directions:

1. In a large heavy-bottomed skillet or wok, heat 2 tablespoons of the olive oil over medium heat. Add the broccoli, sprinkle with salt and pepper, and stir. Add the water, cover, and steam for 5 minutes. Stir, then cover and steam for an additional 5 minutes, or until the broccoli is fork-tender. Set aside.

2. While the broccoli is steaming, season the steak strips generously with salt and pepper.

3. In a large heavy-bottomed skillet or wok, heat the remaining tablespoon of olive oil. Add the steak and cook for 5 minutes, turning halfway through.

4. Make the sauce: In a bowl, whisk together the coconut aminos, sesame oil, garlic, ginger, and sugar. In a separate small bowl, whisk together the arrowroot flour and water to create a slurry. Add the slurry to the sauce and mix.

5. Return the broccoli to the skillet or wok. Add the sauce and mix to coat evenly. Reduce the heat and simmer for 3 minutes.

6. Serve hot over rice, garnished with sliced scallions and sesame seeds.

variation:

Slow Cooker Beef & Broccoli. Whisk together the ingredients for the sauce (minus the arrowroot flour and water slurry) and add it to the slow cooker. Add ½ cup of beef broth, then add the sliced beef and mix until completely coated with the sauce. Cover with the lid and cook on high for 3 hours or on low for 5 to 6 hours, until the meat is cooked through and tender. When the beef is done, steam the broccoli following Step 1 above. Add the slurry to the slow cooker and toss to combine, then add the steamed broccoli and toss everything to combine. Cook on low for 5 minutes, then serve.

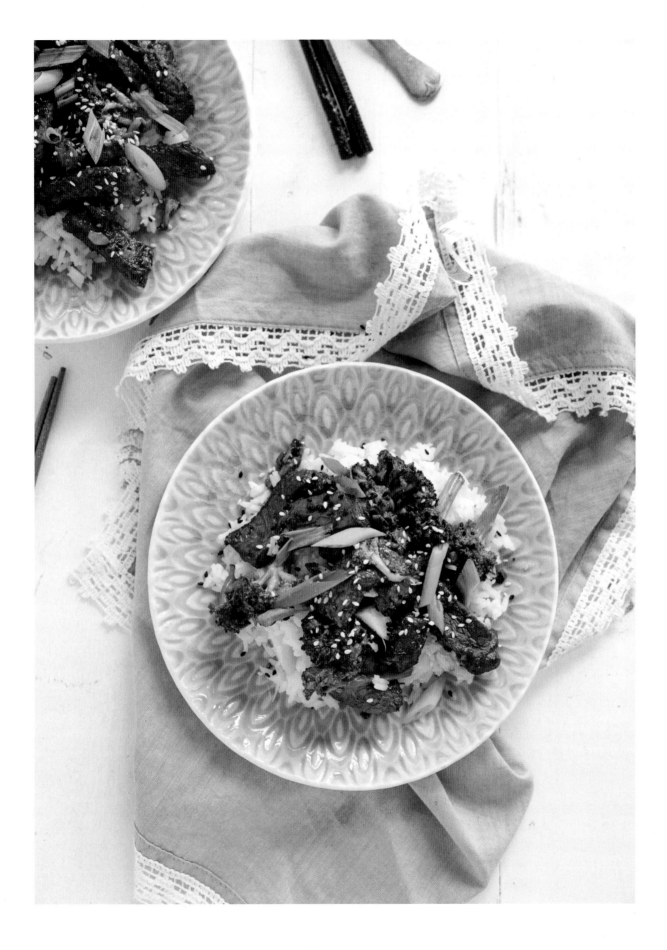

PASTA WITH MEAT SAUCE

serves 4   *prep time* 10 minutes, plus time to make noodles   *cook time* 40 minutes

EGG-FREE / NUT-FREE / DAIRY-FREE OPTION: omit cheese
PALEO-FRIENDLY OPTION: omit cheese

Since I love Italian food, this dish is a frequent dinner in my house. I promise, you won't miss traditional Italian pasta and meat sauce after making this version. The combination of veggie noodles and meaty red sauce will leave you wanting seconds—or thirds!

ingredients:

FOR THE SAUCE:

1 tablespoon extra-virgin olive oil

1 onion, finely diced

3 cloves garlic, minced

1 pound ground beef

1 (24-ounce) jar tomato sauce

1 (6-ounce) can tomato paste

1 teaspoon Italian seasoning

½ teaspoon dried oregano leaves

½ teaspoon garlic powder

½ teaspoon onion powder

¼ teaspoon cracked black pepper, or more as desired

2 pinches of red pepper flakes, or more as desired

½ teaspoon fine sea salt, or more as desired

1 teaspoon coconut sugar

Handful of fresh basil leaves, chopped

FOR THE "PASTA":

1 batch cooked zucchini noodles or spaghetti squash noodles (page 248)

OPTIONAL GARNISHES:

Additional fresh basil leaves

2 tablespoons freshly grated Parmesan cheese

directions:

1. In a large skillet, heat the oil over medium heat and sauté the onion and garlic for 2 minutes until the mixture is fragrant and the onion is beginning to soften.

2. Add the ground beef and cook until browned, about 4 minutes, stirring frequently to break up the meat into small clumps.

3. Add the tomato sauce, tomato paste, spices, salt, sugar, and chopped basil. Mix to incorporate.

4. Lower the temperature and simmer for 30 minutes. Taste and adjust the seasoning and spices as desired.

5. While the sauce simmers, prepare the zucchini or spaghetti squash noodles. Serve immediately with the sauce, garnished with fresh basil and Parmesan cheese, if desired.

notes: The longer the meat sauce simmers, the more tender and flavorful it will be. If you have an hour, keep it going!

Feel free to add some veggies to the sauce, like chopped carrots, sliced mushrooms, or diced zucchini.

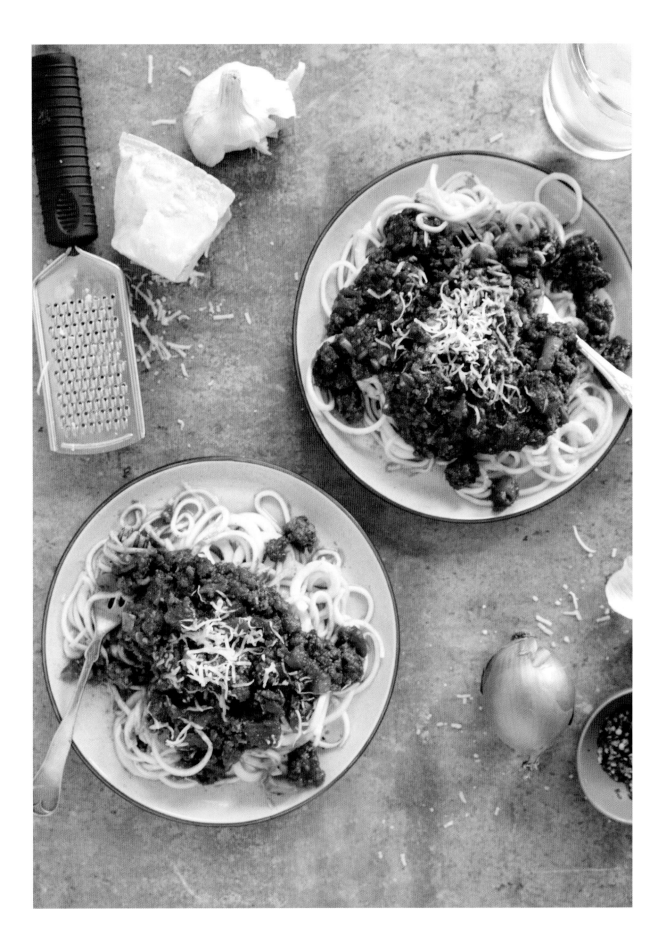

GRILLED STEAK

serves 4 *prep time* 5 minutes *cook time* 15 minutes

EGG-FREE / NUT-FREE / DAIRY-FREE / PALEO-FRIENDLY

Steak on the grill, cooked perfectly to my liking, with a generous slather of chimichurri—that is my kind of dinner! Steak is simple to prepare, and while it can be enhanced with a marinade, it is totally not needed for a fabulously juicy steak. It's all about your prep and timing. I highly recommend buying good-quality meat, seasoning it generously with salt and pepper, watching the cook time, and finally letting the meat rest. And there you have it: a fabulous steak!

ingredients:

4 (1½-inch-thick) beef steaks of choice

Avocado oil

Fine sea salt and freshly ground black pepper

Optional: 1 batch Chimichurri (page 352), for serving

grilling guide:

Rare: 125°F to 130°F

Medium-rare: 130°F to 135°F

Medium: 140°F to 145°F

Well-done: 160°F and higher

directions:

1. Ten to twenty minutes before you plan to grill the steaks, remove them from the refrigerator and let sit, covered, at room temperature.

2. Preheat a grill to high heat. Brush the steaks on both sides with oil and season generously with salt and pepper.

3. Oil the hot grill grates and place the steaks on the grill. Cook until browned and slightly charred, 4 to 5 minutes. Turn the steaks over and continue to grill for 3 to 5 minutes for medium-rare, 5 to 7 minutes for medium, or 8 to 10 minutes for medium to well-done. (For more accurate results, cook to temperature using a meat thermometer following the grilling guide at left.)

4. Transfer the steaks to a plate or cutting board and tent loosely with foil. Let rest for 5 minutes before slicing and serving. Serve with chimichurri, if desired.

serve with:

226
Sweet Potato Truffle Fries

244
Lemon Herb Spring Vegetable Risotto

352
Chimichurri

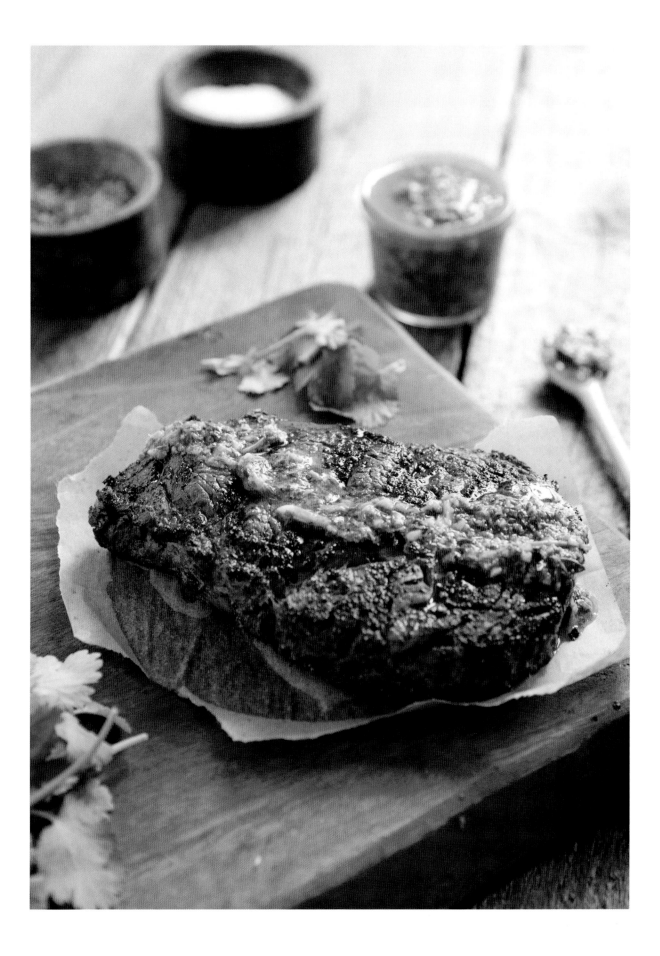

PAD THAI

serves 4 *prep time* 10 minutes *cook time* depends on type of noodle used

....

NUT-FREE / DAIRY-FREE / PALEO-FRIENDLY OPTION: **omit peanuts**

....

This Pad Thai has my heart. I love it with shrimp or chicken, but it's great as a veggie version, too. However you serve it, it makes a hearty and flavorful meal!

ingredients:

FOR THE SAUCE:

¼ cup coconut aminos

1 tablespoon fish sauce

1 teaspoon honey

½ teaspoon unseasoned rice vinegar

Juice of ½ lime

3 cloves garlic, minced

Optional: 4 or 5 dried Thai chiles (omit if you don't like spicy)

1 tablespoon avocado oil or extra-virgin olive oil

1 onion, thinly sliced

1 clove garlic, minced

1 red or green bell pepper, thinly sliced

1 cup shredded green cabbage

¼ cup shredded carrots

1½ cups bean sprouts

2 large eggs, whisked

1 pound peeled and deveined extra-large shrimp (about 18 to 20 shrimp per pound)

8 ounces rice noodles, cooked following package instructions, 3 to 4 cups cooked spaghetti squash noodles (page 248), or 4 cups cooked zucchini noodles (page 248)

FOR GARNISH:

4 lime wedges

2 tablespoons crushed peanuts

2 scallions, chopped

Chopped fresh cilantro or Thai basil

directions:

1. In a bowl, whisk together the sauce ingredients and set aside.

2. Heat the oil in a large skillet over medium heat. Add the onion, garlic, and bell pepper and sauté for 5 minutes, until the veggies begin to soften.

3. Add the cabbage, carrots, and bean sprouts and sauté for 2 minutes.

4. Create a well in the center of the veggie mixture. Pour in the whisked eggs and let set. Once curds have formed and the eggs are no longer liquidy, begin to fold them into the veggies.

5. Add the shrimp and sauté for about 2 minutes, until they begin to turn opaque.

6. Add the sauce and mix to combine.

7. Add the noodles and toss to completely coat with the veggies and sauce.

8. Garnish with the lime wedges, crushed peanuts, chopped scallions, and chopped cilantro. Serve immediately.

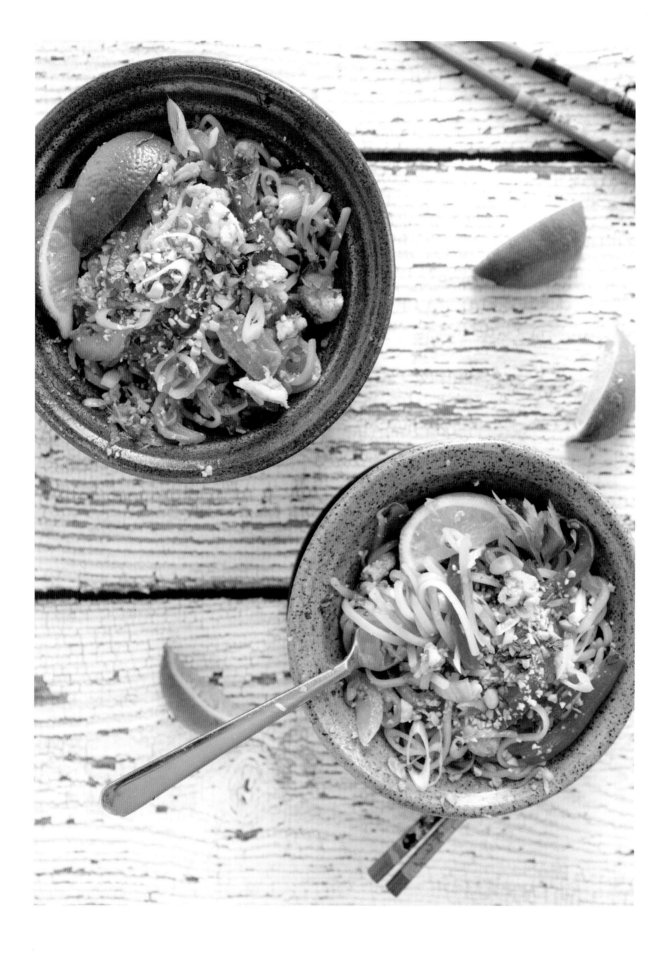

BAKED EGGPLANT PARMESAN

serves 4   *prep time* 15 minutes   *cook time* 50 minutes

....

DAIRY-FREE OPTION: omit cheese / PALEO-FRIENDLY OPTION: omit cheese
VEGAN OPTION: omit cheese

....

Eggplant Parmesan is my all-time favorite Italian dish. I'll tell you, my eggplant
Parm standards are HIGH, and I promise this version will not disappoint! Since
I can do a bit of dairy, I always opt to make this recipe with cheese, but you can
leave it out if you prefer.

ingredients:

1 large eggplant (about 2 pounds),
   sliced ½ inch thick

2 large eggs

1 teaspoon water

1 cup blanched almond flour

Optional: 1 tablespoon freshly
   grated Parmesan cheese

1 tablespoon Italian seasoning

1 teaspoon garlic powder

½ teaspoon onion powder

Pinch of red pepper flakes

½ teaspoon fine sea salt

1 tablespoon extra-virgin olive oil

3 cups marinara sauce, homemade
   (page 338) or store-bought

Optional: 8 ounces mozzarella
   cheese, thinly sliced

Optional: Freshly grated Parmesan
   cheese

Fresh basil leaves

directions:

1. Preheat the oven to 375°F and grease a rimmed baking sheet.

2. Sprinkle the eggplant slices with salt.

3. In a bowl, whisk together the eggs and water.

4. In a separate bowl, combine the almond flour, Parmesan cheese (if using), spices, and salt.

5. Dip the eggplant slices into the egg wash, then into the flour mixture until completely coated. Place on the greased baking sheet. Drizzle the breaded eggplant with the olive oil.

6. Bake for 30 minutes or until golden, flipping halfway through.

7. Spoon ½ cup of the marinara sauce into a 9 by 13-inch baking dish, then add a layer of eggplant slices, sauce, mozzarella cheese (if using), Parmesan cheese (if using), and basil leaves. Repeat the layers, ending with mozzarella and Parmesan.

8. Cover with foil and bake for 20 minutes. Remove the foil and bake for an additional 10 minutes, until the cheese is melted and bubbling. Broil on high for 2 minutes, until the cheese is golden brown.

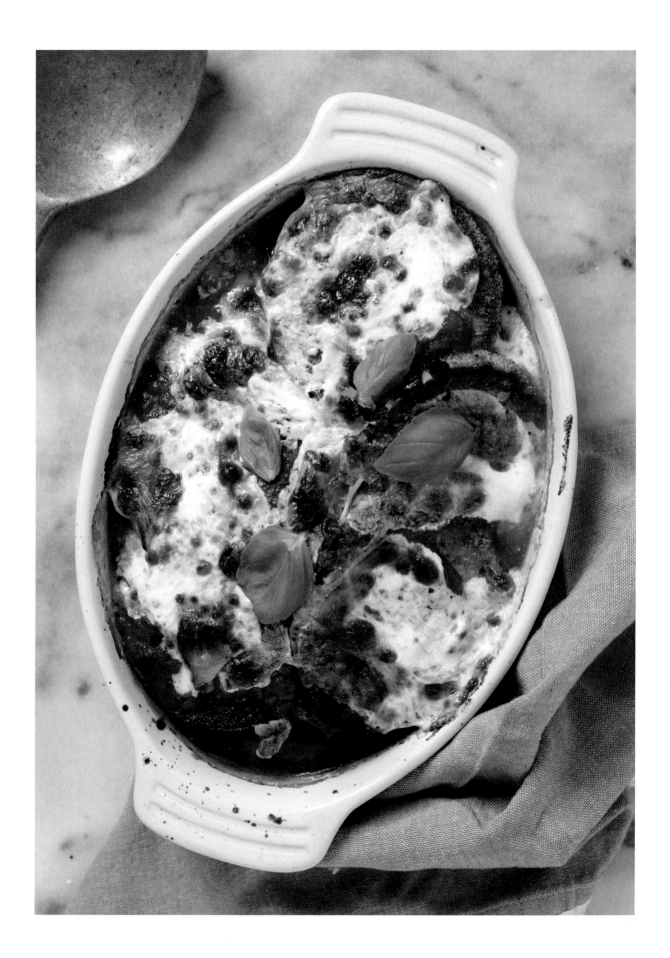

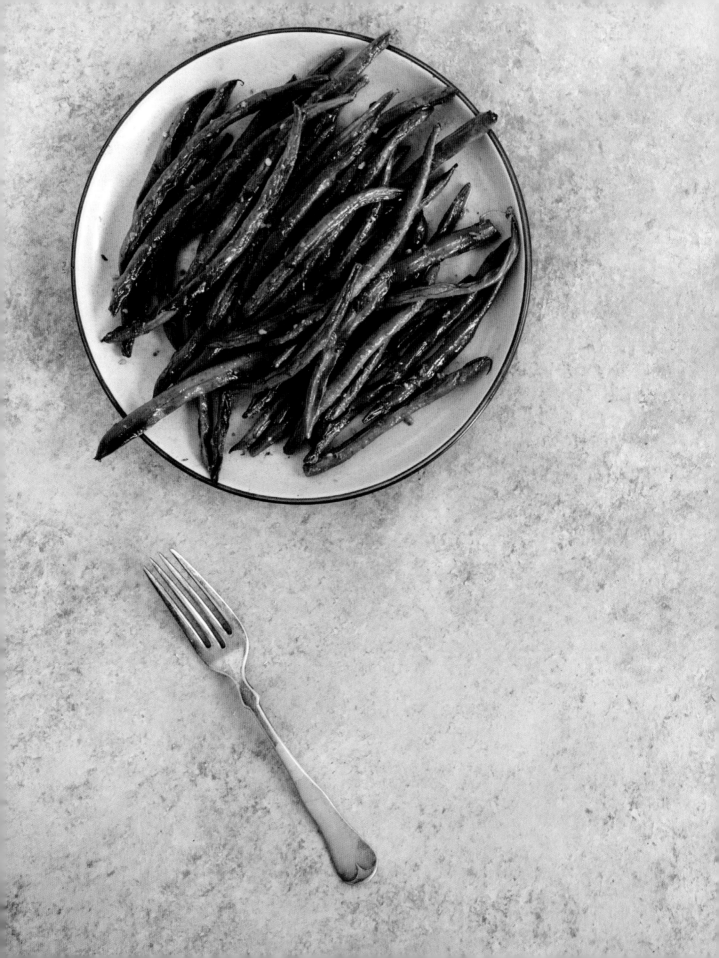

chapter 6

ON THE SIDE

CARAMELIZED BUTTERNUT SQUASH

serves 2 to 4   *prep time* 10 minutes   *cook time* 50 minutes

EGG-FREE / NUT-FREE / DAIRY-FREE OPTION: use coconut oil instead of butter or ghee
PALEO-FRIENDLY OPTION: use ghee or coconut oil instead of butter
VEGAN OPTION: use coconut oil instead of butter or ghee

The perfect accompaniment to any meal!

ingredients:

1 medium butternut squash (about 2 pounds)

2 tablespoons unsalted butter, ghee (page 350), or coconut oil, melted, plus more for the pan

1 tablespoon coconut sugar

½ teaspoon ground cinnamon, plus more for garnish

½ teaspoon fine sea salt

¼ teaspoon freshly ground black pepper

Coarse sea salt, for garnish

directions:

1. Preheat the oven to 375°F and grease a rimmed baking sheet.

2. Peel the squash and slice it in half lengthwise. Remove the seeds and cut into 1-inch cubes. (You should have about 6 cups.)

3. In a large bowl, combine the melted butter, coconut sugar, cinnamon, salt, and pepper. Pour the melted butter mixture over the squash and toss to coat.

4. Place the squash on the greased baking sheet and bake for 40 to 50 minutes, tossing every 15 minutes or so to avoid burning, until caramelized and fork-tender. Garnish with additional cinnamon and coarse sea salt. Serve immediately.

serve with:

Maple-Crusted Salmon   186

Chicken in Mushroom Sauce   172

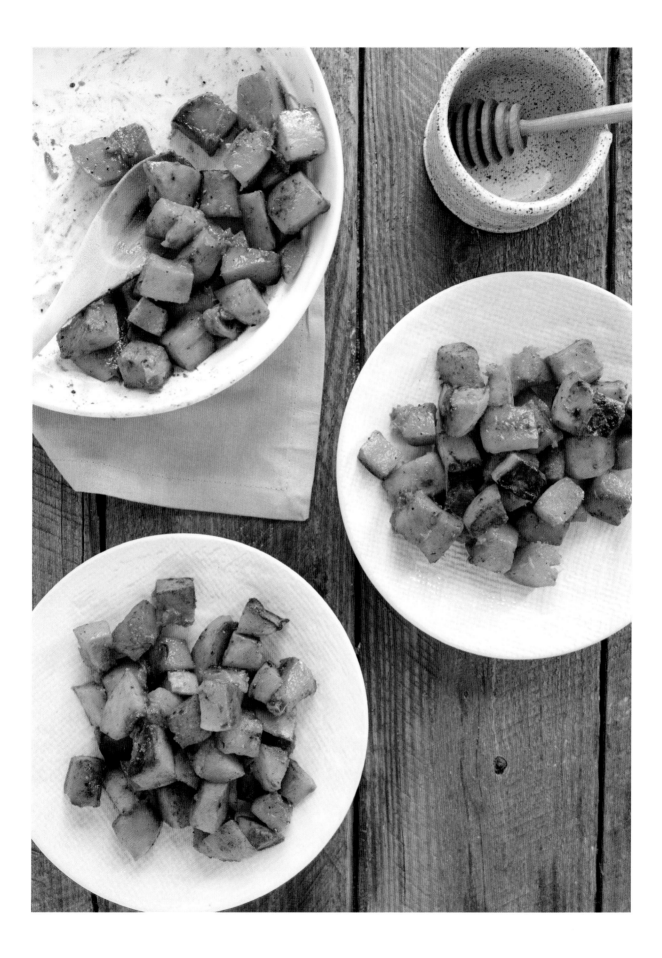

KUNG PAO CAULIFLOWER

serves 2 to 4 *prep time* 10 minutes *cook time* 40 minutes

DAIRY-FREE / PALEO-FRIENDLY

I love this vegetable side! It is reminiscent of a favorite Chinese takeout dish, only it's made with cauliflower instead of the usual chicken. Serve it with any of your favorite mains for a crowd-pleasing side that will fly off the table. (It does in my home!)

ingredients:

1 large head cauliflower, cored and cut into florets

1 cup blanched almond flour

1 teaspoon garlic powder

½ teaspoon fine sea salt

½ teaspoon freshly ground black pepper

1 large egg

1 teaspoon water

1 tablespoon extra-virgin olive oil

FOR THE SAUCE:

¼ cup coconut aminos

1 tablespoon honey

1 teaspoon Sriracha sauce

1 teaspoon grated fresh ginger

2 cloves garlic, smashed with the side of a knife

Optional: 3 to 5 dried chiles (about ½ inch long)

½ teaspoon arrowroot flour

½ teaspoon water

FOR GARNISH:

Sesame seeds

Chopped scallions

directions:

1. Preheat the oven to 400°F. Grease a rimmed baking sheet.

2. In a bowl, mix the almond flour with the garlic powder, salt, and pepper.

3. In a separate bowl, whisk the egg and water.

4. Dip the cauliflower florets into the egg mixture, then into the flour mixture, then place on the baking sheet. Drizzle the coated cauliflower with the olive oil.

5. Bake the cauliflower for 40 minutes or until fork-tender, flipping halfway through.

6. While the cauliflower is baking, prepare the sauce: In a skillet over medium heat, combine the coconut aminos, honey, Sriracha, ginger, garlic, and dried chiles, if using. In a small bowl, mix together the arrowroot flour and water to create a slurry. Add the slurry to the sauce. Bring to a boil, then lower the heat and simmer, stirring constantly, until it becomes thick and sticky, about 2 minutes. Remove from the heat and set aside.

7. Toss the baked cauliflower with the sticky sauce, garnish with sesame seeds and chopped scallions, and serve.

serve with:

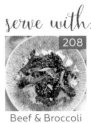

208

Beef & Broccoli Stir-Fry

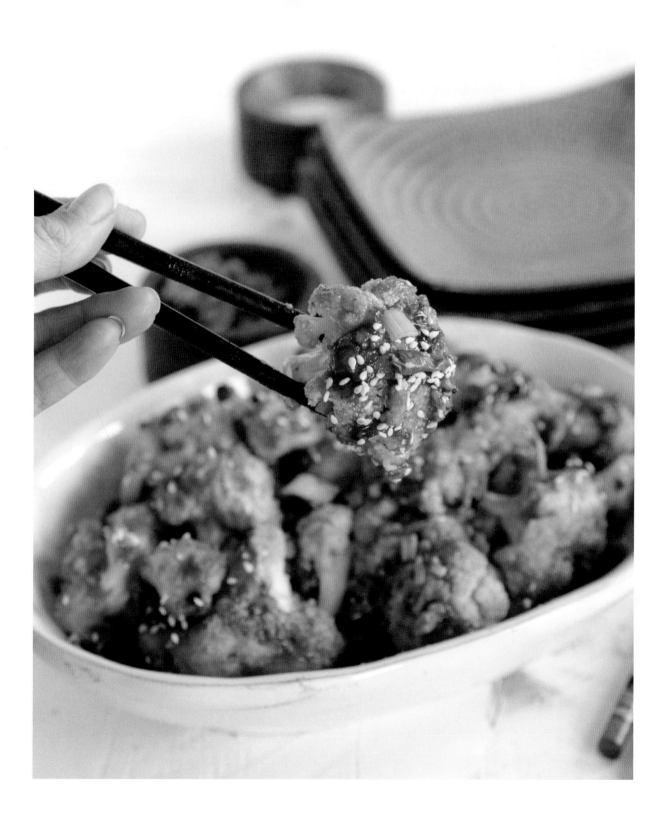

MAPLE BACON BRUSSELS SPROUTS

serves 4 *prep time* 5 minutes *cook time* 30 minutes

EGG-FREE / NUT-FREE / PALEO-FRIENDLY

I love a salty-sweet combination, and these Brussels sprouts hit that nail on the head. This dish will convert almost anyone into a Brussels sprout fan in an instant! You can add more maple syrup if you like them extra sweet, and you can use large Brussels sprouts cut in half or small ones, as I often do!

ingredients:

2 pounds Brussels sprouts, trimmed and sliced in half if large

2 tablespoons extra-virgin olive oil, divided

1 teaspoon fine sea salt

½ teaspoon freshly ground black pepper

½ teaspoon garlic powder

4 strips bacon

1 to 2 tablespoons pure maple syrup

directions:

1. Preheat the oven to 400°F and line a baking sheet with parchment paper.

2. In a large bowl, combine the Brussels sprouts with 1 tablespoon of the olive oil, the salt, pepper, and garlic powder.

3. Place the Brussels sprouts on the parchment-lined baking sheet and bake for 25 to 30 minutes, until fork-tender.

4. While the sprouts are baking, cook the bacon in a large sauté pan over medium heat until crispy, then remove to a plate lined with paper towels to drain. When cool, chop into small pieces. Drain most of the bacon fat from the pan, leaving a little to grease the bottom of the pan.

5. When the Brussels sprouts are done, return the sauté pan with the bacon fat to medium heat and add the remaining tablespoon of olive oil. When the oil is hot, add the baked Brussels sprouts to the pan.

6. Pour 1 tablespoon of maple syrup over the Brussels sprouts and toss to coat evenly with a wooden spoon.

7. Cook over medium heat for 5 minutes, stirring often, until the sprouts are well coated and the maple syrup starts to caramelize them. Remove from the heat and sprinkle with the bacon. Taste, season with additional salt and another tablespoon of maple syrup, if desired, and mix to incorporate. Serve immediately.

serve with:

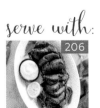

206

Beef Tenderloin with Creamy Horseradish Sauce

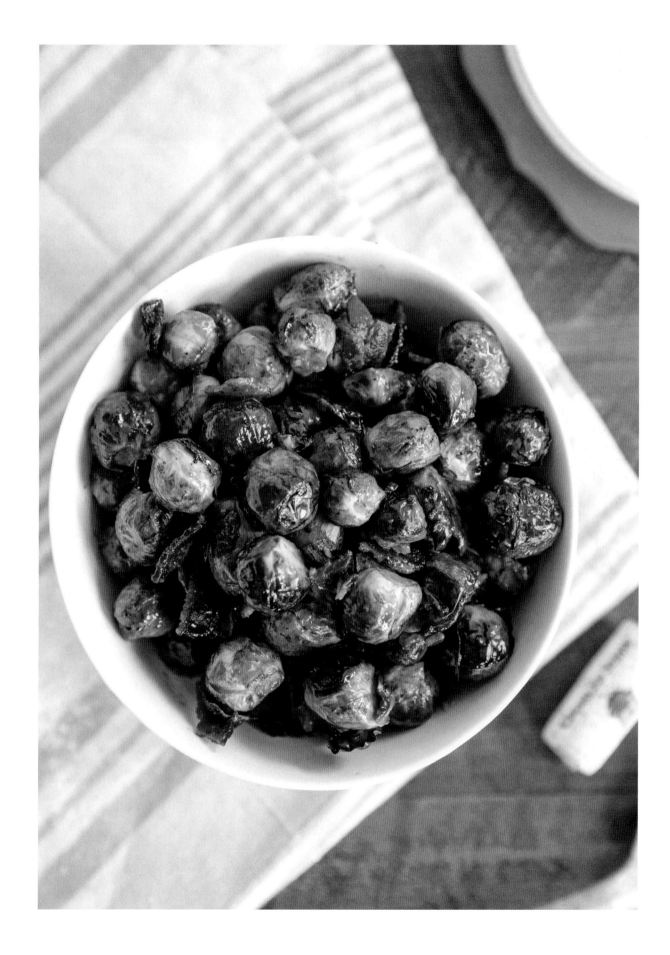

SWEET POTATO TRUFFLE FRIES

serves 2   *prep time* 10 minutes   *cook time* 45 minutes

EGG-FREE OPTION: serve with ketchup instead of mayo / NUT-FREE
DAIRY-FREE OPTION: omit cheese / PALEO-FRIENDLY OPTION: omit cheese
VEGAN OPTION: omit cheese and serve with ketchup instead of mayo

I think we eat these fries once a week, if not more. They are cooked to perfection and tossed with garlic, truffle oil, sea salt, Parmesan cheese, and parsley—a combination that makes for a whole lot of delicious flavor!

ingredients:

1 large Japanese sweet potato or sweet potato variety of choice

1 tablespoon extra-virgin olive oil

1 teaspoon fine sea salt

FOR THE FINISHING SEASONING:

1 tablespoon white truffle oil, or more as desired

2 cloves garlic, minced

1 tablespoon finely chopped fresh flat-leaf parsley

Optional: 2 tablespoons freshly grated Parmesan cheese

Fine sea salt, if needed

FOR SERVING:

Ketchup, homemade (page 342) or store-bought, or mayo, homemade (page 312) or store-bought

directions:

1. Preheat the oven to 400°F.

2. Scrub the potatoes well and dry them thoroughly, then cut them into fries.

3. Toss the fries with the olive oil and 1 teaspoon of salt, then place them on a rimmed baking sheet.

4. Bake the fries for 45 minutes or until crispy, tossing halfway through.

5. Toss the fries with the truffle oil, garlic, parsley, Parmesan cheese (if using), and salt to taste. Serve hot with ketchup, mayonnaise, or both.

note: Japanese sweet potatoes have red skin and a drier white flesh that turns golden when cooked. I find that they are firmer when baked, and I love their subtly sweet flavor.

serve with:

198
All-American Burgers

212
Grilled Steak

196
New England Lobster Rolls

158
Classic Baked Chicken Nuggets

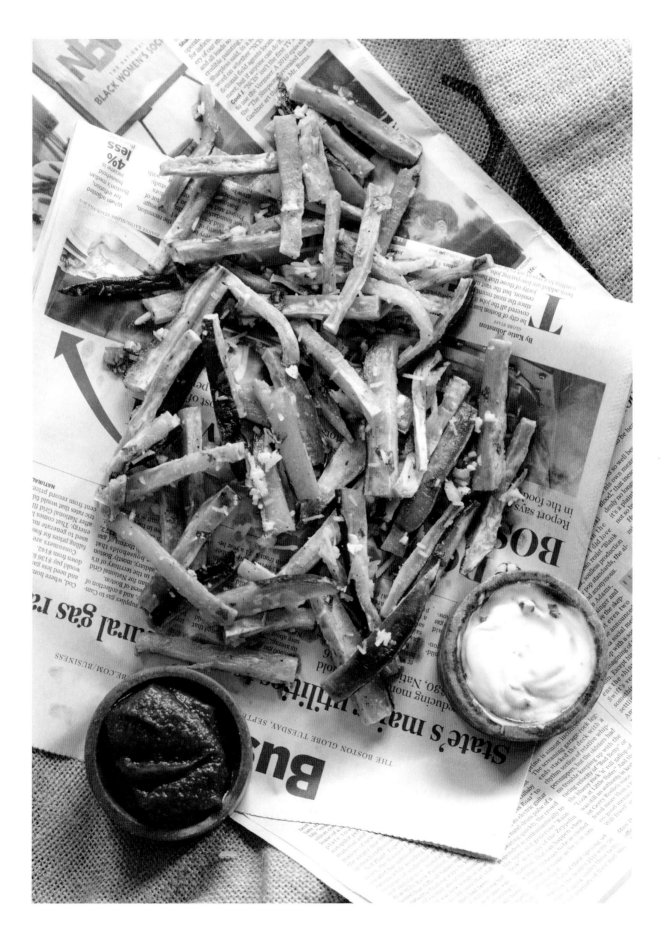

SUMMER'S BEST
GRAINY MUSTARD POTATO SALAD

serves 4   *prep time* 10 minutes   *cook time* 25 minutes

NUT-FREE / DAIRY-FREE / PALEO-FRIENDLY

During the spring and summer, and even throughout the fall, we are outside grilling nonstop. Every BBQ needs a classic potato salad; this is ours!

ingredients:

- 3 pounds mixed potatoes (purple, Yukon Gold, sweet), scrubbed and cut into ½-inch pieces
- 2 large eggs
- 4 strips bacon
- ½ cup mayo, homemade (page 312) or store-bought
- 3 tablespoons whole-grain mustard
- 1 teaspoon apple cider vinegar
- ½ teaspoon lemon juice
- ½ teaspoon garlic powder
- ½ teaspoon coconut sugar or granulated maple sugar
- ½ teaspoon fine sea salt
- ½ teaspoon freshly ground black pepper
- ½ cup chopped scallions

directions:

1. Place the potatoes and a generous pinch of salt in a large stockpot of water and bring to a boil. Boil for 15 to 20 minutes, until the potatoes are fork-tender.

2. While the potatoes are boiling, hard-boil the eggs by boiling or steaming them. (My favorite method is to steam them; see page 66.) Once the eggs are cool, peel and chop them into small pieces and set aside.

3. Fry the bacon in a skillet over medium heat until crispy, 5 to 7 minutes. Remove and let cool, then chop into small pieces and set aside.

4. In a small bowl, whisk together the mayo, mustard, apple cider vinegar, lemon juice, garlic powder, sugar, salt, and pepper.

5. When the potatoes are done, rinse with cold water, pat dry, and transfer to a large bowl. Pour the mayo mixture over the potatoes and gently toss to coat.

6. Top the potatoes with the chopped bacon, hard-boiled eggs, and scallions. Serve immediately or place in the refrigerator to chill before serving. The potato salad will keep in the refrigerator for up to 3 days.

serve with:

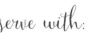

All-American Burgers

Grilled Steak

New England Lobster Rolls

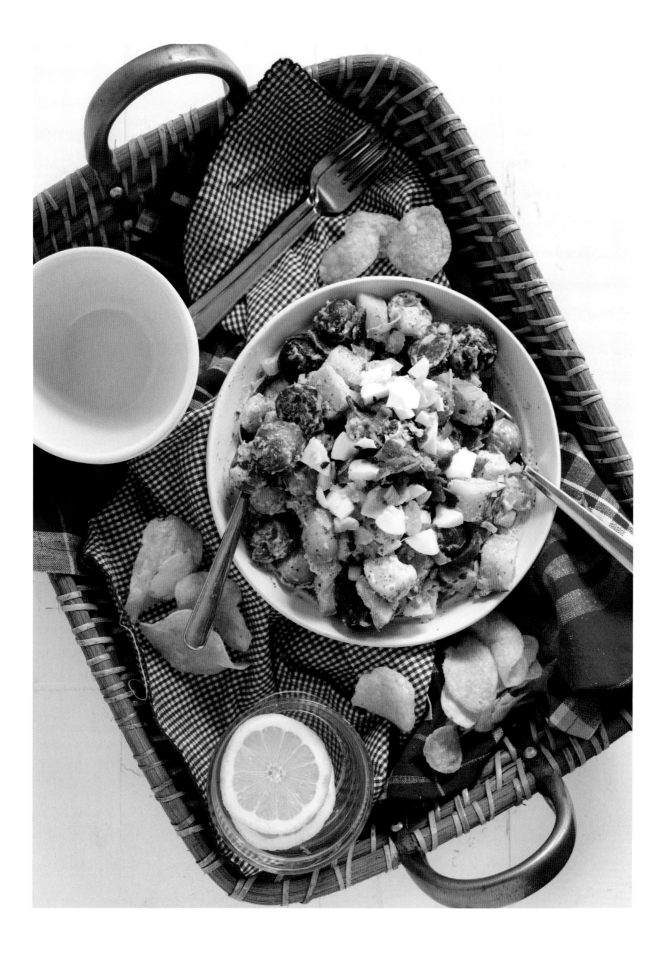

BURNT BROCCOLI

serves 4   *prep time* 5 minutes   *cook time* 45 minutes

EGG-FREE / NUT-FREE / DAIRY-FREE / PALEO-FRIENDLY / VEGAN

Back in New York, where I grew up, we would frequent an Italian restaurant that served up burnt broccoli and burnt green beans, and they're the best things you can imagine. It's not burnt like "ew, inedible burnt," but more like perfectly cooked with a little bit of crisp!

ingredients:

2 large heads broccoli, cut into florets (6 to 8 cups)

3 tablespoons extra-virgin olive oil

4 cloves garlic, minced

1 teaspoon fine sea salt

½ teaspoon freshly ground black pepper

directions:

1. Preheat the oven to 400°F and line a rimmed baking sheet with parchment paper.

2. Toss the broccoli florets with the oil, garlic, salt, and pepper.

3. Place the broccoli on the lined baking sheet and roast for 40 minutes, until tender and starting to get crispy.

4. After 40 minutes, set the broiler to high and broil for 5 minutes, until the broccoli is fully crispy and the edges are starting to brown.

serve with:

186
Maple-Crusted Salmon

192
Scallops Provençal

212
Grilled Steak

158
Classic Baked Chicken Nuggets

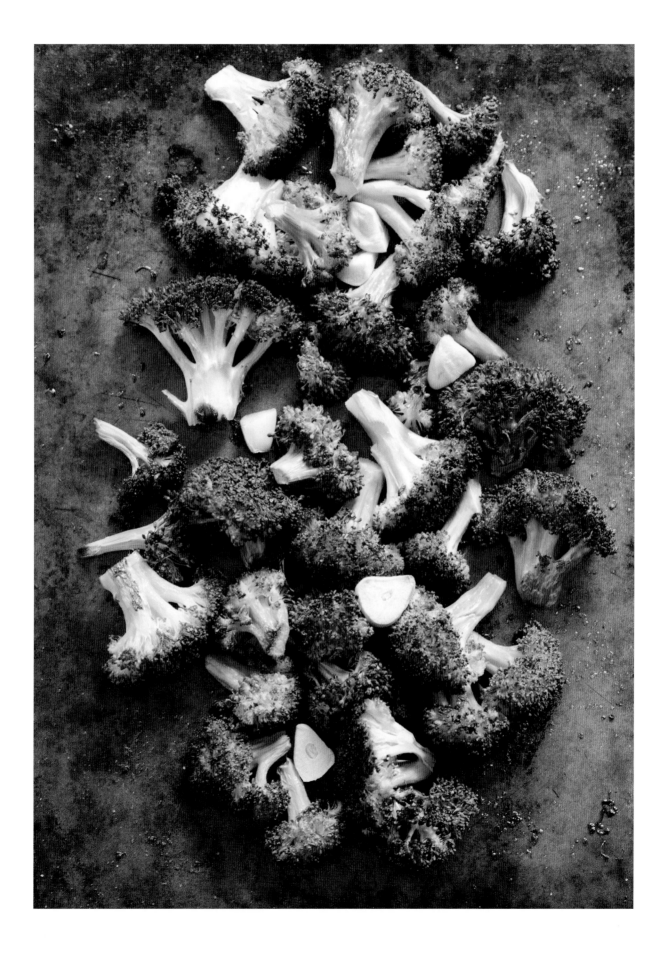

ASIAN SUMMER SLAW

serves 6   *prep time* 20 minutes   *cook time* 5 minutes

EGG-FREE / DAIRY-FREE OPTION: use avocado oil instead of butter or ghee
PALEO-FRIENDLY OPTION: use ghee instead of butter
VEGAN OPTION: use avocado oil instead of butter or ghee

Another must-have addition to any BBQ lunch or dinner is a good slaw. This unique slaw is packed with Thai flavors and is absolutely delicious! I love it because it makes so much, so it's the perfect addition to any party or gathering.

ingredients:

1 (32-ounce) bag coleslaw mix (see note)

⅓ cup avocado oil or extra-virgin olive oil

¼ cup unseasoned rice vinegar or white vinegar

¼ cup coconut aminos

3 tablespoons coconut sugar

1 tablespoon toasted sesame oil

½ teaspoon fine sea salt

1 tablespoon unsalted butter or ghee (page 350)

½ cup slivered almonds, or more as desired

1 tablespoon sesame seeds

¼ cup chopped scallions

Optional: ½ cup raisins, or more as desired

note: To make your own slaw mix, toss together 5 cups of shredded green cabbage (about 1 medium head), 2 cups of shredded red cabbage (about ½ small head), and ½ cup of julienned carrots (about 1 large).

directions:

1. Place the coleslaw mix in a mixing bowl.

2. Make the dressing: In a separate bowl, whisk together the avocado oil, vinegar, coconut aminos, coconut sugar, sesame oil, and salt.

3. Pour the dressing over the cabbage and toss to coat.

4. Heat the butter in a small saucepan over medium heat for 30 seconds. Add the slivered almonds and sesame seeds and sauté for 3 to 4 minutes, until fragrant and beginning to turn golden brown.

5. Remove from the heat and let sit for 5 minutes. Add to the slaw bowl along with chopped scallions and raisins, if adding. Mix to combine and serve immediately.

variation:

Asian Summer Slaw with Shredded Chicken. Add 3 cups of shredded cooked chicken (see "How to Make Easy Shredded Chicken" on page 152) to the coleslaw mix in Step 1 and toss to combine. Continue with the recipe as written. *Serves 6 to 8.*

serve with:

198
All-American Burgers

158
Classic Baked Chicken Nuggets

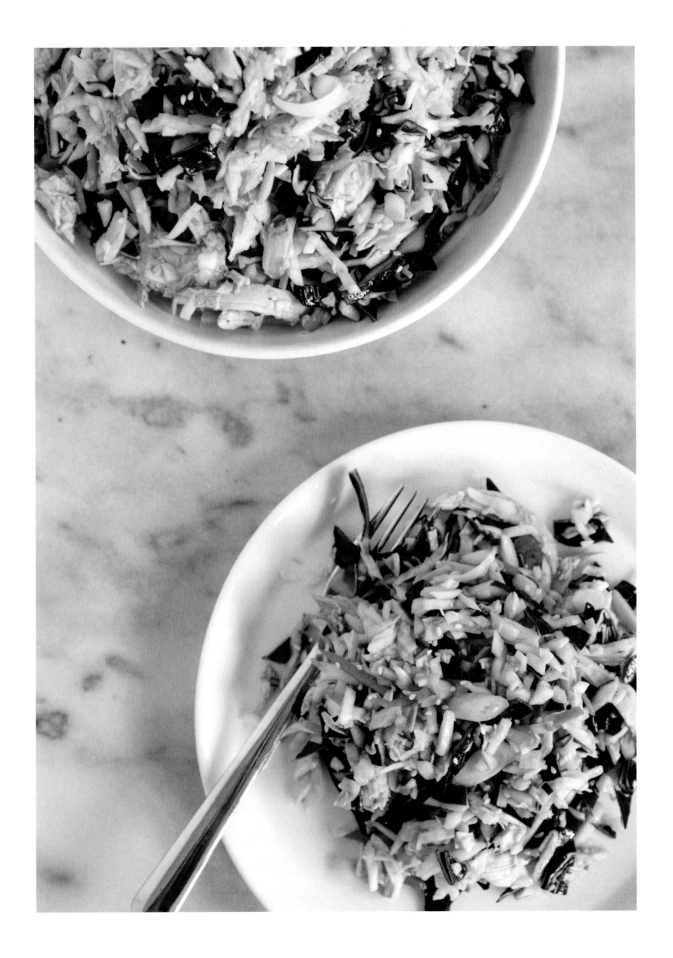

GARLICKY BLISTERED GREEN BEANS

serves 2   *prep time* 5 minutes   *cook time* 20 minutes

EGG-FREE / NUT-FREE / DAIRY-FREE OPTION: use extra-virgin olive oil instead of ghee or butter
PALEO-FRIENDLY OPTION: use ghee instead of butter
VEGAN OPTION: use extra-virgin olive oil instead of ghee or butter

Crispy, flavorful, garlicky green beans cooked just right—a once-a-week type of side dish!

ingredients:

- ¼ cup ghee (page 350) or unsalted butter
- 8 cloves garlic, sliced
- 2 pounds green beans, trimmed
- 1 teaspoon fine sea salt
- ½ teaspoon freshly ground black pepper

directions:

1. In a large oven-safe skillet, heat the ghee over medium heat for 1 minute.

2. Add the garlic and sauté for 2 minutes, until fragrant, stirring to avoid burning.

3. Add the green beans and sauté, stirring often, for about 10 minutes, until fork-tender. Sprinkle with the salt and pepper.

4. Place an oven rack in the center of the oven and turn the broiler to high.

5. Place the skillet in the oven and broil the green beans for 3 to 5 minutes, until slightly crispy and browned, watching to avoid burning.

serve with:

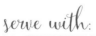

Balsamic Braised Short Ribs — 204

Thai BBQ Salmon — 188

Loaded Italian Meatballs — 182

Beef Tenderloin with Creamy Horseradish Sauce — 206

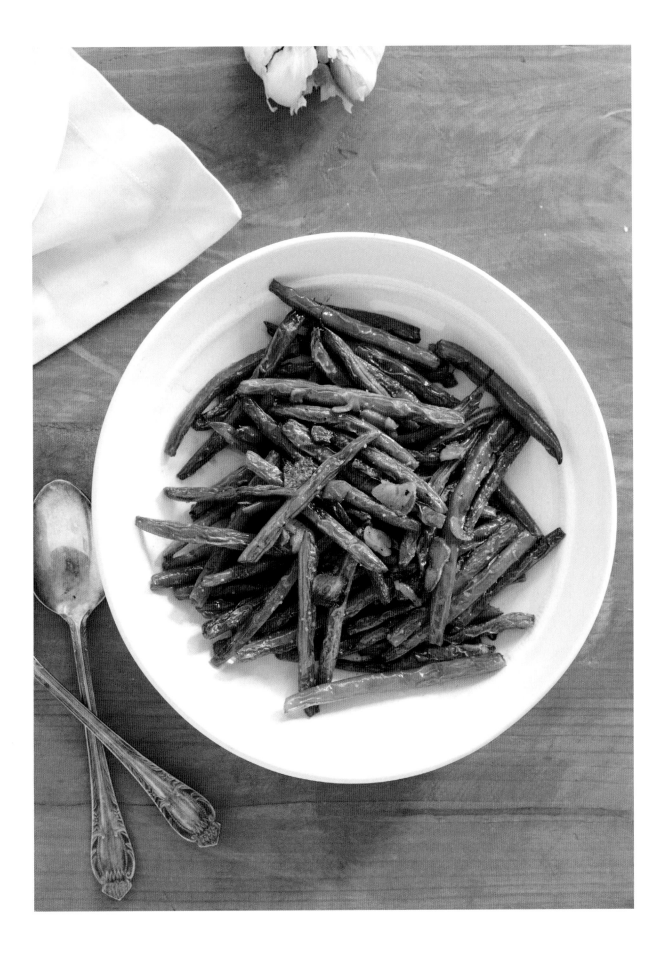

PORK BELLY BRUSSELS SPROUTS WITH LEMON DRESSING

serves 4   *prep time* 10 minutes   *cook time* 25 minutes

EGG-FREE / NUT-FREE / DAIRY-FREE / PALEO-FRIENDLY

This isn't your average, boring Brussels sprouts side dish! If you've never dressed cooked Brussels sprouts with thick and crispy pieces of pork belly and a lemon dressing, you are missing out.

ingredients:

FOR THE DRESSING:

3 tablespoons extra-virgin olive oil or avocado oil

2 tablespoons lemon juice

1 teaspoon Dijon mustard

½ teaspoon honey

Pinch of fine sea salt

2 pounds Brussels sprouts, trimmed, kept whole if small or sliced in half if large

3 tablespoons extra-virgin olive oil, divided

1 teaspoon fine sea salt

½ teaspoon freshly ground black pepper

1½ pounds pork belly, finely diced

directions:

1. Whisk together the ingredients for the dressing and set aside.

2. Preheat the oven to 400°F and line a rimmed baking sheet with parchment paper.

3. In a large bowl, toss the Brussels sprouts with 2 tablespoons of the olive oil and the salt and pepper.

4. Place the Brussels sprouts on the parchment-lined baking sheet and bake for 30 minutes, until fork-tender.

5. While the sprouts are roasting, heat the remaining tablespoon of olive oil in a medium-sized skillet for 1 minute. Add the diced pork belly and cook, stirring often, until crispy, about 15 minutes. Set aside on a plate lined with a paper towel to cool.

6. When the Brussels sprouts are done, toss them in a bowl with the pork belly and lemon dressing. Serve immediately.

serve with:

Scallops Provençal

Nanny's Potted Chicken

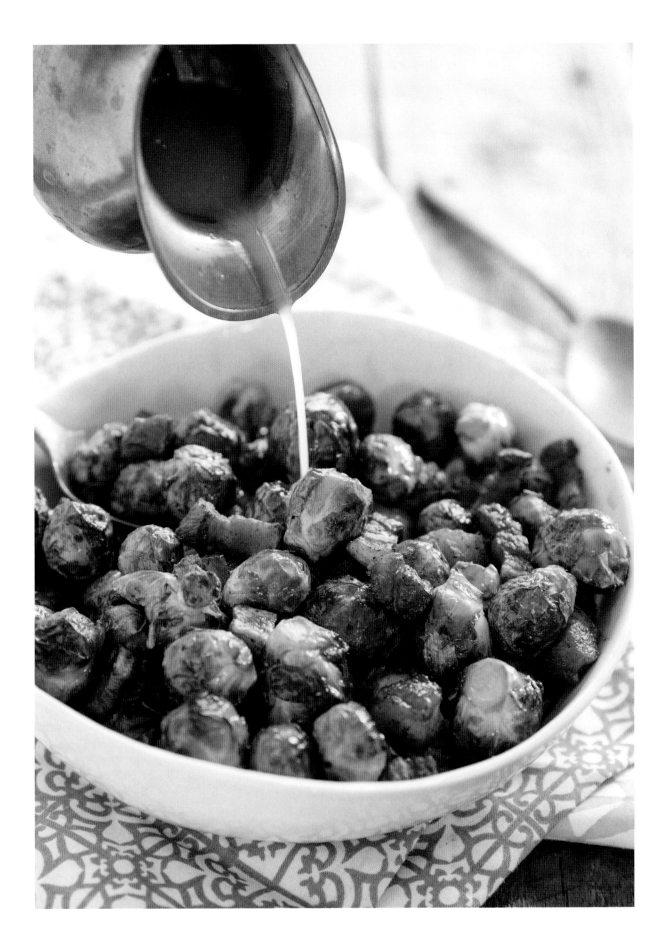

CREAMY MASHED ROOTS TWO WAYS

serves 2 *prep time* 5 minutes *cook time* 20 minutes

EGG-FREE / PALEO-FRIENDLY OPTION: use ghee instead of butter

You don't need heavy cream and all that jazz to make creamy and flavorful mashed roots! With these two options, you'll have a creamy mash that pairs beautifully with just about any dish.

ingredients:

FOR GARLIC MASHED PARSNIPS:

1 pound parsnips, peeled and cubed

¼ to ½ cup unsweetened almond milk, homemade (page 266) or store-bought, or more as needed

3 tablespoons unsalted butter or ghee (page 350)

2 cloves garlic, crushed to a paste

1 teaspoon fine sea salt

½ teaspoon freshly ground black pepper

Optional: 1 tablespoon fresh rosemary, chopped

FOR MASHED SWEET POTATOES:

1 pound sweet potatoes (1 to 2 large), peeled and cubed

¼ to ½ cup unsweetened almond milk, homemade (page 266) or store-bought, or more as needed

3 tablespoons unsalted butter or ghee (page 350)

1 teaspoon fine sea salt

½ teaspoon ground cinnamon

directions:

GARLIC MASHED PARSNIPS:

1. Place the cubed parsnips in a large saucepan and add water to cover. Cook over medium heat until the parsnips are fork-tender, about 20 minutes.

2. Drain the parsnips and pat dry, then return them to the saucepan.

3. To the pan with the parsnips, add ¼ cup of the almond milk, the butter, garlic, salt, pepper, and rosemary, if using. Using a potato masher, mash the parsnips until they're broken down. Add more almond milk as needed to reach your desired creaminess. Transfer the mixture to a blender, or leave it in the pan and use an immersion blender, and blend until completely smooth. Or, if you like your mash more rustic and slightly chunky, omit the blender step and use the potato masher to mash until it reaches your desired consistency. Taste and add additional salt and pepper, if desired. Serve immediately.

MASHED SWEET POTATOES:

1. Place the cubed sweet potatoes in a large saucepan and add water to cover. Cook over medium heat until the potatoes are fork-tender, about 20 minutes.

2. Drain the sweet potatoes and pat dry, then return them to the saucepan.

3. To the pan with the sweet potatoes, add ¼ cup of the almond milk, the butter, salt, and cinnamon. Using a potato masher, mash for about 1 minute, until the ingredients begins to combine. Add more almond milk as needed to reach your desired creaminess. Transfer the mixture to a blender, or leave it in the pan and use an immersion blender, and blend until completely smooth. Taste and add additional cinnamon and salt, if desired. Serve immediately.

serve with:

 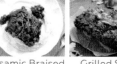

Balsamic Braised Short Ribs Grilled Steak

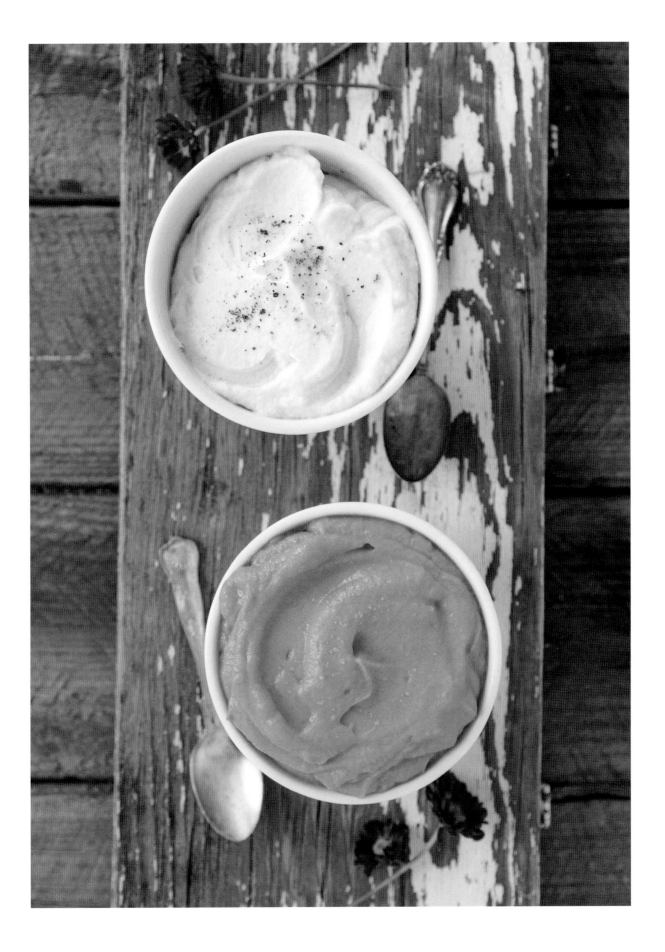

BETTER-THAN-TAKEOUT CHICKEN & PINEAPPLE FRIED RICE

serves 4 as a side, 2 as a main *prep time* 10 minutes *cook time* 20 minutes, plus time to cook rice

NUT-FREE / DAIRY-FREE OPTION: use extra-virgin olive oil instead of ghee or butter
PALEO-FRIENDLY OPTION: use ghee instead of butter

Fried rice is the perfect side dish, and it can easily be made into a full meal when lots of protein is added, as it is here! This dish captures all the flavor of restaurant fried rice, but without the junk and guilt. Plus, cooked pineapple is divine. I highly recommend it!

ingredients:

FOR THE SAUCE:

2 tablespoons coconut aminos

1 teaspoon fish sauce

1 teaspoon Sriracha sauce

½ teaspoon toasted sesame oil (see note)

½ teaspoon coconut sugar

½ teaspoon garlic powder

Pinch of freshly ground black pepper

2 tablespoons ghee (page 350) or unsalted butter

2 cloves garlic, minced

1 onion, diced

1 shallot, finely diced

2 large carrots, diced

½ cup frozen peas

1 cup mushrooms, chopped

1 pound boneless, skinless chicken breasts, cubed

Fine sea salt and freshly ground black pepper

2 large eggs, whisked

2 cups Basic White Rice (page 247) or riced cauliflower (see page 246)

1½ cups diced fresh pineapple

⅓ cup sliced scallions, for garnish

1 tablespoon sesame seeds, for garnish

directions:

1. Combine the sauce ingredients in a small bowl and set aside.

2. Warm the ghee in a large skillet over medium heat, then add the garlic, onion, and shallot and sauté for 2 minutes, until fragrant.

3. Add the carrots, peas, and mushrooms and sauté for 5 to 7 minutes, until the vegetables begin to soften.

4. Season the cubed chicken with two or three pinches each of salt and pepper, then add to the skillet. Cook the chicken for 5 to 7 minutes, stirring often, until it is golden on all sides.

5. Make a space in the middle of the skillet and pour in the whisked eggs. Let them set for 1 minute, then gently scramble in the center until dry. Mix to incorporate the eggs with the vegetables.

6. Add the cooked white rice or raw riced cauliflower and the pineapple. Season the entire mixture with salt and pepper to taste, then mix to fully incorporate and cook until the rice begins to brown, 2 to 4 minutes.

7. Pour in the sauce and mix to fully combine. Taste and add additional salt and pepper, if desired. Garnish with the scallions and sesame seeds.

note: If you don't have toasted sesame oil on hand for the sauce, you can omit it, but it does add a wonderful flavor!

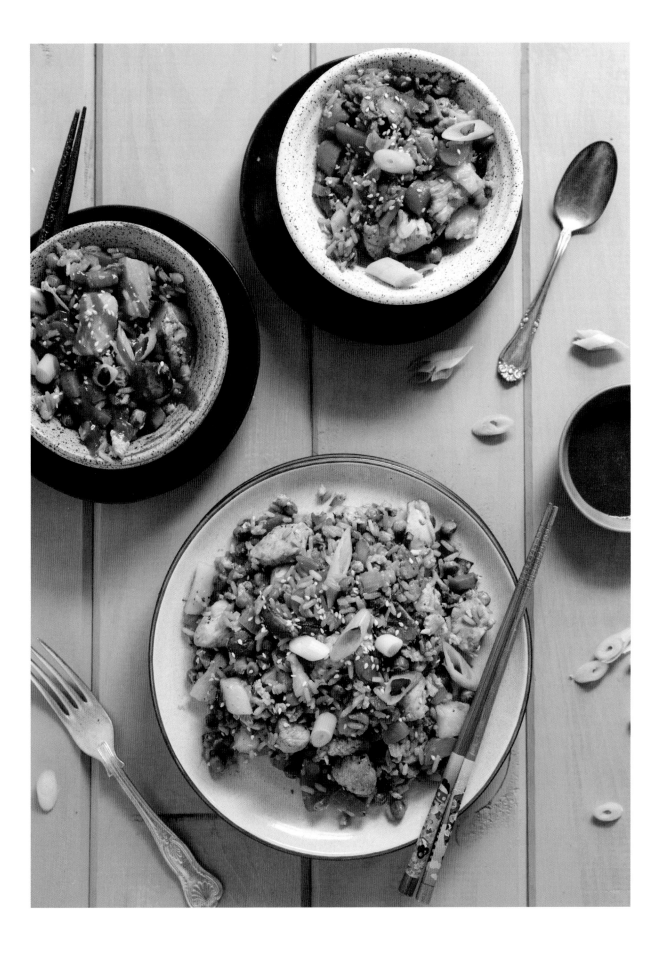

STIR-FRIED VEGGIES

serves 4   *prep time* 10 minutes   *cook time* 20 minutes

EGG-FREE / NUT-FREE / DAIRY-FREE / PALEO-FRIENDLY / VEGAN OPTION: **omit fish sauce**

These stir-fried veggies are a wonderful way to mix up your veggie side dish rotation. They are delicious with grilled or baked chicken, meat, or fish and will elevate an ordinary meal to a next-level one!

ingredients:

FOR THE STIR-FRY SAUCE:

2 tablespoons rice vinegar

2 tablespoons coconut aminos

1 teaspoon fish sauce

1 teaspoon toasted sesame oil

½ to 1 teaspoon chili paste, or more as desired for spicier sauce

1 (½-inch) chunk fresh ginger, grated

¼ teaspoon freshly ground black pepper

½ teaspoon garlic powder

1 tablespoon extra-virgin olive oil or toasted sesame oil

2 cloves garlic, minced

2 cups broccoli florets

1 red bell pepper, sliced

1 yellow or orange bell pepper, sliced

1 green bell pepper, sliced

1 cup mushrooms, chopped

1 red onion, sliced

1 cup snap peas

3 heads baby bok choy, chopped

1 cup bean sprouts

¼ cup sliced scallions, for garnish

2 teaspoons black and/or white sesame seeds, for garnish

Optional: Chopped fresh Thai basil leaves, for garnish

directions:

1. Combine the sauce ingredients in a small bowl and set aside.

2. In a large skillet or wok over medium heat, heat the olive oil until hot, about 1 minute. Add the garlic, broccoli, bell peppers, mushrooms, onion, and snap peas and cook for 8 to 10 minutes, stirring often, until the vegetables soften.

3. Add the bok choy and bean sprouts and sauté for 2 minutes, until the bok choy begins to wilt.

4. Pour in the sauce and stir to combine. Reduce the heat to medium-low and simmer for 5 minutes.

5. Garnish with the scallions, sesame seeds, and Thai basil, if using, and serve immediately.

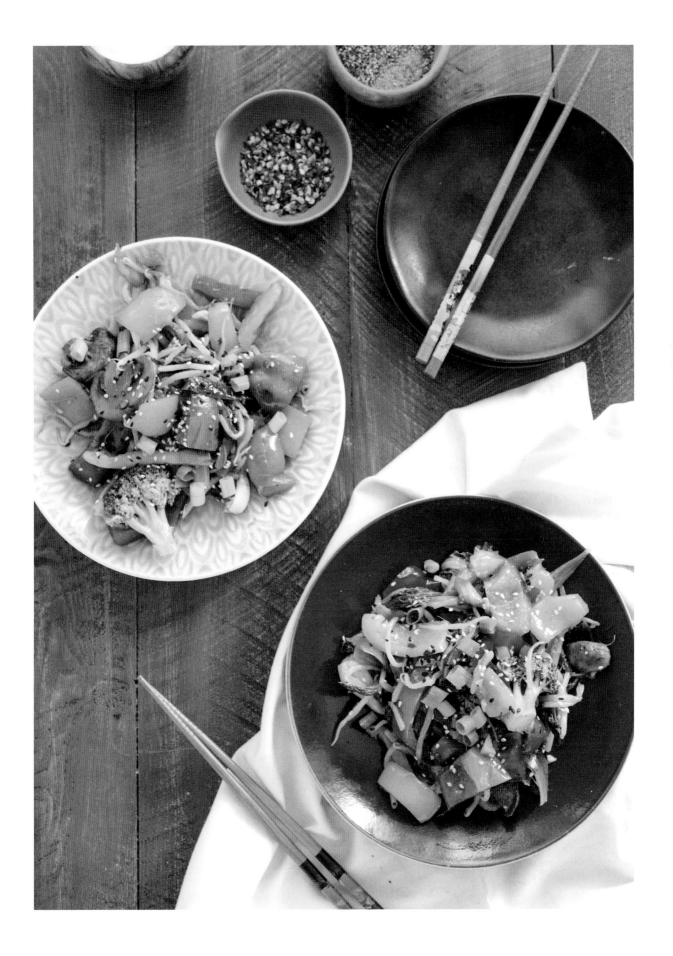

LEMON HERB SPRING VEGETABLE RISOTTO

serves 4   *prep time* 10 minutes   *cook time* 45 minutes

EGG-FREE OPTION: omit poached eggs / NUT-FREE
DAIRY-FREE OPTION: omit cheese and use extra-virgin olive oil instead of ghee or butter
PALEO-FRIENDLY OPTION: omit cheese and use ghee instead of butter
VEGAN OPTION: omit cheese and eggs; use oil instead of ghee or butter and vegetable broth (page 356) instead of chicken broth

Risotto sounds intimidating, right? I promise, you've got this! Whip up this dish and impress your family, friends, and guests.

ingredients:

2 tablespoons ghee (page 350) or unsalted butter

2 cloves garlic, minced

1 onion, finely diced

1 bunch asparagus, tough ends removed, cut into 2- to 3-inch pieces

1 cup Arborio rice

Juice of 1 lemon

4 to 6 cups heated chicken broth, homemade (page 354) or store-bought, divided

¼ cup chopped fresh flat-leaf parsley, plus extra for garnish

¼ cup chopped scallions, plus extra for garnish

Grated zest of 1 lemon

1 teaspoon fine sea salt

1 teaspoon freshly ground black pepper

Pinch of red pepper flakes

Optional: 1 to 2 tablespoons freshly grated Parmesan cheese, as desired

Optional: 1 poached egg per serving (see page 66)

directions:

1. Heat the ghee in a large, deep sauté pan over medium heat. Add the garlic and onion and sauté for about 2 minutes, until fragrant and translucent, then add the asparagus and sauté for an additional minute.

2. Add the rice and stir to incorporate it into the garlic, onion, and asparagus mixture, then add the lemon juice.

3. Add 1 cup of the broth and, stirring constantly, simmer until almost all the broth has been absorbed. Add another cup of the broth and repeat the process. Continue adding broth, 1 cup at a time, until the rice is tender, thick, and creamy. (You may need only 4 cups of broth.)

4. Fold in the parsley, scallions, lemon zest, salt, black pepper, red pepper flakes, and Parmesan cheese, if using.

5. Top with additional parsley, scallions, salt, and pepper—and a poached egg, if desired—and serve immediately!

variation:

Lemon Herb Spring Vegetable Risotto with Truffle Oil. Make it truffled! In Step 4, add 1 to 2 teaspoons of white truffle oil and mix to combine.

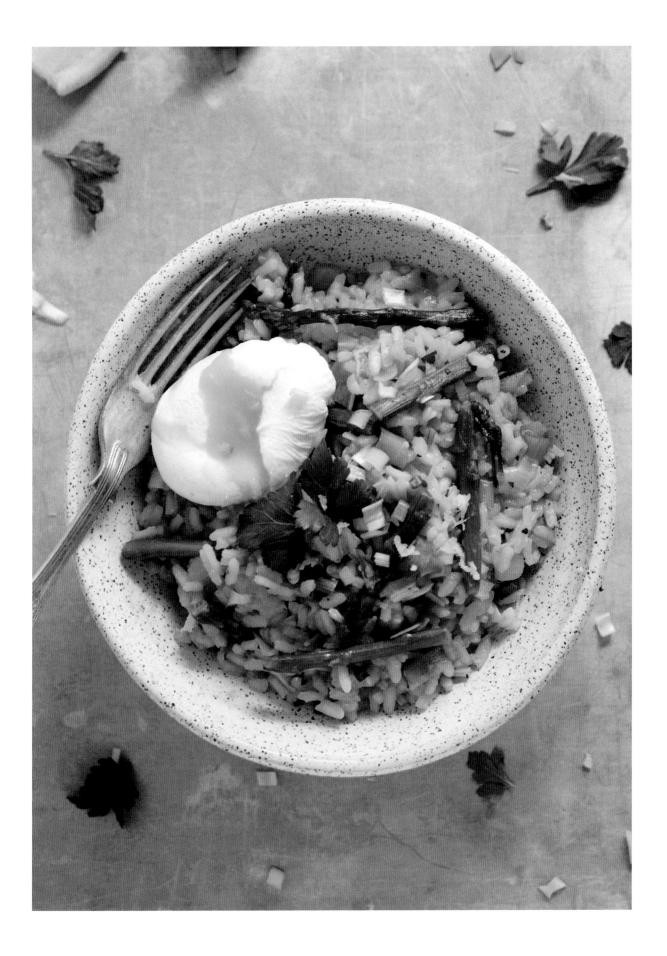

RICE FOUR WAYS

HOW TO MAKE BASIC CAULIFLOWER RICE:

makes about 2 cups rice

....

EGG-FREE / NUT-FREE
DAIRY-FREE OPTION: use avocado oil or extra-virgin
olive oil / PALEO-FRIENDLY OPTION: use ghee or oil
VEGAN OPTION: use oil

....

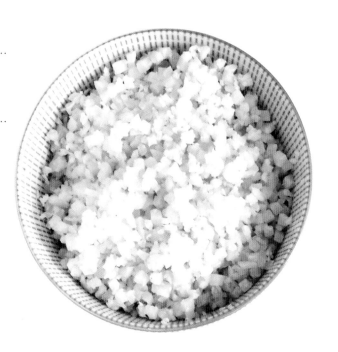

ingredients:

1 head cauliflower, cut into florets

1 tablespoon ghee (page 350), unsalted butter,
   avocado oil, or extra-virgin olive oil

Fine sea salt

directions:

1. Rice the cauliflower: Pulse the cauliflower
florets, in batches, in a food processor until
they are the consistency of rice.

2. Cook the cauli rice: Warm the ghee in a
large skillet over medium heat, then add the
riced cauliflower and sauté for 5 minutes,
until soft and golden brown. Season with
salt to taste.

variation:

Curried Cauliflower Rice. Follow the recipe
above, but in Step 2 add 1 teaspoon of curry
powder, ½ teaspoon of garlic powder, ½
teaspoon of onion powder, a pinch of salt,
a pinch of black pepper, and a pinch of red
pepper flakes.

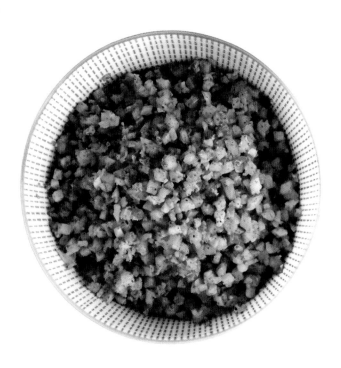

HOW TO MAKE BASIC WHITE RICE:

makes 3 cups rice

....

EGG-FREE / NUT-FREE / DAIRY-FREE OPTION: **use
avocado oil or extra-virgin olive oil** / PALEO-FRIENDLY
OPTION: **use ghee or oil** / VEGAN OPTION: **use oil and
replace chicken broth with water**

....

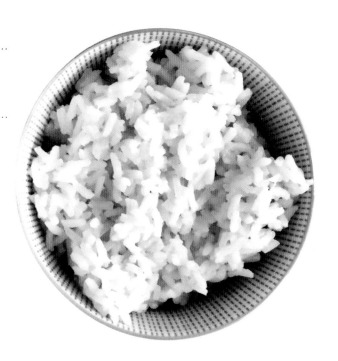

ingredients:

1 cup white jasmine rice

1 tablespoon ghee (page 350), unsalted butter,
   avocado oil, or extra-virgin olive oil

1½ cups chicken broth, homemade (page 354)
   or store-bought

directions:

1. Combine the rice, ghee, and broth in a pot
and bring to a boil.

2. Cover with a tight-fitting lid, reduce the
heat to low, and simmer for 15 minutes.

3. Remove from the heat and let sit for 5 to
10 minutes. Fluff the rice with a fork.

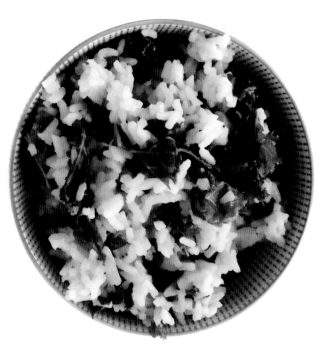

variation:

Loaded Veggie Rice. In a large skillet over
medium heat, heat 1 tablespoon of oil with
½ cup of chopped kale, ¼ cup of chopped
garlic scapes, and any other greens you have
on hand. Sauté until the kale is wilted, then
mix into the cooked rice. Add salt, pepper, and
red pepper flakes as desired.

PASTA ALTERNATIVES

RICE NOODLES

To cook rice noodles, follow the instructions on the package. Rice noodles should always be cooked before being used in the recipes in this book. Make sure that the only ingredient is rice—nothing else added!

Yield: 8 ounces of uncooked rice noodles makes 2½ cups of cooked noodles, serving about 4 people

KELP NOODLES

Serve raw in salads or boil to soften slightly for use as noodles.

Yield: 8 ounces of uncooked kelp noodles makes 1 cup of cooked noodles, serving about 2 people

SPAGHETTI SQUASH NOODLES

Preheat the oven to 400°F. Cut the spaghetti squash in half lengthwise and scrape out the seeds. Drizzle the cut sides of the squash with 1 tablespoon of extra-virgin olive oil and sprinkle with salt and pepper. Place the squash halves facedown on a rimmed baking sheet and add 2 tablespoons of water to speed up the baking time. Bake for 35 to 40 minutes, until the squash is fork-tender and the skin gives when you press it. Remove from the oven and set aside to cool. Using two forks, shred the spaghetti squash threads, then transfer them to a bowl and set aside. Use right away or store in the fridge for up to 5 days.

Yield: 1 large spaghetti squash (about 7 pounds) makes 7 cups of cooked noodles, serving 4 to 5 people

SPIRAL-SLICED VEGGIE NOODLES

I usually use zucchini to make veggie noodles because zucchini noodles are easy, light, and fairly neutral, but many other vegetables can be used. Some other good options are carrots, summer squash, parsnips, broccoli stems, sweet potatoes (need to be cooked), and butternut squash (needs to be cooked).

To make veggie noodles, peel the vegetable of your choice (if desired or needed), then cut off the ends. If it is longer than 6 inches, slice the vegetable in half crosswise. Then use a spiral slicer (also called a Spiralizer) or mandoline fitted with the desired blade to slice the vegetable, or use a vegetable peeler or julienne peeler to shave the vegetable into noodles.

To cook veggie noodles, heat oil (about 1 tablespoon for 2 cups of raw noodles) in a skillet over medium heat with a pinch of red pepper flakes, if desired. Add the veggie noodles and cook for 2 minutes, just until they begin to soften. Don't overcook or the noodles will become too soft and watery! Use cooked veggie noodles right away or store in the fridge for up to 2 days. Raw spiral-sliced veggie noodles will keep in the fridge for up to 4 days.

Yield: 3 large zucchini (about 1½ pounds) make about 6 cups of raw noodles or 3 cups of cooked noodles, serving about 4 people or enough for 1 cup of sauce

zucchini noodles

rice noodles

kelp noodles

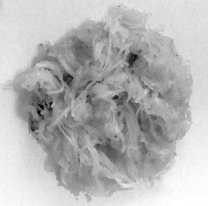

squash noodles

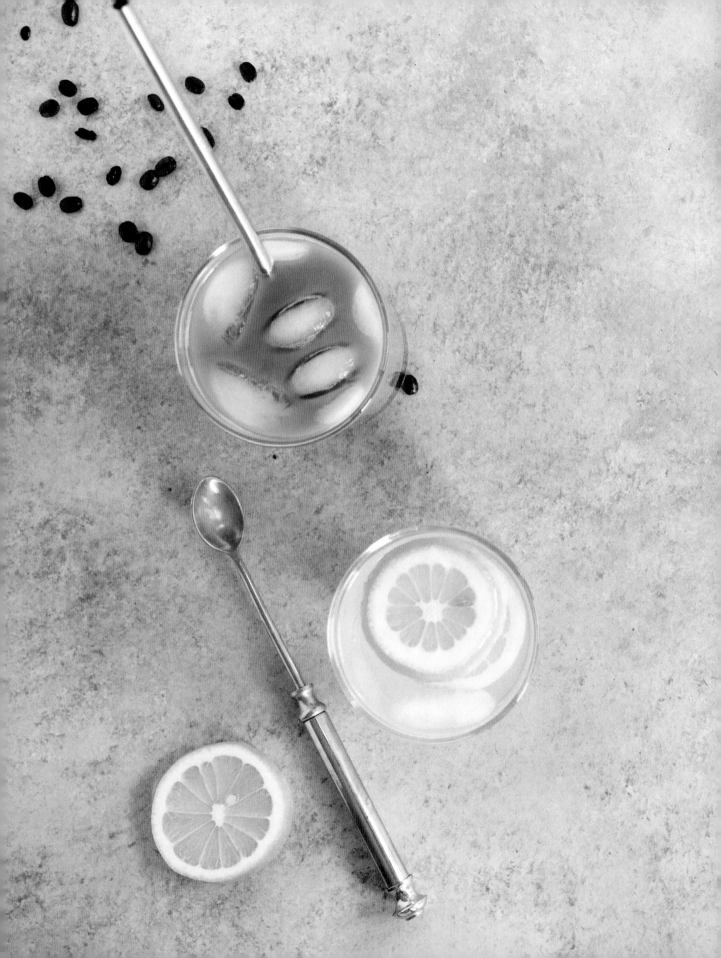

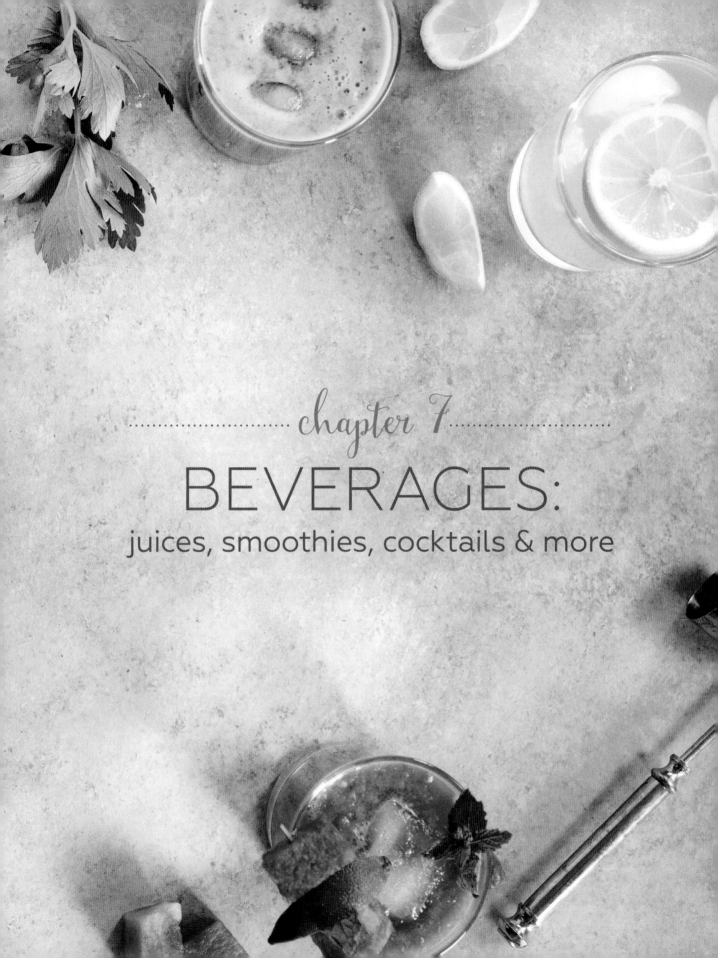

chapter 7

BEVERAGES:
juices, smoothies, cocktails & more

CLASSIC MARGARITA

makes one 6-ounce serving   *prep time* 5 minutes

....

EGG-FREE / NUT-FREE / DAIRY-FREE / VEGAN

....

Margaritas are one of my favorite cocktails when they are done right. Often they are loaded with sour mix and too much sweetener, so I love to make my own! A bartender here in Boston named Carlos is the margarita master and generously taught me his method to share with all of you. This recipe is just right—it's the perfect drink for one or can be doubled or tripled to serve more.

ingredients:

FOR THE LIME SALT RIMMER:

2 tablespoons coarse sea salt

Grated zest of 1 lime

1 small lime wedge

FOR THE MARGARITA:

2 cups ice cubes, preferably purchased bagged cubes (see notes)

1½ ounces silver tequila

1 ounce Cointreau or triple sec (see notes)

¾ ounce lime juice

Squeeze of lemon juice

Optional: Lime slice or wedge, for garnish

directions:

1. On a small plate, mix together the coarse sea salt and lime zest. Rub the rim of a tumbler or rock glass with the lime wedge to dampen it, then dip it into the lime salt rimmer mixture.

2. Put the ice in a cocktail shaker. Add the tequila, Cointreau, lime juice, and lemon juice. Shake vigorously about 60 times (yes, 60 times!), until the shaker is cold and almost frosted.

3. Pour the margarita with the ice cubes into the rimmed glass. Garnish with a slice or wedge of lime, if desired, and serve immediately.

notes: Carlos taught me that bagged ice is essential for quality cocktails!

I use Cointreau when making margaritas. It is an orange liqueur made in the style of triple sec, but it is less sweet than the typical triple sec. If you opt for triple sec, you may want to add an extra squeeze of lemon juice.

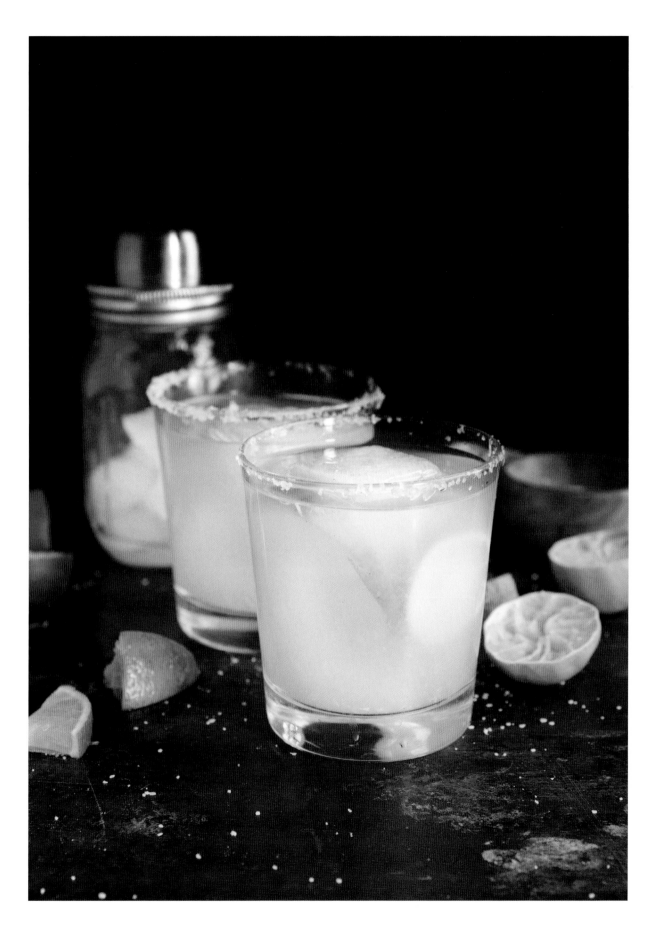

CLASSIC SANGRIA

makes ten 11-ounce servings   *prep time* 15 minutes

EGG-FREE / NUT-FREE / DAIRY-FREE / VEGAN

Classic sangria is always a must for a party, and you won't go wrong serving this one up. It's delicious, without all the junk.

ingredients:

2 green apples, cored and sliced

2 oranges, sliced

2 lemons, cut in half

1 lime, cut in half

2 (750-ml) bottles Spanish red wine, such as Garnacha

3 cups orange juice

1½ cups soda water

⅓ cup pure maple syrup

2 ounces spiced rum, such as Sailor Jerry's

Juice of ½ lemon

½ teaspoon ground cinnamon

¼ teaspoon ginger powder

Ice cubes, preferably purchased bagged cubes, for the pitcher and glasses

GARNISH OPTIONS:

Lime wedges

Lemon wedges

Orange wedges

directions:

1. Place all of the ingredients in a gallon-size pitcher and add 2 cups of ice. Stir well.

2. Serve immediately in large glasses of ice. Garnish each glass with lime, lemon, and/or orange wedges.

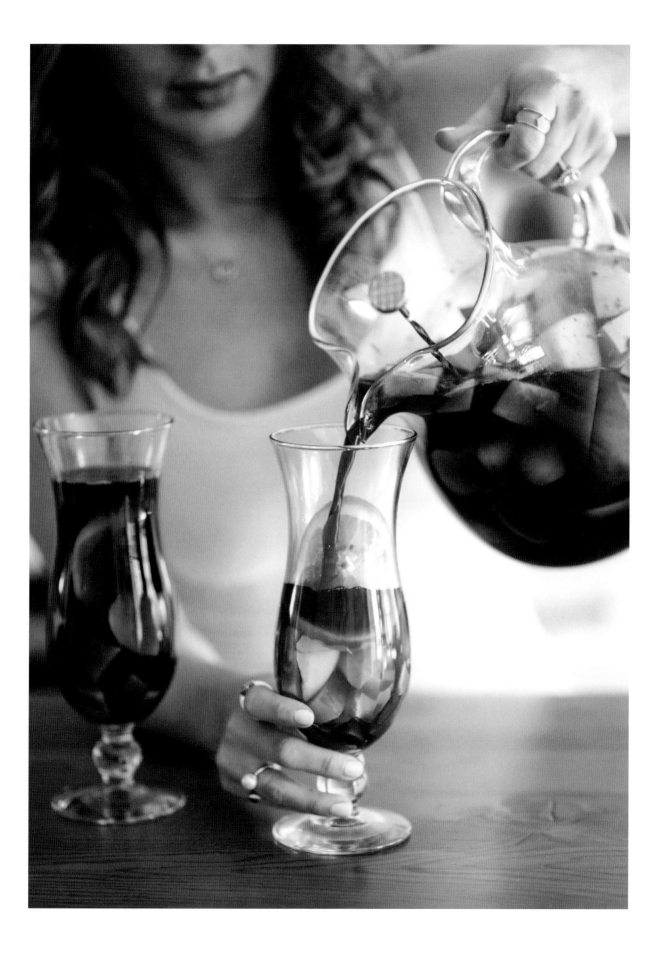

APPLE CIDER SANGRIA

makes eight 8-ounce servings   *prep time* 15 minutes

EGG-FREE / NUT-FREE / DAIRY-FREE / VEGAN

Wondering what to do with the fresh apple cider and all of the apples from a morning spent apple picking or shopping at your local farmer's market? Make this sangria, of course! In the fall, this is my go-to drink to whip together for family and friends. It gets rave reviews; it's got just the right amount of sweetness and *all* of the autumn flavors you love!

ingredients:

2 green or red apples or one of each, cored and sliced

1 orange, peeled and segmented

¼ cup pomegranate seeds

1 (750-ml) bottle white wine, such as Pinot Grigio

2½ cups apple cider

1 cup soda water

1 tablespoon honey

2 cinnamon sticks

½ teaspoon ground cinnamon

Optional: 1 (1-inch) chunk fresh ginger, peeled and sliced

4 ounces gluten-free vodka

Ice cubes, preferably purchased bagged cubes, for serving

directions:

1. Place the apples, orange, and pomegranate seeds in a large pitcher.

2. Add the wine, apple cider, soda water, honey, cinnamon sticks, ground cinnamon, and ginger, if using, and stir to combine.

3. Add the vodka, stir, and taste. Adjust by adding more cinnamon, honey, apple cider, or vodka, if desired.

4. Store covered in the refrigerator until ready to serve. For the best flavor, let it chill for about 2 hours to allow the flavors to blend.

5. Mix before serving and serve over ice. This sangria is best if used soon after being made but will last in the fridge for up to 2 days.

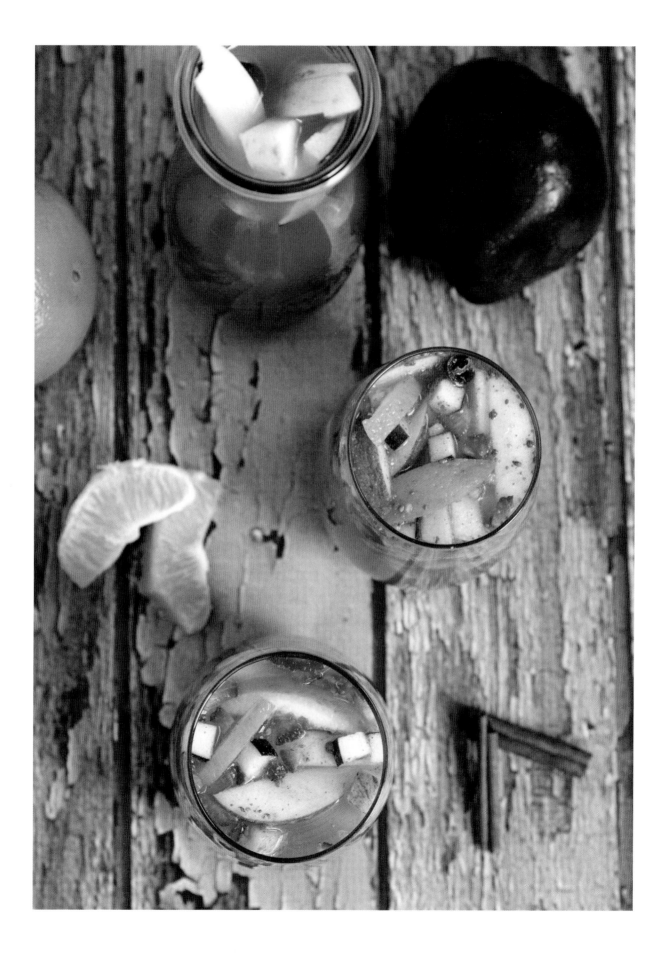

SUNDAY BRUNCH BLOODY MARYS

makes six to eight 8-ounce servings   *prep time* 10 minutes

EGG-FREE / NUT-FREE / DAIRY-FREE / VEGAN OPTION: omit shrimp and bacon garnishes

I have to confess, I'm more of a Mimosa lady than a Bloody Mary lady. But Mike and all of our friends love a good Bloody, so I made it my mission to create a squeaky-clean mix that they would love. Whip up a batch of this mix for your next weekend brunch and make a little Bloody Mary bar that everyone can swoon over!

ingredients:

FOR THE BLOODY MARY MIX:

1 (48-ounce) can or jar tomato juice

¼ heaping cup prepared horseradish, homemade (page 346) or store-bought

2 tablespoons plus 1 teaspoon hot sauce, such as Tabasco or Frank's RedHot, or more as desired

Juice of ½ orange

1 teaspoon lemon juice

1 teaspoon freshly ground black pepper

1½ teaspoons celery salt

½ teaspoon celery seed

½ teaspoon fine sea salt

¼ teaspoon paprika

Dash of cracked black peppercorns

Optional: 3 tablespoons Sweet & Smoky BBQ Sauce (page 328)

Optional: Cayenne pepper, to taste

FOR THE SPICY SALT RIMMER:

1 teaspoon smoked paprika

¼ teaspoon chili powder

1 teaspoon coarse sea salt

1 small lemon or lime wedge

FOR THE CELERY SALT RIMMER:

1 tablespoon celery salt

1 tablespoon coarse sea salt

1 small lemon or lime wedge

Ice cubes, preferably purchased bagged cubes, for serving

12 to 16 ounces gluten-free vodka, such as Tito's or Ciroc

GARNISH OPTIONS:

Celery sticks

Cheese cubes

Cooked and peeled shrimp

Cooked bacon strips

Lemon slices or wedges

Lime slices or wedges

Olives

Pepperoncini

Pickle spears

Pickled jalapeños

tip: I like to step it up and add a teaspoon or two of freshly grated horseradish root to each serving!

variation:

Virgin Bloody Marys. This one is easy! Simply omit the vodka.

directions:

1. In a pitcher, combine the ingredients for the Bloody Mary mix. The mix is best if served immediately but can be stored in the refrigerator for up to 2 days.

2. Rim the glasses: Mix together the rimmer ingredients of your choice on a small plate. Rub the rim of an 8-ounce glass with a lime or lemon wedge to dampen it, then dip it into the rimmer mixture to coat.

3. Assemble the drinks: Fill the rimmed glasses with ice. Add 2 ounces of vodka to each glass, then top with Bloody Mary mix. Stir to combine.

4. Garnish as desired and serve.

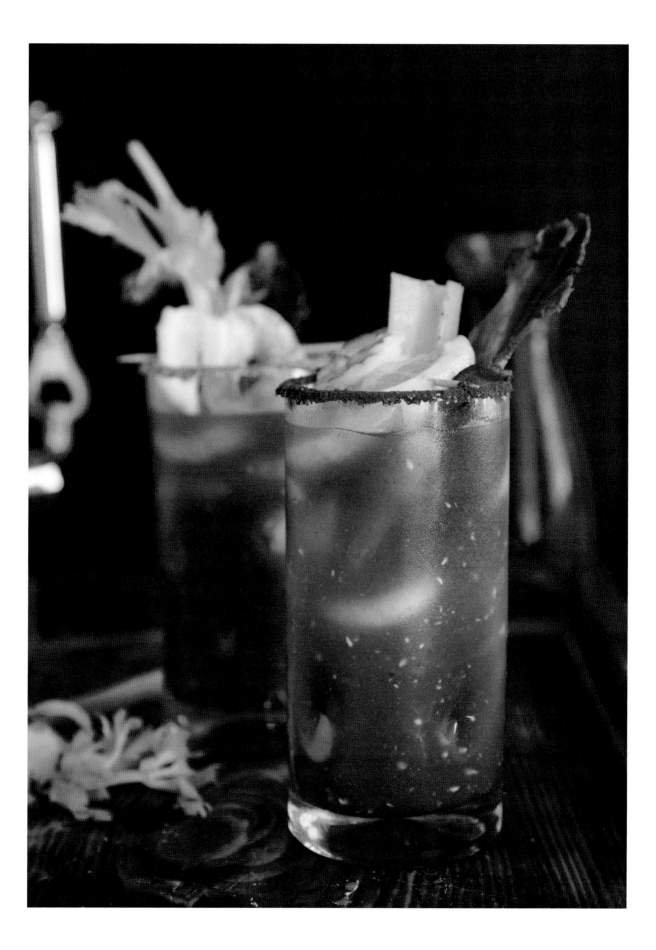

WATERMELON MOJITO

makes one 8-ounce serving   *prep time* 5 minutes

EGG-FREE / NUT-FREE / DAIRY-FREE / VEGAN

Come summertime, the Watermelon Mojitos are flowing! Watermelon and mint are the perfect combination in this delicious and refreshing cocktail.

ingredients:

4 to 6 fresh mint leaves

1 tablespoon granulated maple sugar or coconut sugar

Juice of ½ lime

½ cup cubed watermelon, plus more for garnish

Ice cubes, preferably purchased bagged cubes

1½ ounces white rum

Soda water

Fresh mint leaves, for garnish

SPECIAL EQUIPMENT:
Muddler (or use a wooden spoon)

directions:

1. In a tall glass, muddle the mint leaves, sugar, and lime juice together until the sugar dissolves.

2. Add the cubed watermelon and muddle until pureed. Alternatively, you can puree the watermelon in a blender, then add it to the glass.

3. Fill the glass with ice, then add the rum and stir to combine.

4. Top with soda water and garnish with watermelon and mint leaves. Serve immediately.

note: This recipe works well with raspberries, too!

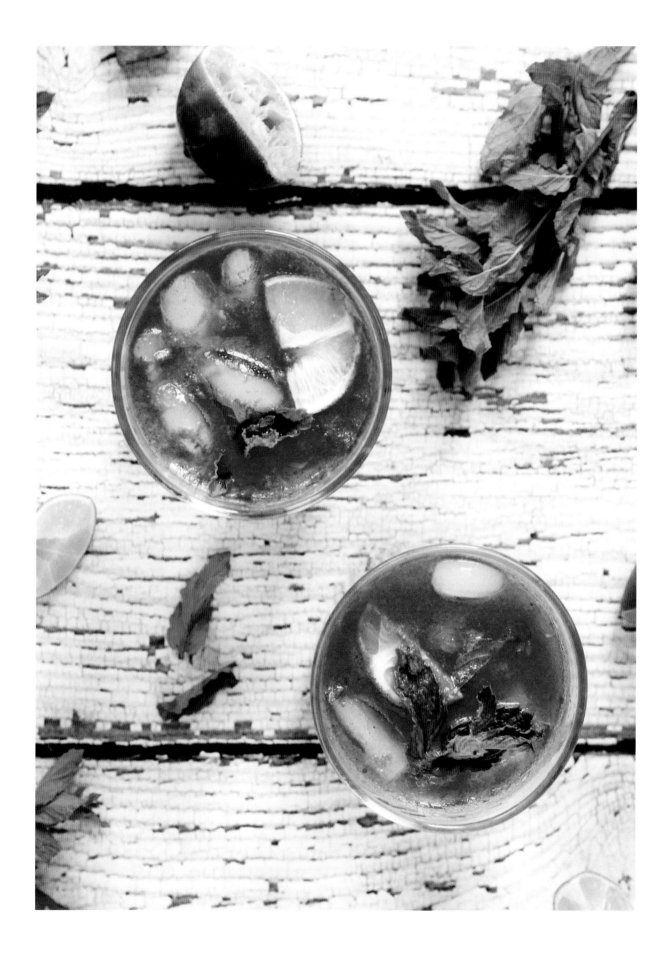

REFRESHING LEMONADE

makes six to eight 14-ounce servings   *prep time* 15 minutes

EGG-FREE / NUT-FREE / DAIRY-FREE / PALEO-FRIENDLY / VEGAN

The arrival of BBQ season means eating meals outside and taking in the gorgeous weather. There's no better way to add to that than with a big batch of refreshing lemonade, reminiscent of childhood lemonade stands.

ingredients:

FOR THE SUGAR WATER:
¾ cup granulated maple sugar
2 cups water

3 cups lemon juice (about 16 lemons)
1 gallon water
2 lemons, sliced

make it boozy: Add 4 to 6 ounces of gluten-free vodka to the pitcher.

give it a zing: Add 1 thinly sliced jalapeño pepper to the pot in Step 1. Strain the jalapeño before pouring the sugar water into the pitcher in Step 2. Garnish with additional jalapeño slices.

directions:

1. In a medium-sized pot over medium heat, combine the maple sugar with the 2 cups of water and stir until the sugar is dissolved. Set aside to cool for 5 minutes.

2. Pour the sugar water and lemon juice into a large pitcher.

3. Fill with ice and about 1 gallon of water. Add the lemon slices to the pitcher.

4. Pour into glasses and serve immediately.

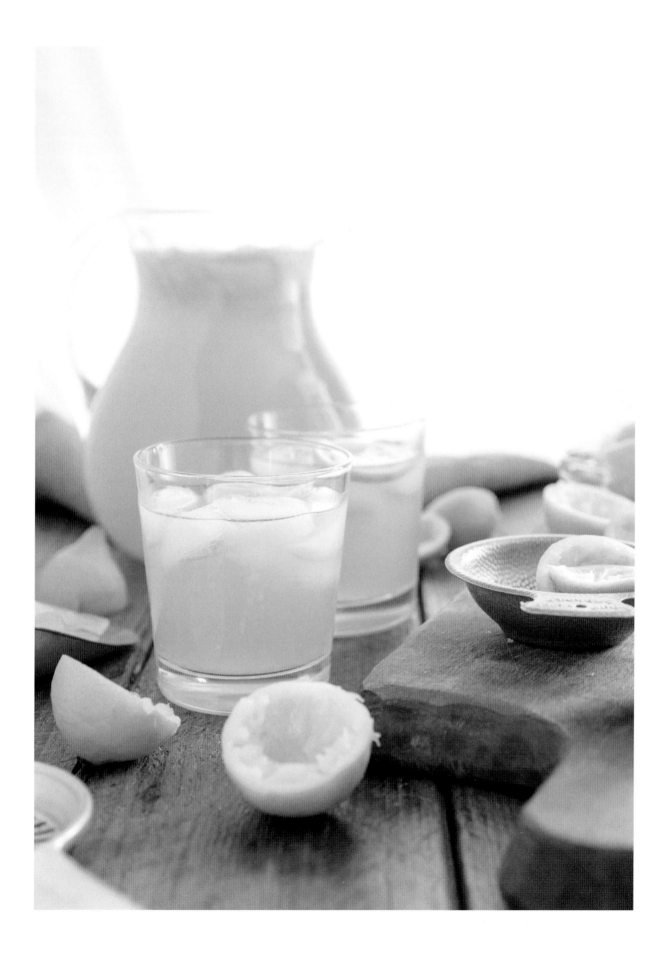

COLD-BREW CONCENTRATE

makes about 2 quarts concentrate   *prep time* 5 minutes, plus time to steep coffee grounds

EGG-FREE / DAIRY-FREE / PALEO-FRIENDLY / VEGAN

There comes a point in the year when it's all about iced coffee for me. I whip up batches of this delicious cold-brew concentrate with my favorite ground coffee and enjoy delicious cold-brew iced coffee for a fraction of the price that I'd pay at a coffee shop. Plus, adding a little of this concentrate to my Buttercream Frosting is a winning idea!

ingredients:

1¾ cups ground coffee

4 cups filtered water

FOR SERVING:

Ice cubes

Optional: Almond milk, homemade (page 266) or store-bought

SPECIAL EQUIPMENT:

Cheesecloth

Sieve

directions:

1. Dump the ground coffee into a pitcher. Pour in the water and stir.

2. Cover with a lid or plastic wrap and let steep in the refrigerator for 12 hours.

3. After 12 hours, pour the concentrate through a cheesecloth-lined sieve into a wide-mouth quart-size mason jar.

4. To serve, fill a tall 8-ounce glass with ice, then add equal amounts of water and coffee concentrate and stir to blend. Top with some almond milk, if desired. Store the concentrate in the refrigerator for up to 1 week.

use in:

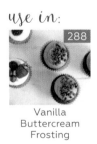

288

Vanilla Buttercream Frosting

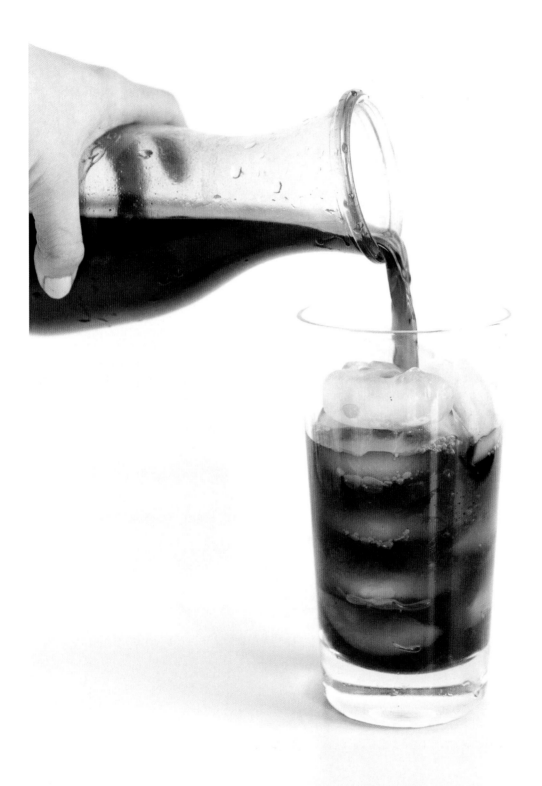

ALMOND MILK

makes 1 quart　*prep time* 10 minutes, plus time to soak almonds

EGG-FREE / DAIRY-FREE / PALEO-FRIENDLY / VEGAN

If you've never made your own almond milk, I understand. I mean, it's easier to just buy a jug at the store, right? But the taste—oh, the taste! There's nothing like fresh homemade almond milk. That's a promise. Don't be intimidated to make this; I guarantee that it's way easier than you think! You can use this same method to make any type of nut milk. Try it with hazelnuts, cashews, or walnuts!

ingredients:

1 cup raw almonds
7 cups filtered water, divided

SPECIAL EQUIPMENT:
High-speed blender
Cheesecloth

directions:

1.　Place the almonds and 3 cups of the filtered water in a container, cover, and let soak in the refrigerator overnight.

2.　Drain the water. Place the soaked almonds and the remaining 4 cups of water in a high-speed blender and blend for about 1 minute, until smooth.

3.　Once blended, place a cheesecloth-lined sieve over a bowl, then pour the almond milk through the sieve.

4.　Pick up the sides of the cheesecloth and squeeze out any remaining liquid from the pulp (all you should be left with is thick pulp). Discard the pulp. Store the almond milk in the refrigerator for up to 1 week.

variation:

Sweetened or Unsweetened Vanilla-Flavored Almond Milk. In Step 2, add to the blender the seeds scraped from 1 whole vanilla bean and, if you prefer the milk sweetened, 1 tablespoon of maple syrup.

use in:

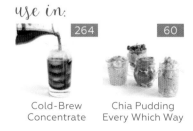

264 Cold-Brew Concentrate

60 Chia Pudding Every Which Way

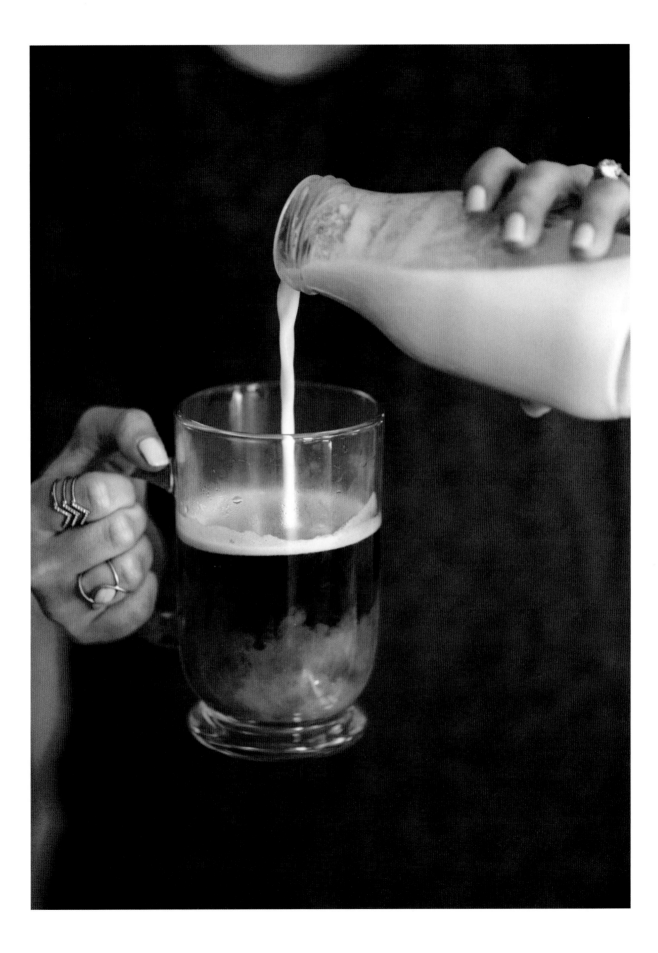

CREAMY HOT CHOCOLATE WITH MARSHMALLOW TOPPING

serves 2   *prep time* 5 minutes   *cook time* 10 minutes

EGG-FREE / DAIRY-FREE / PALEO-FRIENDLY
VEGAN OPTION: use whipped cream instead of meringue for garnish

On a cool evening or a snowy day, there's nothing dreamier than cozying up with family or a good book and enjoying some hot cocoa. Without all the added junk, and with some delicious toppings, this hot cocoa will become a family staple!

ingredients:

3 cups plain or vanilla-flavored almond milk, homemade (page 266) or store-bought

Seeds scraped from 1 whole vanilla bean or 1 teaspoon vanilla extract

2 teaspoons granulated maple sugar

Pinch of ground cinnamon

Pinch of fine sea salt

1 cup dark chocolate chips (see note)

OPTIONAL GARNISHES:

Marshmallow Meringue (page 280) or Salted Vanilla Bean Whipped Cream (page 282)

Cinnamon sticks

Cocoa powder or shaved chocolate

directions:

1. In a medium-sized heavy-bottomed saucepan, heat the almond milk, vanilla bean seeds, maple sugar, cinnamon, and salt until boiling.

2. Once boiling, whisk in the chocolate; continue whisking until the chocolate is melted and the milk is frothy, about 2 minutes.

3. Serve immediately with the garnish(es) of your choice.

note: If you use very dark chocolate chips, you may want to add a little extra sweetener. Different chocolates will alter the taste.

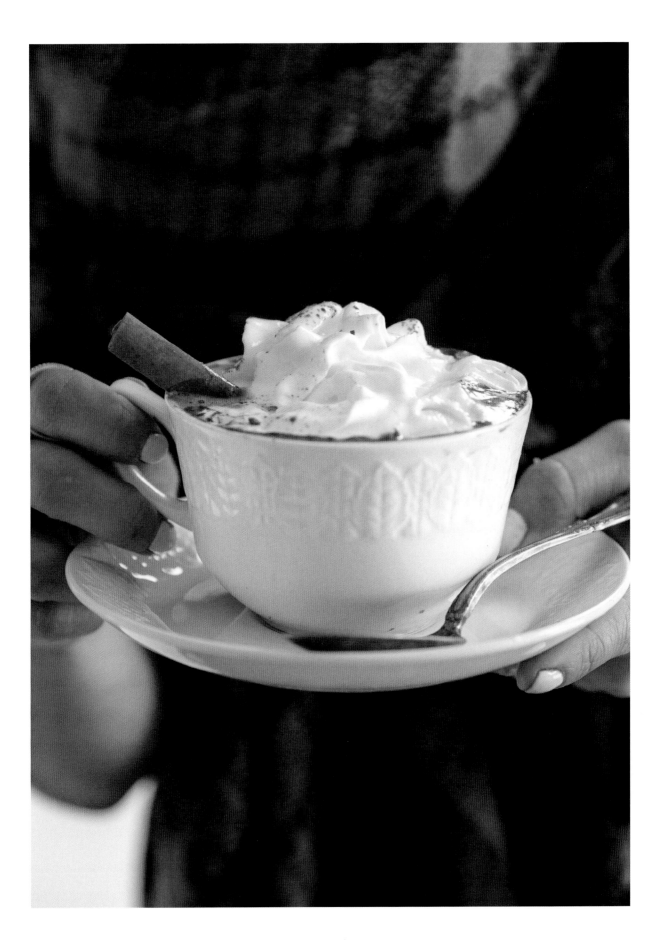

BANANA COFFEE SMOOTHIE

serves 1   *prep time* 5 minutes, plus time to freeze banana and brew and chill coffee or make concentrate

EGG-FREE / DAIRY-FREE / PALEO-FRIENDLY / VEGAN OPTION: use vegan protein powder

This smoothie is my absolute favorite. When you're in the mood for a creamy, dessert-like smoothie with a pick-me-up, this is your answer. I like to save half of my morning cup of coffee and make this smoothie as a mid-morning snack! Don't forget to have a banana already frozen when you're ready to make this smoothie. I always keep a stash of chunked bananas in the freezer so that I can make a smoothie whenever the mood strikes.

ingredients:

1 large banana, cut into chunks and frozen

½ cup vanilla-flavored almond milk, homemade (page 266) or store-bought

½ cup freshly brewed coffee, cooled, or ¼ cup Cold-Brew Concentrate (page 264) mixed with ¼ cup water

1 teaspoon pure maple syrup

½ teaspoon chia seeds

Handful of ice cubes

Pinch of ground cinnamon

Optional: 1 scoop protein powder

directions:

Place all of the ingredients in a blender and blend until completely smooth, about 30 seconds. Serve immediately.

note: Adding a scoop of protein powder will give your smoothie a little more substance!

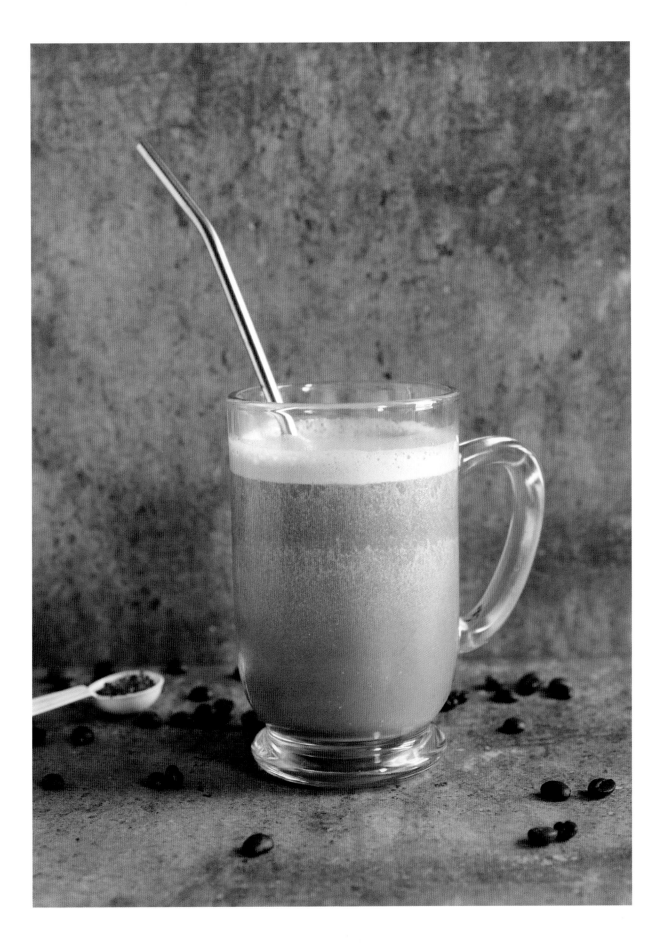

ISLAND BLAST GREEN SMOOTHIE

makes two 8-ounce servings   *prep time* 5 minutes

EGG-FREE / NUT-FREE / DAIRY-FREE / PALEO-FRIENDLY / VEGAN

Mike and I first had a variation of this oh-so-refreshing smoothie while on a trip to Jamaica in 2015 (right after we got engaged!). I fell in love with the flavor combination and the nice healthy dose of good-for-you ingredients that are packed into it.

ingredients:

1 cup coconut water, preferably chilled

1 stalk celery

1 small banana

½ cucumber

1 cup frozen pineapple chunks

⅓ cup fresh flat-leaf parsley stems and leaves (from 1 small bunch)

1 (¼- to ½-inch) chunk fresh ginger, peeled

Optional: 1 tablespoon fresh mint leaves

directions:

Place all of the ingredients in a high-speed blender and blend until completely smooth, about 30 seconds. Divide between two glasses and serve immediately.

note: If you don't have a high-speed blender, you can make this smoothie in a regular blender. To do so, coarsely chop the celery, cut the cucumber into chunks, and finely chop or grate the ginger before adding them to the blender.

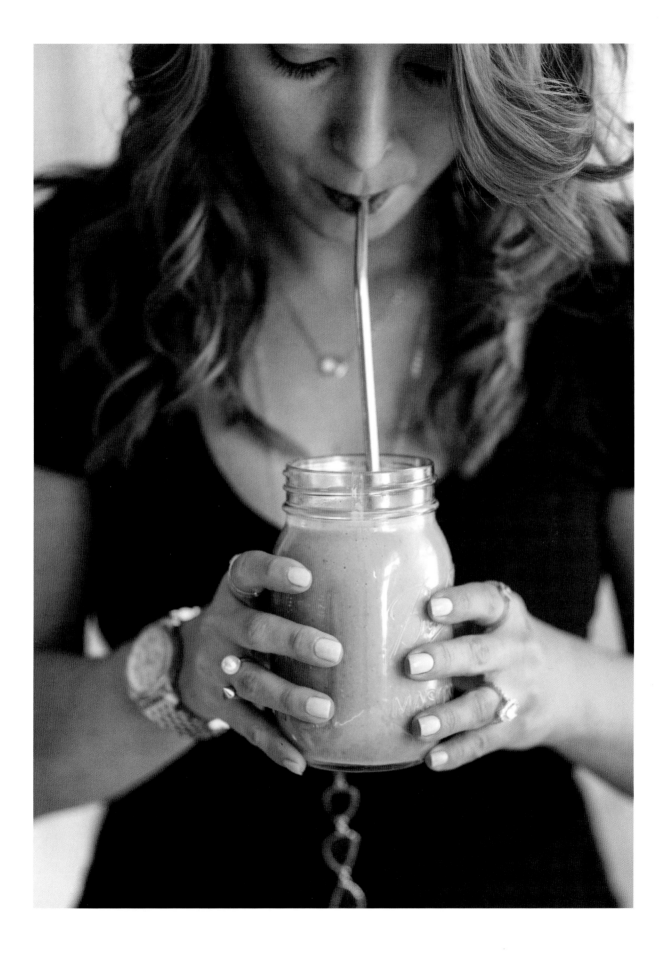

VANILLA CHAI SPICE SMOOTHIE

makes one 12-ounce or two 6-ounce servings   *prep time* 5 minutes

EGG-FREE / DAIRY-FREE / PALEO-FRIENDLY
VEGAN OPTION: use maple syrup instead of honey and use vegan protein powder

Chai flavors are so unique and comforting. They come together in this tasty shake/smoothie to bring you a unique twist on a chai latte!

ingredients:

1 cup almond milk, homemade (page 266) or store-bought

1 large banana, cut into chunks and frozen

½ teaspoon honey or pure maple syrup, or more as desired

½ teaspoon chia seeds

½ teaspoon ground cinnamon, plus more for garnish

¼ teaspoon vanilla extract

Seeds scraped from ½ vanilla bean

⅛ teaspoon ground cardamom

⅛ teaspoon ground cloves

⅛ teaspoon ground nutmeg

Optional: 1 scoop protein powder

Salted Vanilla Bean Whipped Cream (page 282), for garnish

directions:

Place all of the ingredients in a blender and blend until completely smooth, about 30 seconds. Serve immediately, garnished with whipped cream and a dusting of cinnamon.

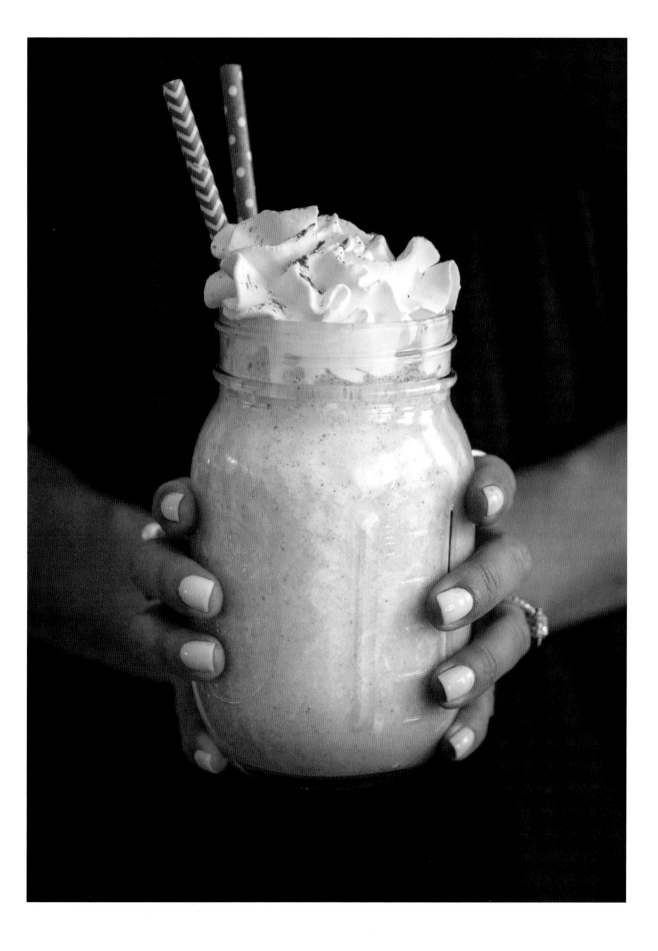

JUICING AT HOME FOUR WAYS

makes two 8-ounce servings (per recipe) *prep time* 5 minutes

EGG-FREE / NUT-FREE / DAIRY-FREE / PALEO-FRIENDLY / VEGAN

I have to admit, I'm new to the juicing world. To be honest, I always thought it was wasteful and that you weren't getting all of the benefits of the fruits and veggies. But I've discovered the powers of juicing. Juicing is a great way to get additional nutrients into your diet, absorb immune-boosting nutrients, and access digestive enzymes that are naturally found in veggies and herbs. Here are four of my favorite at-home juicing recipes; you can also use the handy guide on page 365 to build your own! In most cases, the peels of the fruit are not removed, and the cores and seeds can be left in as well. For this reason, it's particularly important to buy organic produce for juicing (though I recommend buying organic whenever possible).

GREEN PEAR JUICE

ingredients:

4 Bartlett pears
1 large handful kale (about 5 ounces)
1 red apple
3 sprigs fresh mint

directions:

1. Run the ingredients for the juice of your choice through a juicer, following the instructions for your machine.

2. Pour into two glasses and serve. The juice is best if served immediately, but can be stored in an airtight container in the fridge for up to 24 hours.

note: It's helpful to use a kitchen scale to weigh ingredients when juicing if you are trying to replicate flavors and make a specific serving size. But you can guesstimate here if you are so inclined!

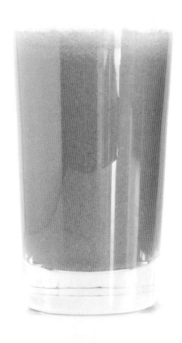

TROPICAL CARROT JUICE

ingredients:

4 large carrots (about 12 ounces)

¼ lemon, peeled

1 (1-inch) chunk fresh ginger

1 orange, peeled

1 green apple

BEET GODDESS JUICE

ingredients:

3 small/medium beets (about 13 ounces), trimmed and halved

½ cup fresh strawberries, hulled

1 red apple

1 (1-inch) chunk fresh ginger

1 cucumber (about 8 ounces)

5 ounces watermelon rind

¼ lemon, peeled

GREEN MACHINE JUICE

ingredients:

2 ounces celery (1 or 2 stalks)

2 green apples

1 handful kale (about 4 ounces)

1 cucumber (about 8 ounces)

1 small handful spinach (about 2 ounces)

1 (1-inch) chunk fresh ginger

8 ounces fresh pineapple chunks

⅛ lemon, peeled

SPECIAL EQUIPMENT: Juicer

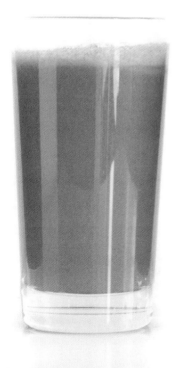

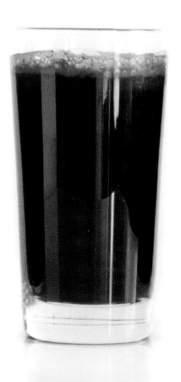

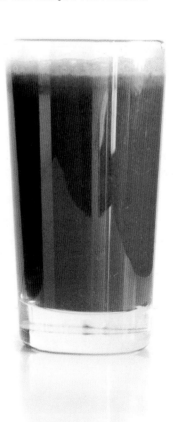

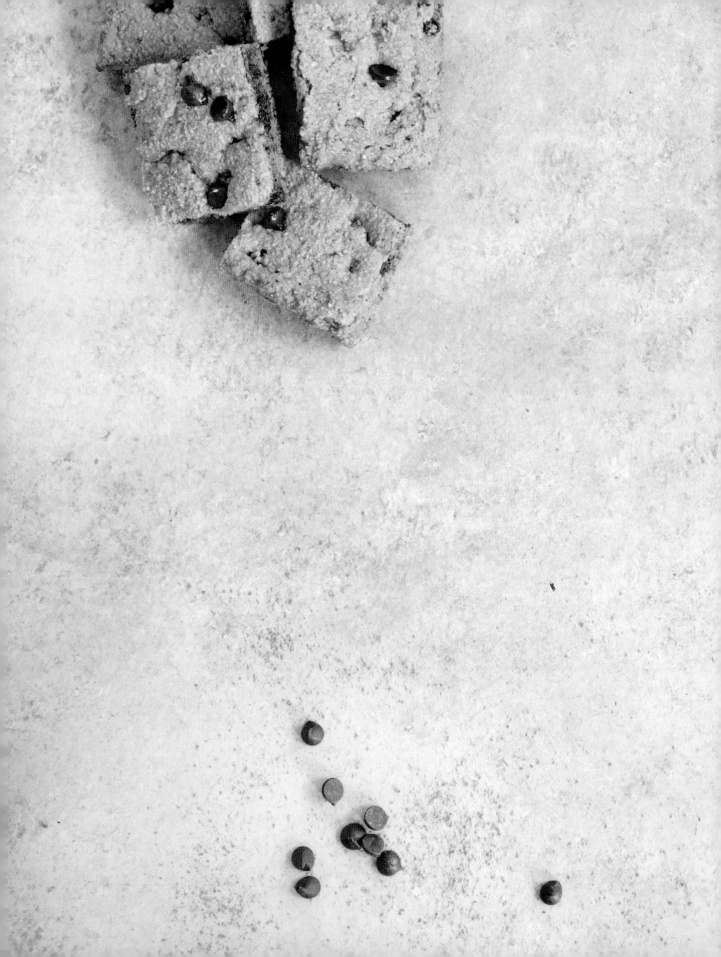

chapter 8

SOMETHING SWEET:
desserts & treats

S'MORES POTS DE CRÈME

serves 6   *prep time* 5 minutes, plus time to chill (not including graham cracker crumbs)   *cook time* 10 minutes

DAIRY-FREE OPTION: use oil instead of butter or ghee in graham cracker crumbs
PALEO-FRIENDLY OPTION: use ghee or oil instead of butter in graham cracker crumbs

I have and always will be obsessed with all things s'mores. I just love the graham cracker + marshmallow + chocolate combination. It screams summer nights by the fire pit, which are another thing I'll never tire of. Once you've made my homemade faux graham cracker crumbs, you don't have to turn on the oven again (unless you want to get fancy and broil the tops of the marshmallow meringue). And once these rich s'mores cups are assembled, you won't be able to keep your hands off them!

ingredients:

1 batch graham cracker crumbs
  (page 78)

FOR THE CHOCOLATE CUSTARD
PUDDING:

Cream scooped from the top of
  1 chilled (13½-ounce) can full-fat
  coconut milk

⅓ cup granulated maple sugar or
  coconut sugar

2 tablespoons arrowroot flour

Pinch of fine sea salt

1 (10-ounce) bag dark chocolate
  chips

1 teaspoon vanilla extract

FOR THE MARSHMALLOW MERINGUE:

2 large egg whites

½ teaspoon fresh lemon juice

⅓ cup honey

directions:

1. Place the baked and cooled crackers in a food processor and pulse until fine. Set aside.

2. Make the pudding: In a medium-sized saucepan over medium heat, whisk together the coconut cream, sugar, arrowroot flour, and salt. Bring the mixture to a boil, then reduce the heat to medium-low and whisk vigorously for 2 minutes. Add the chocolate chips and vanilla and whisk until the chocolate is completely melted and the mixture has thickened to the consistency of pudding.

3. Pour the pudding into six 8-ounce glass jars or cups, then place in the refrigerator to chill. (If you plan to brown the tops of the s'mores, be sure to use heatproof jars or cups.)

4. Make the marshmallow meringue: In a stand mixer fitted with the whisk attachment, whip the egg whites with the lemon juice until soft peaks form, about 1 minute.

5. In a small saucepan, heat the honey until it reaches 130°F on a candy thermometer and is bubbling, about 1 minute.

6. With the mixer running on medium speed, slowly pour the heated honey into the bowl with the egg whites, increase the speed to high, and beat until stiff, glossy peaks form, about 2 minutes.

7. To assemble: Take the jars of pudding out of the refrigerator. Add 2 tablespoons (or more) of the graham cracker crumbs. Then spoon 2 to 4 tablespoons of the meringue into each jar. If you have a kitchen torch, brown the tops, if desired. If you don't have a torch, you can preheat the broiler to high and place oven-safe glass jars under the broiler until the top of the meringue is golden, 1 to 2 minutes, watching carefully to avoid burning.

8. Garnish with additional graham cracker crumbs, then set in the refrigerator to chill for at least 2 hours, or up to 12 hours, before serving. Leftovers will keep in the fridge for 1 to 2 days.

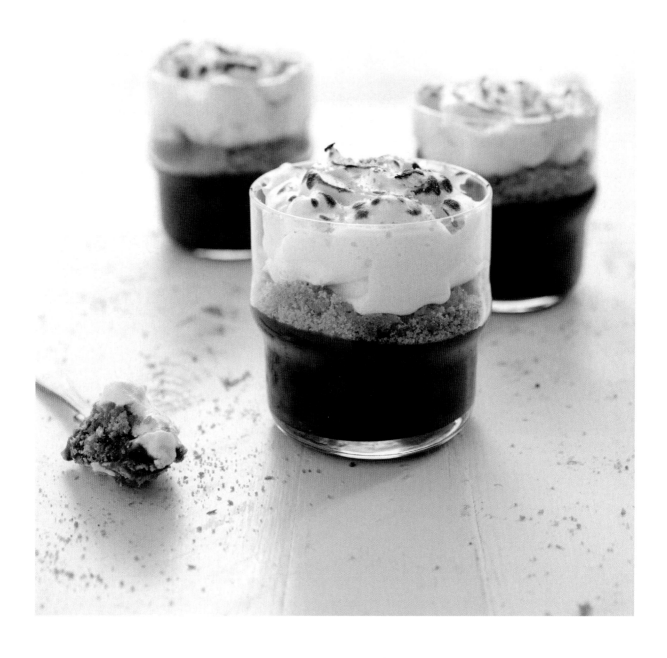

CARIBBEAN DESSERT PARFAITS

serves 2   *prep time* 15 minutes (not including graham cracker crumbs)

DAIRY-FREE OPTION: use oil instead of butter or ghee in graham cracker crumbs
PALEO-FRIENDLY OPTION: use ghee or oil instead of butter in graham cracker crumbs

No baking required! A delicious and light fruit dessert reminiscent of island life.

ingredients:

FOR THE SALTED VANILLA BEAN WHIPPED CREAM:

Cream scooped from the top of 1 chilled (13½-ounce) can full-fat coconut milk (see note)

2 tablespoons pure maple syrup

½ teaspoon vanilla extract

Seeds scraped from 1 vanilla bean

½ teaspoon coarse sea salt, or more as desired

2 kiwis, peeled and sliced

3 mandarin oranges, peeled and segmented

1½ cups strawberries, hulled and sliced

1 banana, sliced

2 fresh figs, quartered

½ cup unsweetened coconut flakes, toasted, for garnish

½ batch graham cracker crumbs (page 78), for garnish

directions:

1. Make the Salted Vanilla Bean Whipped Cream: In a stand mixer fitted with the whisk attachment, whip the ingredients for the whipped cream until smooth and soft peaks form, about 3 minutes. Taste and add additional salt and sweetener, if desired.

2. To assemble: Place about one-quarter of the fruit, except for the figs, in two 14-ounce glass jars or cups. Pipe or spoon some whipped cream into each cup, then add another layer of fruit, reserving a few pieces of mixed fruit and the fig quarters for garnish. Top each cup with additional whipped cream, the fig quarters, and the reserved fruit pieces and garnish with toasted coconut and graham cracker crumbs.

3. Serve immediately.

note: If you tolerate dairy, you can use 1 cup of heavy cream (local if possible) in place of the coconut milk.

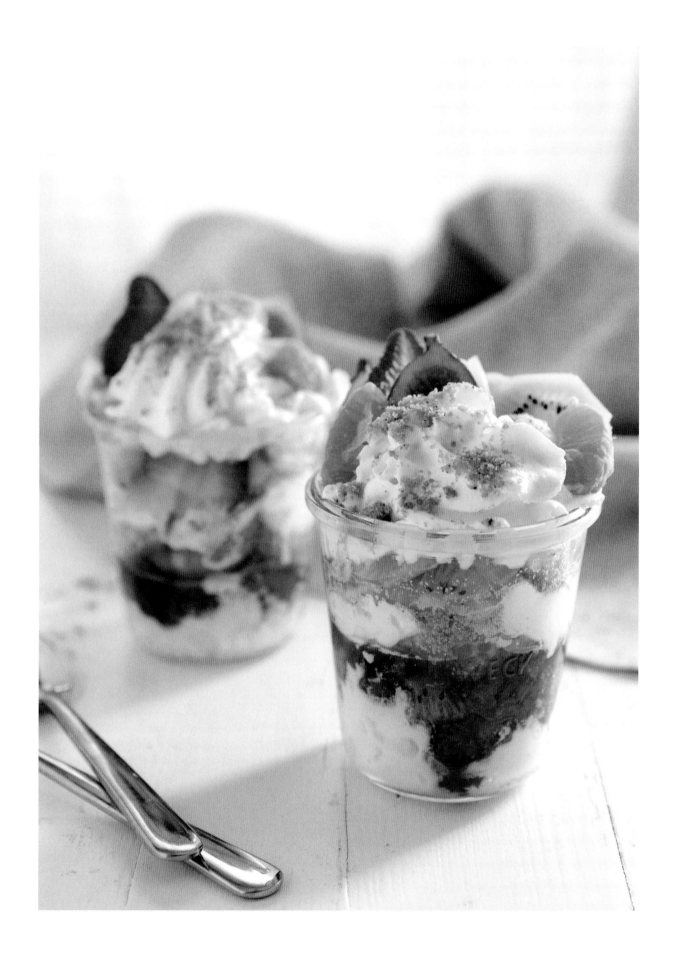

NO-BAKE SEA SALT COOKIE DOUGH CUPS

makes about 25 mini cups or 10 regular-sized cups
prep time 10 minutes, plus time to soak cashews and for cups to set

EGG-FREE / DAIRY-FREE / PALEO-FRIENDLY / VEGAN

Another no-bake treat—because sometimes you just don't feel like baking or cooking! I have to tell you, having these sweet treats in the freezer has been a highlight of my nights. (Is that sad? Let's go with no.) I love these because they *"ain't your average"* chocolate cups. They are the perfect bite-sized treats filled with a creamy vegan "cookie dough" that packs just the right amount of sweetness!

ingredients:

FOR THE COOKIE DOUGH:

2 cups raw cashews

2 tablespoons coconut oil, melted

2 tablespoons pure maple syrup

1 teaspoon vanilla extract

Pinch of fine sea salt

⅓ cup mini dark chocolate chips

1 (10-ounce) bag dark chocolate chips

Coarse sea salt, for garnish

tip: Don't have a double boiler? You can create your own double boiler setup with a saucepan and a heatproof bowl that fits snugly over the top and doesn't allow steam to escape. Just be sure that the bottom of the bowl doesn't touch the simmering water below it!

directions:

1. Make the cookie dough: Soak the cashews in a bowl of cold water for a minimum of 2 hours or up to 12 hours.

2. Drain the water and transfer the soaked cashews to a food processor or high-speed blender. Add the coconut oil, maple syrup, vanilla, and salt. Blend until completely smooth, about 1 minute. Taste and add additional salt or maple syrup, if desired.

3. Mix in the mini chocolate chips by hand and set the cookie dough aside.

4. Melt the chocolate: Place water in the bottom of a double boiler so that the water level is ½ inch below the upper pan. Pour the bag of chocolate chips into the upper pan, then place the double boiler over low heat. Stir the chocolate constantly until it is melted. Do not allow the water in the bottom of the double boiler to come to a boil while the chocolate is melting.

5. Place 25 mini or 10 regular-sized parchment paper baking liners on a rimmed baking sheet.

6. Spoon about 1 heaping teaspoon of chocolate into each liner, then use a small brush or the back of a spoon to swirl the chocolate around to coat the bottom and almost all the way up the sides. You want the filling to be completely enclosed in the chocolate shell, so make sure that the liners are well coated.

7. Spoon half a tablespoon of cookie dough into the center of each chocolate-lined baking liner, then cover the cookie dough with the remaining chocolate and smooth it out to seal the edges. Sprinkle with coarse sea salt, then place in the fridge or freezer to set (about 30 minutes in the fridge or 15 minutes in the freezer).

8. Store in the refrigerator for up to 1 week or in the freezer for up to 1 month.

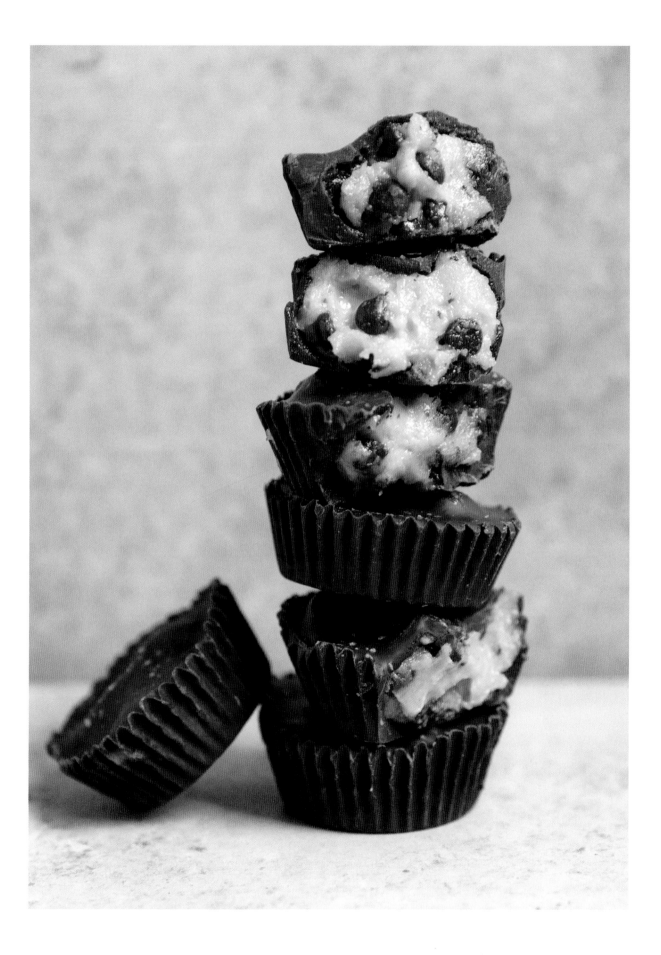

CARROT CAKE BARS

makes 9 to 12 bars   *prep time* 10 minutes (not including frosting)   *cook time* 25 minutes

DAIRY-FREE / PALEO-FRIENDLY

Know a carrot cake lover? I think we all do, because carrot cake is delicious! These Carrot Cake Bars are moist, flavorful, and sweetened just right.

ingredients:

1 cup sifted blanched almond flour

⅓ cup coconut sugar

1 teaspoon baking powder

¼ teaspoon baking soda

¼ teaspoon ground cinnamon

⅛ teaspoon fine sea salt

2 large eggs

¼ cup unsweetened applesauce

1 teaspoon vanilla extract

Optional: 2 teaspoons grated fresh ginger or ½ teaspoon ginger powder

⅓ cup grated carrots

⅓ cup chopped raw walnuts, plus more for garnish (garnish optional)

¼ cup raisins

Optional: 3 tablespoons dark chocolate chips

1½ cups Vanilla Buttercream Frosting (page 288), or more as desired

directions:

1. Preheat the oven to 350°F and line an 8-inch square baking dish with parchment paper.

2. In a bowl, whisk together the almond flour, coconut sugar, baking powder, baking soda, cinnamon, and salt until well blended. Whisk in the eggs, applesauce, vanilla, and ginger, if using, until smooth.

3. Fold in the carrots, walnuts, raisins, and chocolate chips, if using.

4. Pour the batter into the baking dish, smooth out the top, and bake for about 25 minutes, until a toothpick comes out clean when inserted in the middle.

5. While the cake is baking, make the frosting and set aside.

6. When the cake is done, let it cool completely in the pan before frosting or cutting.

7. Spread the frosting evenly across the top of the cake and garnish with extra chopped walnuts, if desired. Cut into 9 to 12 bars to serve.

8. Store the bars in a closed container in the refrigerator for up to 5 days.

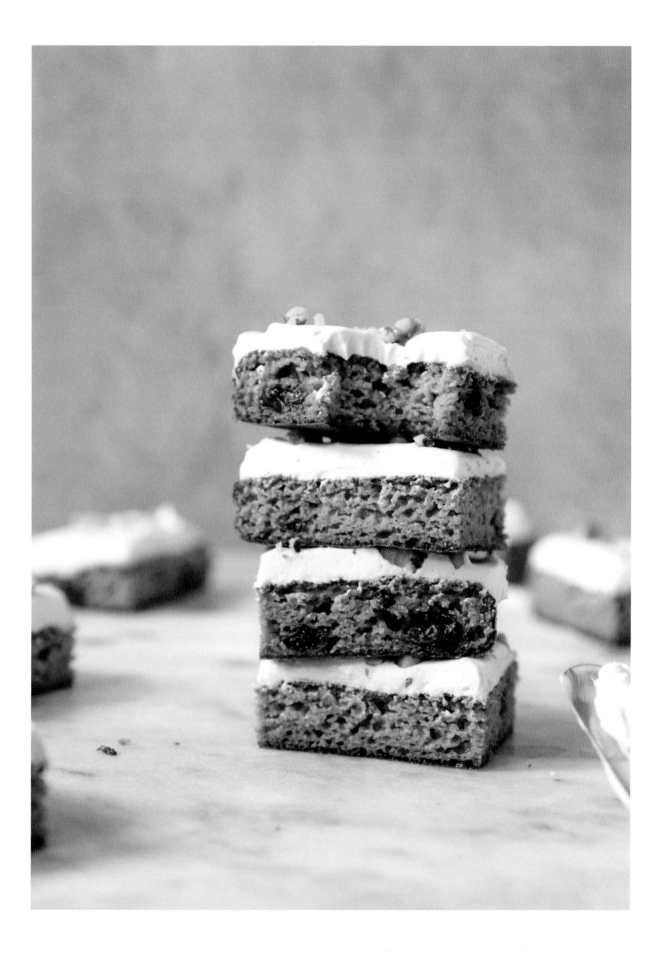

VANILLA BUTTERCREAM FROSTING

makes about 2 cups   *prep time* 10 minutes

EGG-FREE

Classic buttercream frosting, because sometimes we just need to celebrate!

ingredients:

1 cup (2 sticks) unsalted butter, softened

3 cups powdered sugar, sifted

1 teaspoon vanilla extract

1 to 2 tablespoons almond milk, homemade (page 266) or store-bought

directions:

1. In the bowl of a stand mixer fitted with the whisk attachment, mix the butter for 1 minute.

2. Add the sugar and mix on low speed until well blended. Increase the speed to medium and beat until fluffy, another 1 to 2 minutes.

3. Add the vanilla and 1 tablespoon of the almond milk and continue to beat on medium speed for 3 to 5 minutes, until fluffy and lighter in color, adding the additional tablespoon of almond milk (or more) if needed to achieve a spreading consistency. If making the frosting ahead, store in the refrigerator and rewhip before using.

variations:

Chocolate Buttercream Frosting. Add 1 cup of cocoa powder in Step 2.

Coffee Buttercream Frosting. Add 1 tablespoon of Cold-Brew Concentrate (page 264) and ½ teaspoon of cocoa powder in Step 3.

Strawberry Buttercream Frosting. Place ¼ cup of whole freeze-dried strawberries in a small food processor or grinder and grind until powdery, then add to the frosting in Step 2.

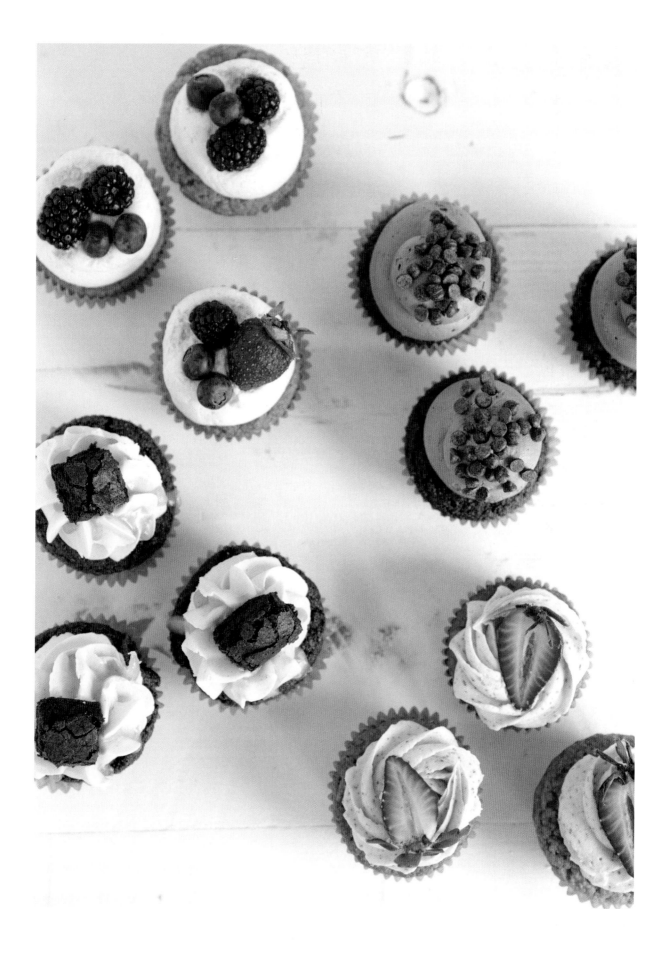

PEAR TARTLETS

serves 4   *prep time* 15 minutes (not including tart crust dough)   *cook time* 40 minutes

Hello, gorgeous! When pears are in season, they are my go-to for salads, baking, and so on. They are delicious, with just the right amount of sweetness. I love that these fancy tarts look as mouthwatering as they taste. They are simple to prepare and will impress your friends, family, and guests!

ingredients:

1 batch chilled tart crust dough (page 70)

3 large Bosc pears or 6 small Seckel pears

Juice of ½ lemon

2 tablespoons coconut sugar

FOR THE CRUMBLE TOPPING:

2 tablespoons blanched almond flour

2 tablespoons coconut sugar

3 tablespoons cold unsalted butter, cut into cubes

notes: As shown in the photo, there are many ways to slice and arrange the pears! Try arranging them like a flower, slicing them in quarters, or just tossing them in a random design.

If you prefer, you can use a 9-inch tart pan to make one large tart instead of four tartlets.

directions:

1. Preheat the oven to 350°F. Grease four 4½-inch tart pans.

2. After completing Steps 1 and 2 of the tart crust recipe, press the chilled dough into the bottom and up the sides of the prepared mini tart pans. Using a fork, prick holes in the dough, then par-bake the crusts for 10 minutes, until lightly golden.

3. While the crusts are par-baking, slice the pears to your desired thickness, from razor thin up to ⅓ inch thick. Place the lemon juice in a bowl of cold water, then soak the sliced pears in the lemon water for 5 minutes.

4. Remove the pears from the lemon water, pat them dry, and transfer them to a clean, dry bowl. Gently toss the pears in the coconut sugar and arrange them in the tart crusts just to the top, not overflowing.

5. Make the crumble topping: In a bowl, mix together the flour and sugar, then use a fork or your fingertips to mix in the butter until you create clumps ranging in size from ¼ to ½ inch.

6. Sprinkle the topping mixture over the pears. Bake for 40 minutes or until the pears are soft, bubbling, and cooked and the crumble topping is golden brown.

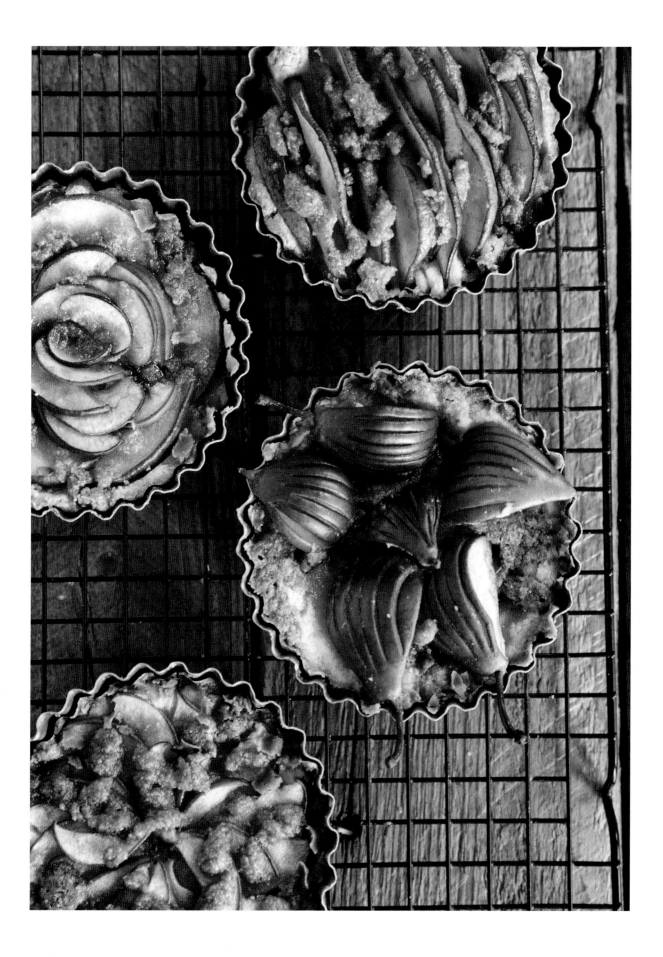

FLOURLESS SKILLET BROWNIES

serves 8   *prep time* 5 minutes   *cook time* 30 minutes

NUT-FREE

Brownies in a pan, brownies in a skillet, brownies made into a sundae with ice cream, brownies cut into little pieces and used as a dessert topping—give me *all* the brownies! With the avocado, you'll even sneak some added healthy fat into everyone's lives with this dessert (you won't taste it, I promise).

ingredients:

1¼ cups dark chocolate chunks, divided

¼ cup (½ stick) unsalted butter

1 ripe avocado, peeled and pitted

2 large eggs

2 tablespoons pure maple syrup

1 teaspoon vanilla extract

⅓ cup granulated maple sugar or coconut sugar

¼ cup cocoa powder

½ teaspoon baking powder

Pinch of fine sea salt

note: You can also bake this batter in an 8-inch square baking dish lined with parchment paper.

directions:

1. Preheat the oven to 350°F and grease a 12-inch cast-iron skillet.

2. Place water in the bottom of a double boiler so that the water level is ½ inch below the upper pan. Place 1 cup of the chocolate chunks and the butter in the upper pan, then set the double boiler over low heat. Stir often until the chocolate is melted. Pour the melted chocolate into a large mixing bowl.

3. In a blender, blend the avocado until smooth. Add the avocado to the melted chocolate and mix until combined.

4. Add the eggs to the chocolate-avocado mixture and whisk to combine. Stir in the maple syrup and vanilla.

5. In a bowl, mix together the sugar, cocoa powder, baking powder, and salt. Add the dry mixture to the wet and mix with a wooden spoon or spatula to combine.

6. Fold in the remaining ¼ cup of chocolate chunks and pour the batter into the prepared skillet.

7. Bake for 25 minutes or until a toothpick comes out clean when inserted in the middle. Let cool completely in the pan before cutting. Store in a container on the counter or in the refrigerator for up to 4 days, or freeze for up to 1 month.

serve with:

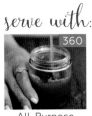

All-Purpose Caramel Sauce

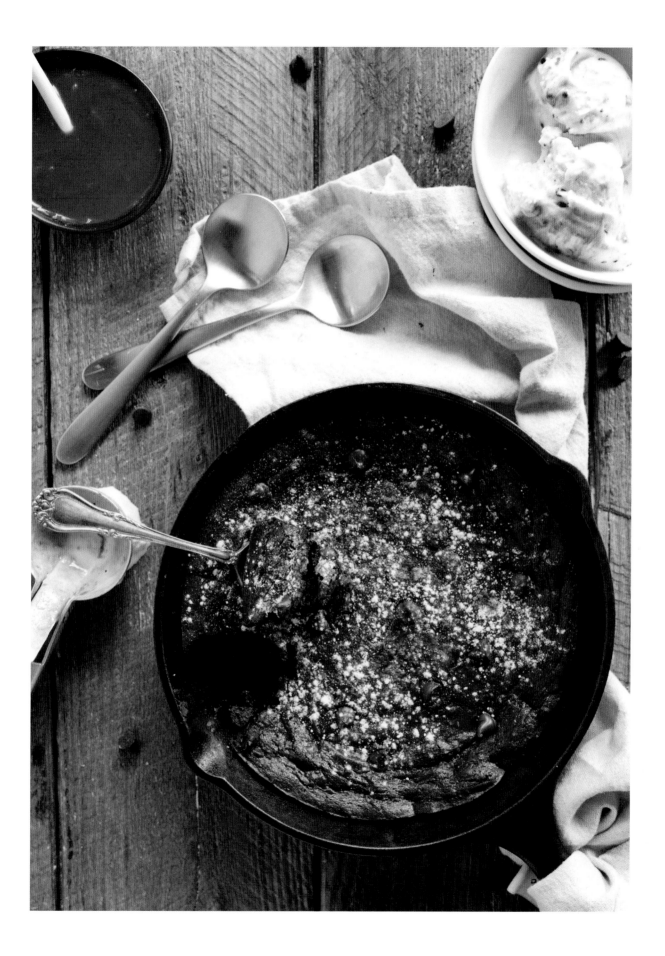

CRUNCHY CHOCOLATE COOKIES

makes 1 dozen cookies   *prep time* 15 minutes   *cook time* about 15 minutes

Sometimes a *crunchy* cookie is a must. These chocolate cookies are reminiscent of those store-bought chocolate sugar cookies that I used to eat as a child. They are the perfect little treats to serve as is or to mix into ice cream or crumble as a crust (see variation below).

ingredients:

1¼ cups dark chocolate chips, divided

3 tablespoons unsalted butter

1 cup sifted blanched almond flour

¼ cup coconut sugar or granulated maple sugar

½ teaspoon baking soda

Pinch of fine sea salt

1 large egg

1 teaspoon vanilla extract

Coarse sea salt, for garnish

directions:

1. Preheat the oven to 350°F and line a baking sheet with parchment paper.

2. Melt the chocolate: Place water in the bottom of a double boiler so that the water level is ½ inch below the upper pan. Place 1 cup of the chocolate chips and the butter in the upper pan, then set the double boiler over low heat. Stir constantly until the chocolate is melted. Do not allow the water in the bottom of the double boiler to come to a boil while the chocolate is melting.

3. In a bowl, whisk the almond flour, coconut sugar, baking soda, and salt until well blended.

4. Add the egg and vanilla to the flour mixture and mix to combine. Then add the melted chocolate mixture and mix until smooth. Fold in the remaining ¼ cup of chocolate chips.

5. Using a medium-sized cookie scoop or a spoon, scoop 1½ tablespoons of cookie dough onto the parchment paper. Leave about 2 inches of space between the cookies, as they will spread.

6. Bake for 12 minutes or until the cookies become flat. Turn off the oven but leave the baking sheet in the oven for 5 more minutes. Gently transfer the cookies to a baking rack to cool.

7. Store in a container on the counter for up to 1 week, or freeze for up to a couple of months.

variation:

Chocolate Cookie Crust. Use these cookies to make a chocolate crust! Finely grind the entire batch in a food processor or high-speed blender. You should get about 1⅓ cups of ground cookie crumbs. Then mix the crumbs with ¼ cup of melted unsalted butter and press into an 8-inch baking dish.

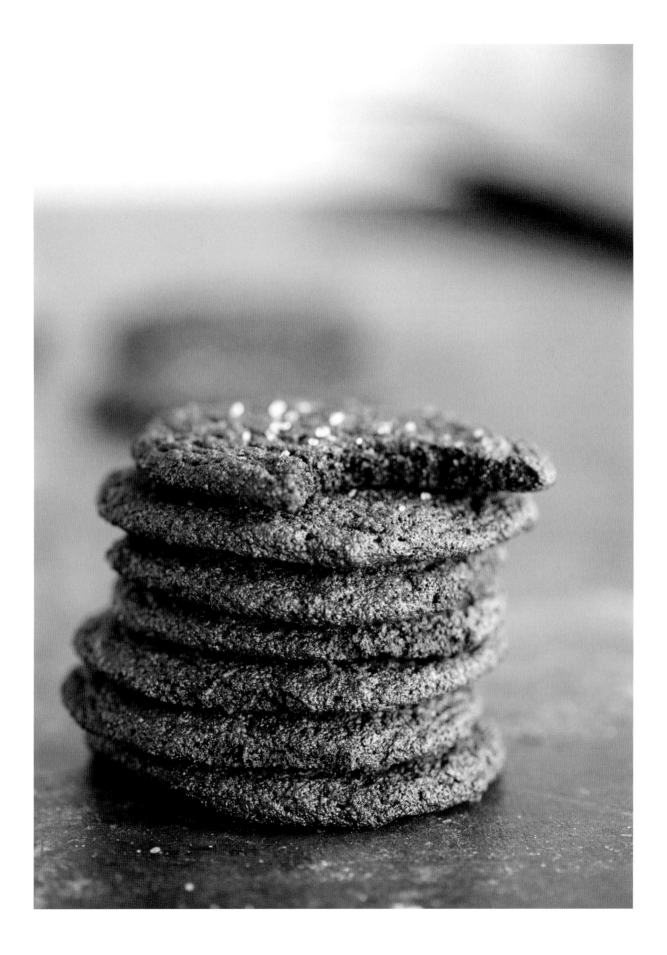

JAM CRUMB BARS

makes 9 large squares   *prep time* 10 minutes (not including jam)   *cook time* 40 minutes

DAIRY-FREE OPTION: replace butter with coconut oil
PALEO-FRIENDLY OPTION: replace butter with coconut oil
VEGAN OPTION: use coconut oil instead of butter in crust and crumb topping, and use maple syrup instead of honey in crust

A buttery shortbread-like crust, bursting with your favorite fruit and a crumb topping for the ultimate fruity dessert bars. Pack them to go, or slice and serve them after dinner or at brunch!

ingredients:

FOR THE CRUST:

2 cups sifted blanched almond flour

2 tablespoons tapioca flour

¼ cup melted unsalted butter

¼ cup pure maple syrup or honey

1 teaspoon vanilla extract

½ teaspoon fine sea salt

FOR THE CRUMB TOPPING:

1 cup blanched almond flour

1 tablespoon unsalted butter, softened

1 teaspoon vanilla extract

1 teaspoon pure maple syrup

Pinch of fine sea salt

FOR THE FILLING:

1 batch Quick & Easy Jam, any flavor (page 330)

directions:

1. Preheat the oven to 350°F and line an 8-inch square baking dish with parchment paper.

2. In a bowl, mix together the crust ingredients until evenly combined and press into the bottom of the prepared pan. Par-bake the crust for 10 minutes.

3. In a small bowl, mix together the ingredients for the crumb topping until they form crumbles.

4. Spread the jam onto the par-baked crust, then drop the crumb topping across the top.

5. Bake for 30 minutes, until the jam is bubbling and the crumb topping is golden brown. Let cool completely in the pan before slicing into squares.

6. Store the bars in the refrigerator for up to 4 days.

variation:

Baked Fruit Crumb Bars. Don't want to make jam? Make these bars with fresh or frozen fruit instead! Combine 3 cups of fresh or frozen berries or cherries (small berries can be left whole and larger ones, like strawberries, cut in half) or diced apples with 2 tablespoons of coconut sugar or granulated maple sugar, 1 tablespoon of arrowroot flour, 2 teaspoons of lemon juice, and 1 teaspoon of vanilla extract. Toss to coat evenly and spread onto the par-baked crust in Step 4, then complete the rest of the recipe as written.

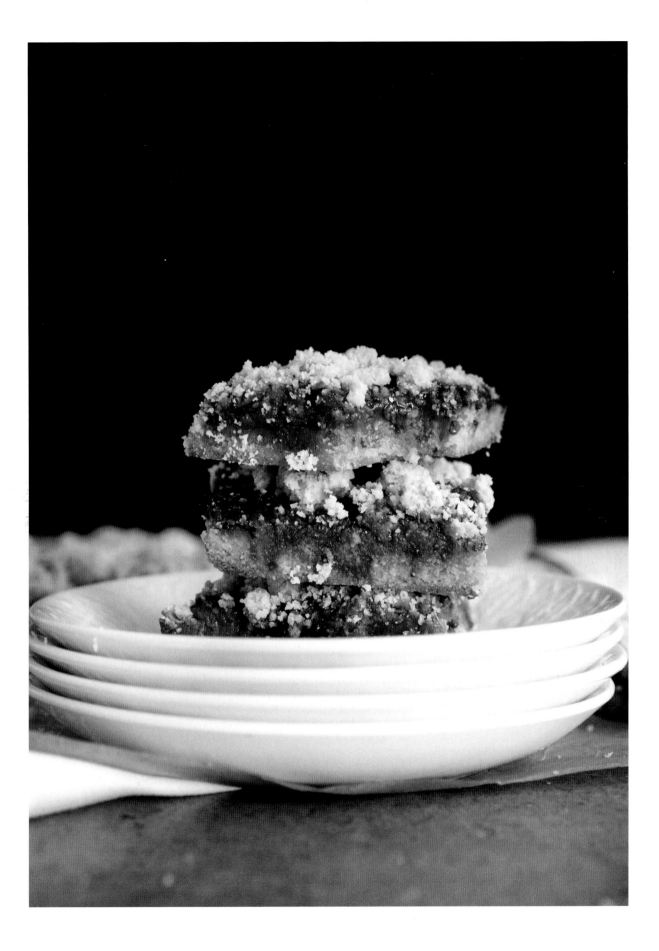

CHOCOLATE CHUNK COOKIE BARS

makes 1 dozen 2 by 2¾-inch bars   *prep time* 10 minutes   *cook time* 20 minutes

DAIRY-FREE / PALEO-FRIENDLY

Cookies in bar form are just wonderful! To satisfy everyone's sweet tooth, you can make these with chocolate chunks or with carrots, walnuts, and cranberries (see variation below). They are the perfect treat to make in a pinch, slice up, and bring with you to any event.

ingredients:

1½ cups blanched almond flour
1 tablespoon coconut flour
½ cup coconut sugar
1 teaspoon baking powder
½ teaspoon baking soda
Pinch of fine sea salt
2 large eggs
2 tablespoons palm shortening
1 teaspoon vanilla extract
½ cup dark chocolate chunks

note: I personally prefer these bars slightly undercooked. Keep an eye on them in the oven and pull them out when they're baked to your liking. Careful: They go quickly from cooked to overcooked!

directions:

1. Preheat the oven to 350°F. Line an 8-inch square baking dish with parchment paper.

2. In a mixing bowl, whisk the almond flour, coconut flour, coconut sugar, baking powder, baking soda, and salt until well combined.

3. Add the eggs, shortening, and vanilla and mix well to combine. Fold in the chocolate chunks.

4. Scoop the batter into the prepared pan and spread it out evenly.

5. Bake for 20 minutes, until the top is golden brown and a toothpick comes out clean when inserted in the middle. Let cool completely in the pan before cutting. The bars will become denser as they cool.

6. Store the bars in a container on the counter for up to 2 days or in the refrigerator for up to 5 days.

variation:

Morning Glory Cookie Bars. Replace the chocolate chunks with ¼ cup of grated carrots, ¼ cup of chopped raw walnuts, and ¼ cup of dried sweetened cranberries.

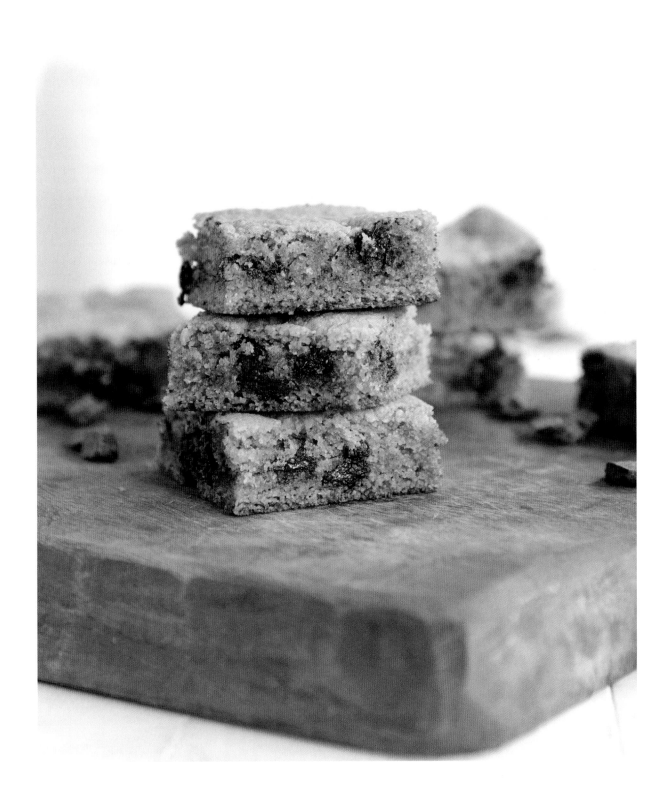

YELLOW BIRTHDAY CAKE

makes one 8-inch round or square, single-layer cake (6 to 8 servings)
prep time 8 minutes (not including frosting)   *cook time* 25 to 30 minutes

....

NUT-FREE / DAIRY-FREE OPTION: frost with whipped cream (page 282) instead of buttercream
PALEO-FRIENDLY OPTION: frost with whipped cream (page 282) instead of buttercream

....

Moist and fluffy, this all-purpose yellow birthday cake will be loved by all.

ingredients:

½ cup sifted coconut flour

½ cup sifted tapioca flour

1 teaspoon baking powder

½ teaspoon baking soda

Pinch of fine sea salt

5 large eggs

½ cup plus 2 tablespoons unsweetened applesauce

⅓ cup honey or pure maple syrup

1 teaspoon vanilla extract

1 batch Buttercream Frosting, flavor of choice (page 288)

GARNISH IDEAS:

Edible flowers

Fresh fruit (throw on some red and blue berries for a festive July Fourth or Memorial Day party!)

Crumbled Cookie Bar pieces (page 298)

directions:

1. Preheat the oven to 350°F and grease an 8-inch round or square cake pan.

2. In a large bowl, whisk the coconut flour, tapioca flour, baking powder, baking soda, and salt until well blended.

3. Add the eggs, applesauce, honey, and vanilla and mix until smooth.

4. Pour the batter into the prepared pan and smooth out the top. Bake for 25 to 30 minutes, until a toothpick comes out clean when inserted in the middle.

5. Let cool completely in the pan, then gently loosen the sides of the cake by running a spatula or knife around the edge of the pan. Remove the cake from the pan.

6. Using a spatula, frost the top of the cake with about half of the frosting, then frost the sides with the rest. Garnish as desired. Store in the refrigerator for up to 1 week or in the freezer for up to 1 month.

note: To make a double-layer cake, as pictured, double the cake and frosting ingredients.

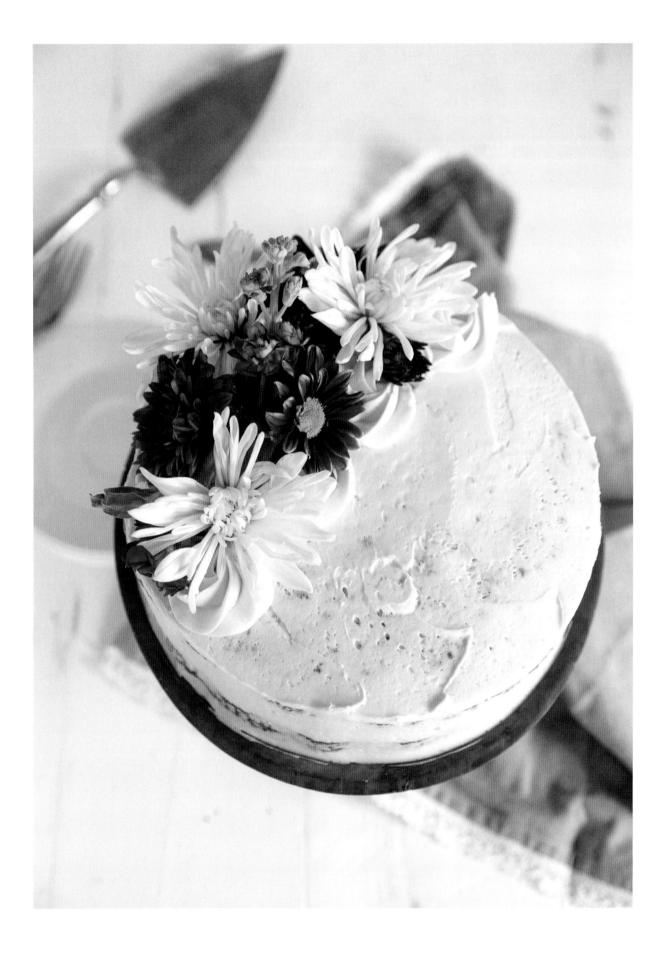

CHOCOLATE BIRTHDAY CAKE

makes one 8-inch round or square, single-layer cake (6 to 8 servings)
prep time 8 minutes (not including frosting)   *cook time* 25 to 30 minutes

....

NUT-FREE / DAIRY-FREE OPTION: frost with whipped cream (page 282) instead of buttercream and use avocado oil instead of butter / PALEO-FRIENDLY OPTION: frost with whipped cream (page 282) instead of buttercream and use avocado oil instead of butter

....

This birthday cake is for the chocolate lover in your family. Additional shaved dark chocolate adds an element of melted chocolate heaven to every bite!

ingredients:

½ cup sifted coconut flour

½ cup sifted tapioca flour

¼ cup cocoa powder

1 teaspoon baking powder

½ teaspoon baking soda

Pinch of fine sea salt

5 large eggs

½ cup plus 2 tablespoons unsweetened applesauce

⅓ cup honey or pure maple syrup

1 tablespoon avocado oil or melted unsalted butter

1 teaspoon vanilla extract

Optional: ⅓ cup shaved dark chocolate

1 batch Buttercream Frosting, flavor of choice (page 288)

Optional: Mini dark chocolate chips, for garnish

directions:

1. Preheat the oven to 350°F and grease an 8-inch round or square cake pan.

2. In a large bowl, whisk the coconut flour, tapioca flour, cocoa powder, baking powder, baking soda, and salt until well blended.

3. Add the eggs, applesauce, honey, oil, and vanilla and mix until smooth. Fold in the shaved dark chocolate, if using.

4. Pour the batter into the prepared pan and smooth out the top. Bake for 25 to 30 minutes, until a toothpick comes out clean when inserted in the middle.

5. Let cool completely in the pan, then gently loosen the sides of the cake by running a spatula or knife around the edge of the pan. Remove the cake from the pan.

6. Using a spatula, frost the top of the cake with about half of the frosting, then frost the sides with the rest. Sprinkle mini chocolate chips on top as desired. Store in the refrigerator for up to 1 week or in the freezer for up to 1 month.

note: To make a triple-layer cake, as pictured, you will need to make a double batch of the batter and bake two cake layers, then make a single batch of batter and bake the third layer. Make a triple batch of the frosting. To decorate the cake, place about ¾ cup of frosting in a piping bag fitted with an extra-large star pastry tip and pipe swirls or rosettes, then sprinkle with mini chocolate chips.

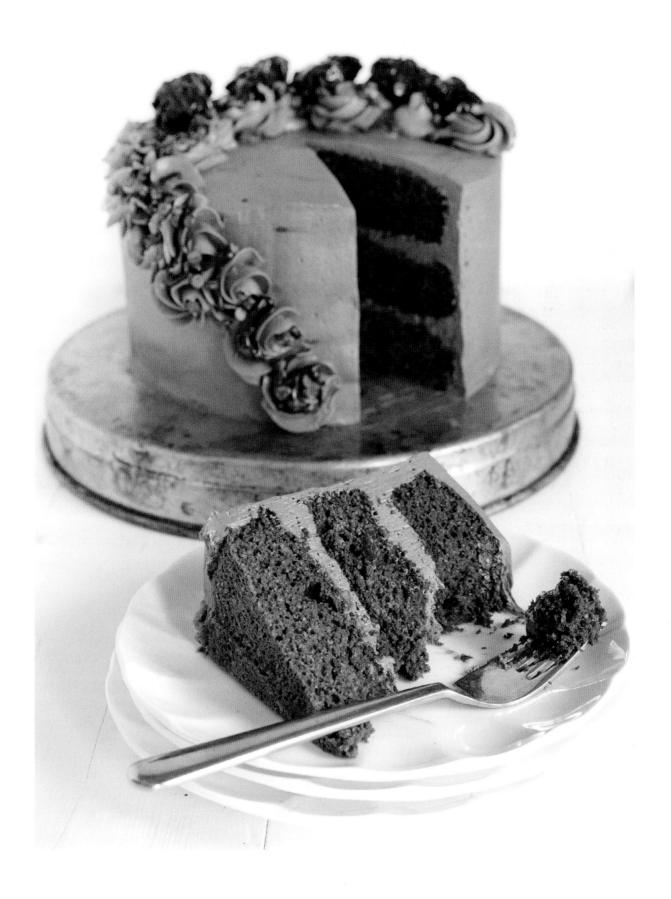

CLASSIC VANILLA CUPCAKES

makes 9 cupcakes   *prep time* 8 minutes (not including frosting)   *cook time* 15 to 20 minutes

DAIRY-FREE OPTION: frost with whipped cream (page 282) instead of buttercream
PALEO-FRIENDLY OPTION: frost with whipped cream (page 282) instead of buttercream

Calling all vanilla fans! Nobody will know that these classic vanilla cupcakes are free of gluten, grains, and refined sugar. This recipe is a must for birthday parties and festive holidays!

ingredients:

1 cup sifted blanched almond flour

1 tablespoon coconut flour

1 teaspoon baking powder

½ teaspoon baking soda

Pinch of fine sea salt

3 large eggs

3 tablespoons honey or pure maple syrup

2 tablespoons unsweetened applesauce

1 teaspoon vanilla extract

1 batch Vanilla Buttercream Frosting (page 288)

Fresh fruit, sliced or quartered (small berries can be left whole), for garnish

directions:

1. Preheat the oven to 350°F and line 9 cups of a standard 12-cup muffin tin with parchment paper liners or silicone liners.

2. In a bowl, whisk together the almond flour, coconut flour, baking powder, baking soda, and salt until well blended.

3. Add the eggs, honey, applesauce, and vanilla and mix until smooth.

4. Pour the batter into the lined muffin cups, filling each cup about three-quarters full. Bake for 15 to 20 minutes, until a toothpick comes out clean when inserted in the middle.

5. Let cool completely before frosting. Apply the frosting with a spatula or, for a pretty presentation, use a piping bag and tip to pipe the frosting. Garnish with fresh fruit. Store in the refrigerator for up to 1 week or in the freezer for up to 1 month. If freezing, add the fresh fruit after defrosting the cupcakes.

variation:

Strawberry Cupcakes. Fold ⅓ cup of finely diced fresh strawberries into the batter in Step 3 and use Strawberry Buttercream Frosting (page 288) to frost the cupcakes. Garnish with fresh strawberries.

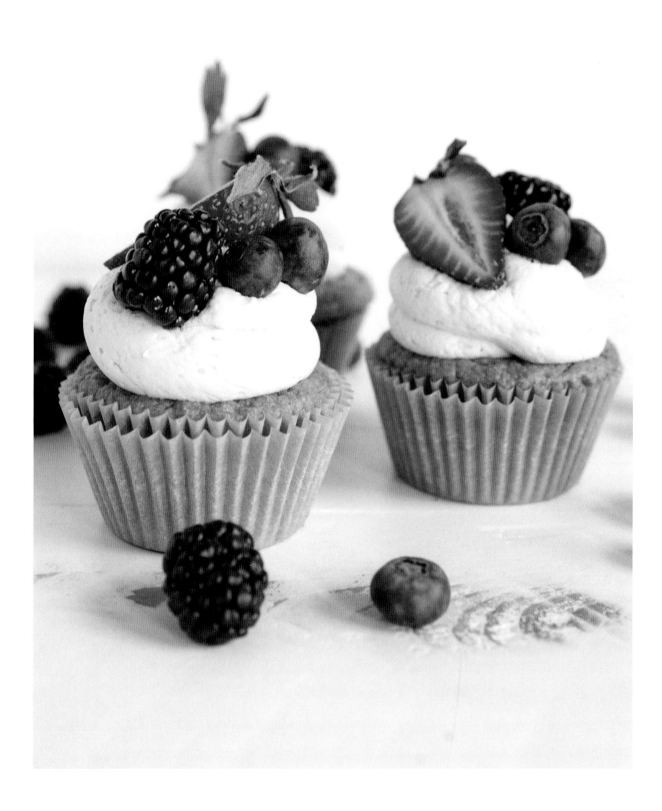

DOUBLE CHOCOLATE CUPCAKES

makes 9 cupcakes   *prep time* 8 minutes (not including frosting)   *cook time* 15 to 20 minutes

DAIRY-FREE / PALEO-FRIENDLY

Are you a chocolate lover? Then these moist, extra-chocolaty cupcakes are for you!

ingredients:

1 cup sifted blanched almond flour

¼ cup cocoa powder

1 tablespoon coconut flour

1 teaspoon baking powder

½ teaspoon baking soda

Pinch of fine sea salt

3 large eggs

3 tablespoons unsweetened applesauce

3 tablespoons honey or pure maple syrup

1 teaspoon vanilla extract

⅓ cup dark chocolate chunks

1 batch Chocolate Buttercream Frosting (page 288)

Mini dark chocolate chips, for garnish

directions:

1. Preheat the oven to 350°F and line 9 cups of a standard 12-cup muffin tin with parchment paper liners or silicone liners.

2. In a bowl, whisk together the almond flour, cocoa powder, coconut flour, baking powder, baking soda, and salt until well blended.

3. Add the eggs, applesauce, honey, and vanilla and mix until smooth. Fold in the chocolate chunks.

4. Pour the batter into the lined muffin cups, filling each cup about three-quarters full. Bake for 15 to 20 minutes, until a toothpick comes out clean when inserted in the middle.

5. Let cool completely before frosting. Apply the frosting with a spatula or, for a pretty presentation, use a piping bag and tip to pipe the frosting. Garnish the frosted cupcakes with mini chocolate chips. Store in the refrigerator for up to 1 week or in the freezer for up to 1 month.

variation:

Caramel Brownie Cupcakes. Top the cupcakes with All-Purpose Caramel Sauce (page 360) and Flourless Skillet Brownies (page 292) cut into ½-inch squares.

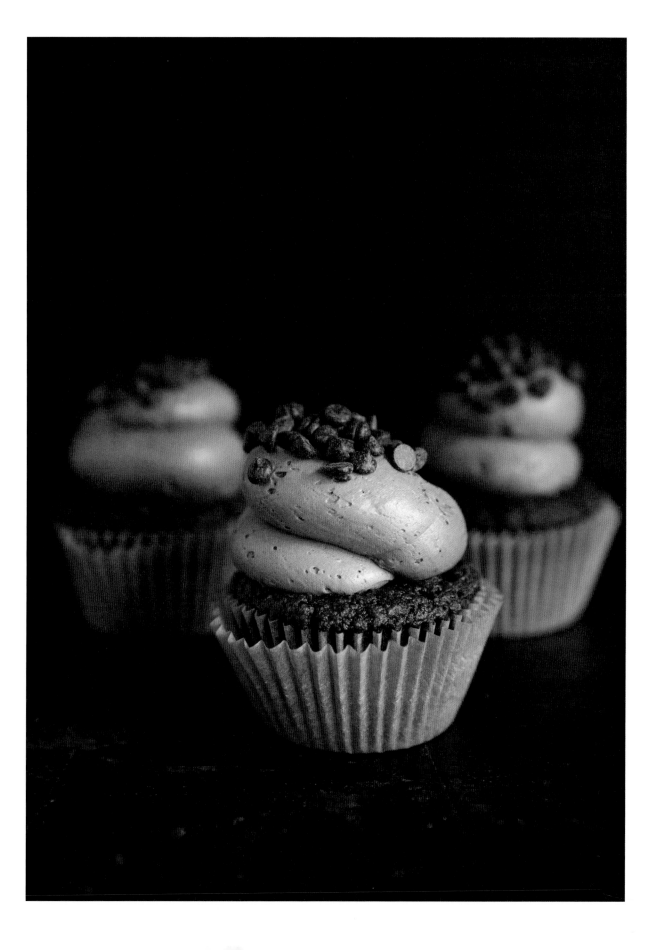

BROWN BUTTER APPLE CRISP

serves 4 *prep time* 10 minutes *cook time* 45 to 55 minutes

EGG-FREE

Here's my perfect fall dessert scenario: a bowl of delicious brown butter apple crisp, made with perfectly tender cooked apples and a fabulous crisp topping, and topped with some homemade caramel sauce and dairy-free ice cream. It doesn't get much better than that in my book!

ingredients:

¼ cup (½ stick) unsalted butter
4 apples, peeled, cored, and sliced
1 teaspoon lemon juice
Seeds scraped from 1 vanilla bean
⅓ cup coconut sugar
1 tablespoon blanched almond flour
1 teaspoon ground cinnamon

FOR THE CRUMB TOPPING:

1 cup blanched almond flour
Optional: ¼ cup sliced raw almonds
3 tablespoons granulated maple
  sugar or coconut sugar
Pinch of fine sea salt
¼ cup (½ stick) unsalted butter
½ teaspoon ground cinnamon
Pinch of fine sea salt

directions:

1. Preheat the oven to 350°F and grease an 8-inch square or 9-inch oval baking dish.

2. In a small saucepan over medium heat, melt the butter. Continue to heat the butter until it comes to a rapid simmer. It will start popping and crackling, and you'll see brown bits starting to separate and fall to the bottom of the pan. Reduce the heat to low, stir, and continue to simmer until the butter becomes brown, about 2 minutes (watch to avoid burning), then immediately remove from the heat. Let cool for 5 minutes.

3. In a large bowl, toss the apples with the lemon juice, vanilla bean seeds, coconut sugar, almond flour, cinnamon, and brown butter, then pour into the prepared baking dish.

4. Mix together the ingredients for the crumb topping and sprinkle over the entire apple mixture.

5. Bake until the apples are bubbling and the crumb topping is golden brown, 40 to 50 minutes.

6. Serve hot. Store leftovers in the refrigerator for up to 1 week.

serve with:

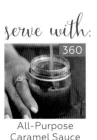

All-Purpose
Caramel Sauce

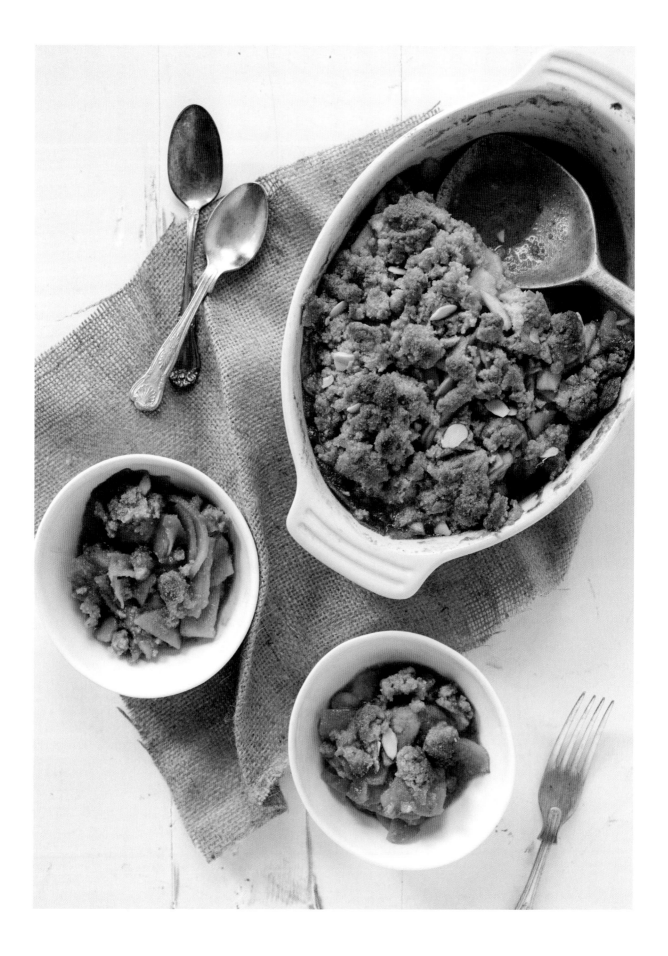

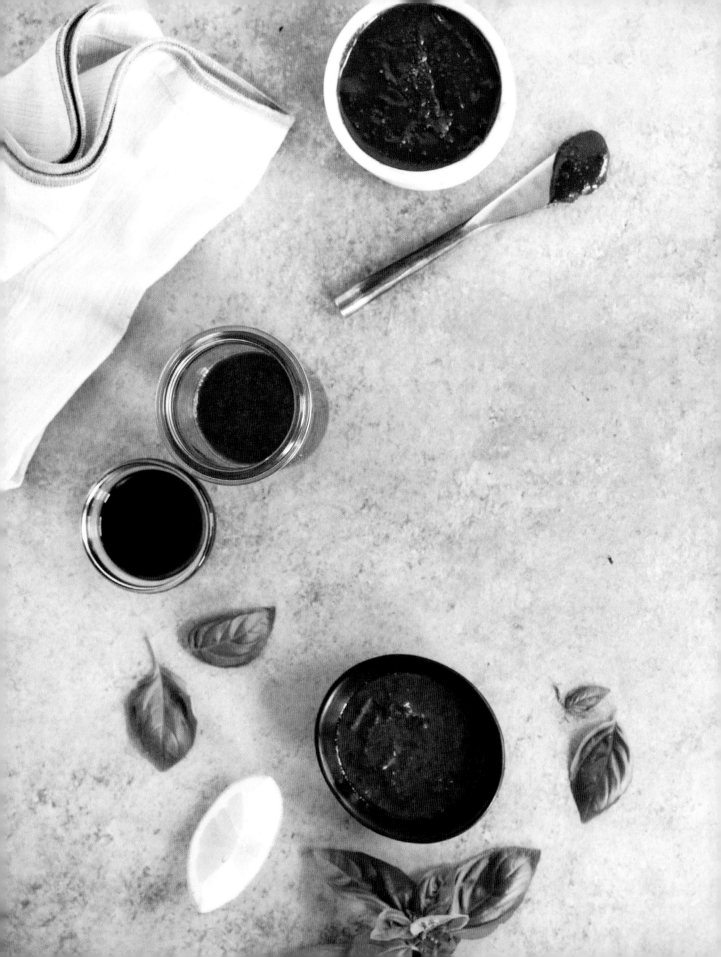

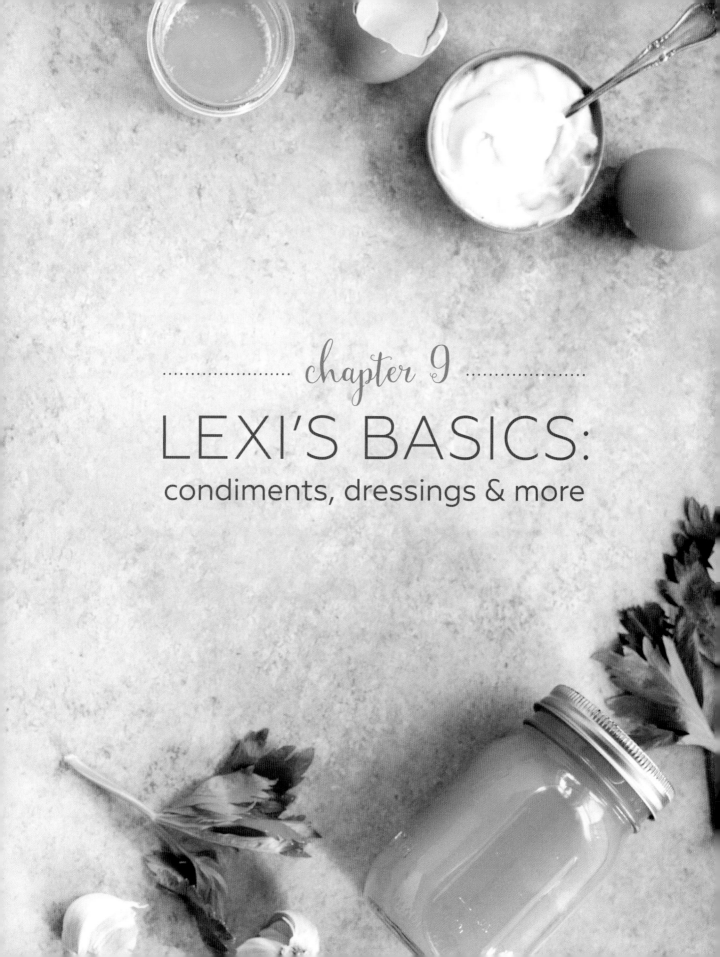

chapter 9

LEXI'S BASICS:
condiments, dressings & more

EASY HOMEMADE MAYO

makes 1 cup (about 8 ounces)   *prep time* 5 minutes

NUT-FREE / DAIRY-FREE / PALEO-FRIENDLY

Homemade mayo is so easy to throw together; it makes you wonder why you ever purchased store-bought mayo! This classic version is delightful and versatile, and it serves as a base for four flavor variations that will add a kick to any dish.

ingredients:

1 large egg, at room temperature

1 teaspoon lemon juice

½ teaspoon dry mustard

Pinch of fine sea salt

Pinch of freshly ground black pepper

1¼ cups avocado oil or light olive oil

directions:

1. In a food processor, pulse the egg, lemon juice, dry mustard, salt, and pepper until combined.

2. With the machine running on medium speed, very slowly pour in the oil until the mayo thickens.

3. Taste and add additional salt, if desired. Store the mayo in a closed container in the refrigerator for up to 2 weeks.

variations:

Spicy Mayo. Add 1 teaspoon of Sriracha sauce to ½ cup of mayonnaise and mix until combined. Taste and add more Sriracha if desired.

Herb Mayo. Add 1 tablespoon of Italian seasoning to ½ cup of mayonnaise and mix until combined.

Truffle Aioli. Crush a clove of garlic to a paste. Add that, along with 2 teaspoons of truffle oil, to ½ cup of mayonnaise and mix until combined.

Horseradish Mayo. Add 3 tablespoons of prepared horseradish (store-bought or homemade, page 346) and a pinch of cayenne pepper to ½ cup of mayonnaise and mix until combined.

use in:

 320

Creamy Caesar Dressing

 198

New England Lobster Rolls

 174

Creamy Chicken Bacon Spaghetti Squash Boats

 178

Creamy Cajun Chicken Pasta

use on:

 198

All-American Burgers

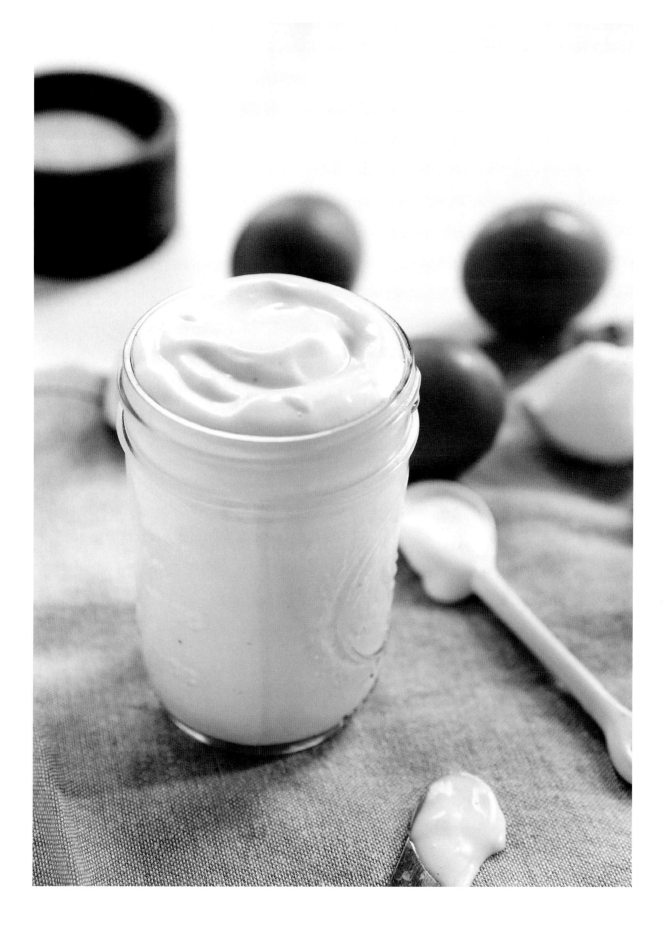

EVERYTHING BAGEL SPREAD

makes ½ cup   *prep time* 2 minutes

NUT-FREE / DAIRY-FREE / PALEO-FRIENDLY

I love a good spread on a hearty sandwich or lettuce wrap, especially one that's a little different from your average condiment, like this one. This everything bagel spread is fantastic on any sandwich, and it reminds me of those bagels that I devoured while growing up. It's also great as a dipping sauce with fries!

ingredients:

½ cup mayo, homemade (page 312) or store-bought
1 teaspoon avocado oil
1 teaspoon white sesame seeds
1 teaspoon black sesame seeds
1 teaspoon dried minced onion
1 teaspoon dried minced garlic
1 teaspoon poppy seeds
Pinch of coarse sea salt

directions:

1. In a bowl, combine all of the ingredients. Mix until well combined and use as desired.

2. Store the spread in an airtight container in the refrigerator for 1 to 2 weeks.

use on:

80

All-Purpose
Sandwich Bread

serve with:

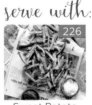
226

Sweet Potato
Truffle Fries

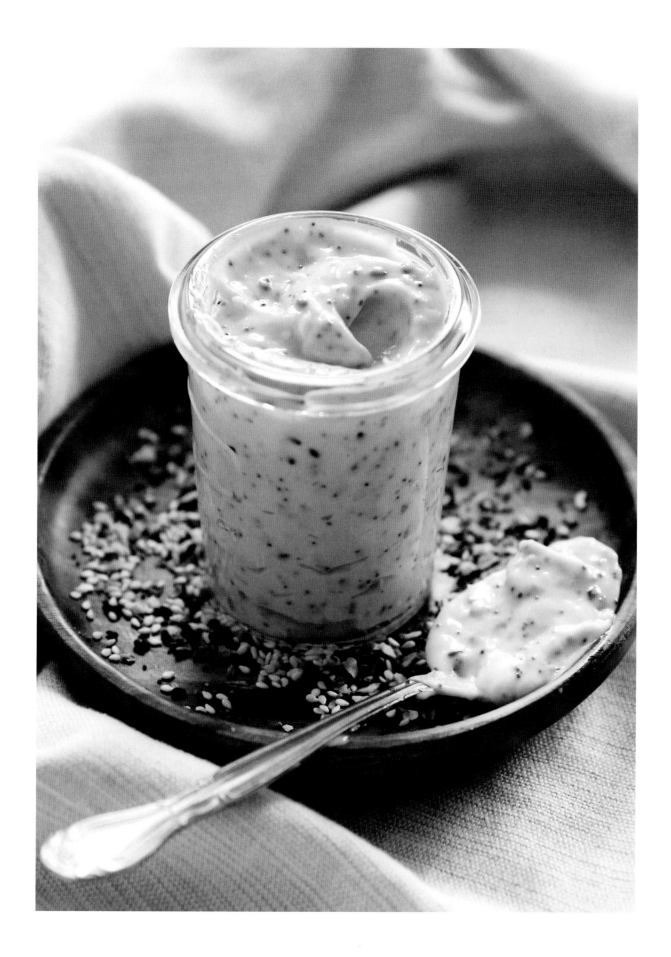

LEXI'S PESTO

makes ½ cup   *prep time* 5 minutes

EGG-FREE / NUT-FREE OPTION: use sunflower seeds
DAIRY-FREE OPTION: omit cheese / PALEO-FRIENDLY OPTION: omit cheese
VEGAN OPTION: omit cheese

This pesto can make a dish, all the while adding some delicious fresh herbs and greens to your meal. I love how creative you can get with pesto: you can mix up the various herbs and greens, as well as the nuts!

ingredients:

1½ cups spinach or roughly chopped kale

1 cup fresh basil leaves

½ cup raw pine nuts, cashews, walnuts, or other nuts of choice

2 cloves garlic, roughly chopped

1 tablespoon freshly grated Parmesan cheese

Pinch of fine sea salt

Pinch of freshly ground black pepper

Optional: ⅛ teaspoon red pepper flakes

⅓ to ½ cup extra-virgin olive oil

Optional: Splash of lemon juice

directions:

1. Place the spinach, basil, nuts, garlic, Parmesan cheese, salt, black pepper, and red pepper flakes, if using, in a food processor or blender. Pulse until the spinach and basil are broken down.

2. With the machine running, pour in the olive oil: Use ⅓ cup if you like a thicker pesto or ½ cup if you like a runnier pesto. Once the pesto reaches your desired consistency, stop, taste, and add additional salt and pepper and/or a splash of lemon juice, if desired.

3. Store the pesto in a closed container in the refrigerator for up to 1 week.

use in: *use on:*

152

Pesto Chicken Salad

248

Zucchini Noodles or Spaghetti Squash Noodles

226

Sweet Potato Truffle Fries

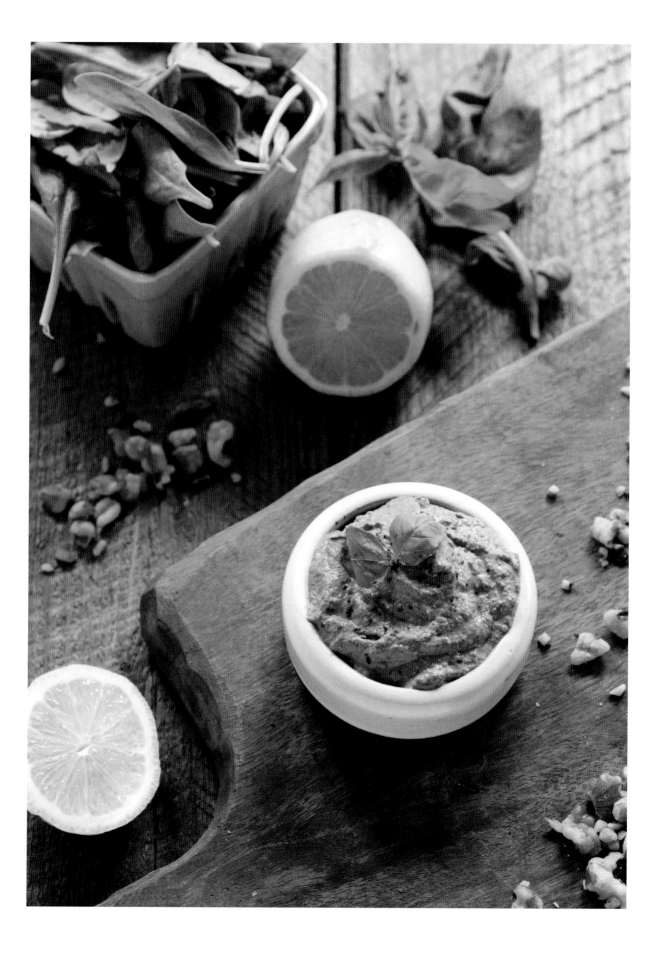

RANCH DRESSING

makes about 1¼ cups *prep time* 5 minutes

....

NUT-FREE OPTION: use coconut milk / DAIRY-FREE / PALEO-FRIENDLY

....

Ranch dressing has so many uses. It kicks things like wings, BBQ chicken pizza, and salad up a notch. But buying it in a store? No thank you! When I can't pronounce multiple ingredients listed on the label, no deal. This homemade ranch is simple to make and simply delicious—all the flavors you want from ranch dressing, without any guilt.

ingredients:

1 cup mayo, homemade (page 312) or store-bought

⅓ cup finely chopped scallions

¼ cup unsweetened, unflavored nondairy milk of choice, homemade (page 266) or store-bought

½ teaspoon dried dill

½ teaspoon dried parsley

½ teaspoon garlic granules

½ teaspoon onion granules

¼ teaspoon fine sea salt

⅛ teaspoon freshly ground black pepper

directions:

1. In a bowl, whisk together all of the ingredients. Taste and adjust the seasoning and spices as desired. Chill before serving.

2. Store the dressing in a closed container in the refrigerator for up to 4 days.

serve with:

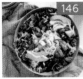
104
Wings

BBQ Chicken Pizza
176

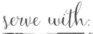

146
Chopped BBQ Chicken Cobb Salad

78
Veggies & crackers as a snack

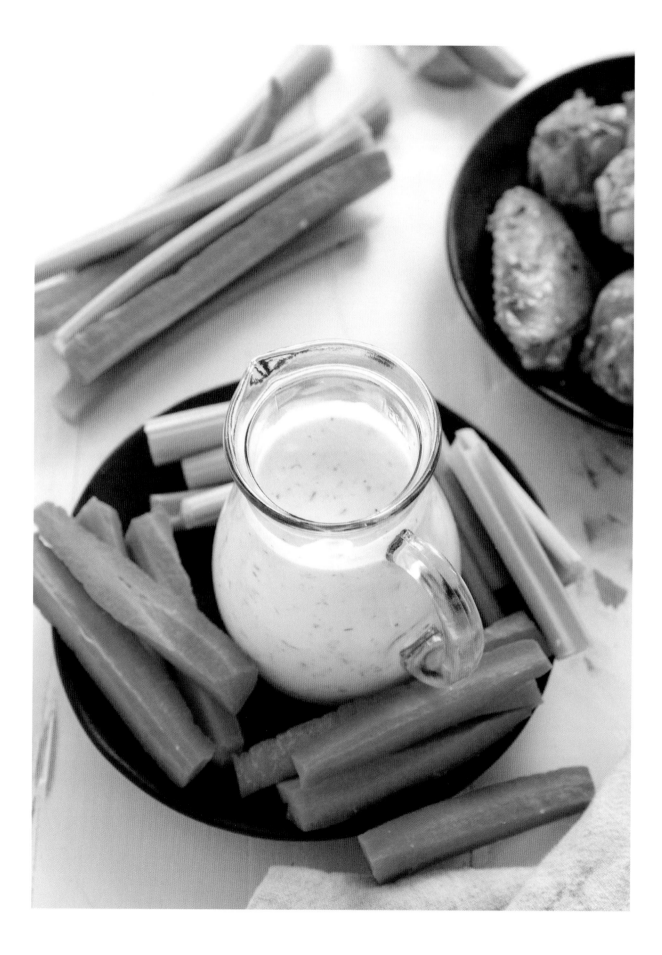

CREAMY CAESAR DRESSING

makes ½ cup   *prep time* 5 minutes

NUT-FREE / DAIRY-FREE / PALEO-FRIENDLY

Caesar dressing—especially *creamy* Caesar dressing—seems naughty. It's one of the first store-bought dressings that I ditched from my diet when I started my journey to clean eating. No more, my friends! This Caesar dressing is made with good-quality ingredients and packs all the flavor of the dressing you love.

ingredients:

- ½ cup mayo, homemade (page 312) or store-bought
- 2 teaspoons avocado oil or extra-virgin olive oil
- 1 clove garlic, roughly chopped
- 1 teaspoon apple cider vinegar
- 1 teaspoon Dijon mustard
- 1 teaspoon lemon juice
- ½ teaspoon anchovy paste
- Pinch of fine sea salt
- Pinch of freshly ground black pepper

directions:

1. Place all of the ingredients in a blender and pulse once (about 5 seconds), just until the dressing is thick and smooth. If you overblend, the dressing will become watery.

2. Taste and add additional salt and pepper, if desired. Serve immediately or store in a closed container in the refrigerator for up to 1 week.

use on:

142

Kale Caesar Salad

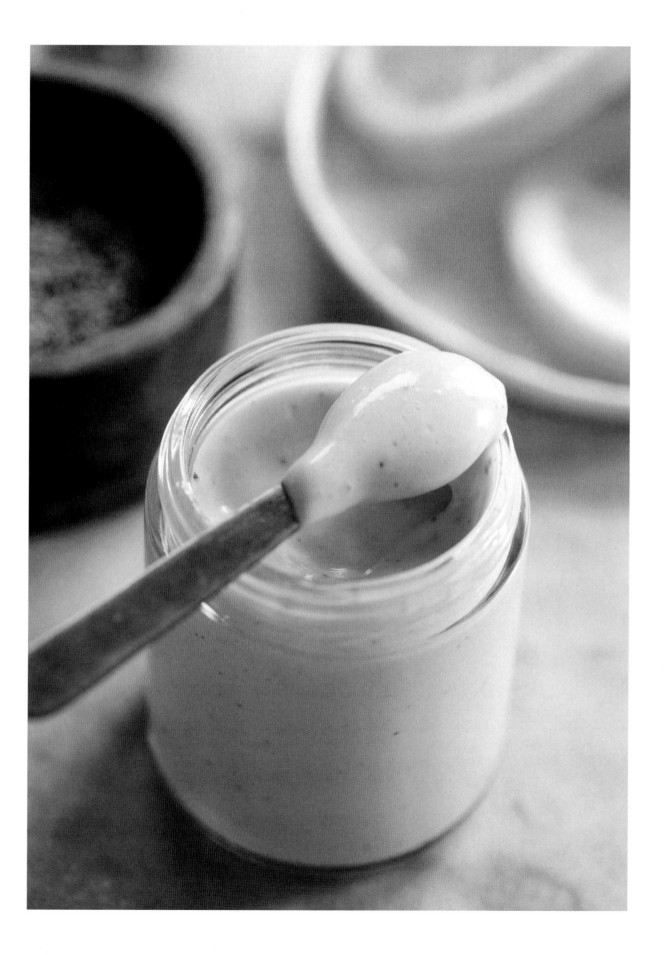

MAPLE BALSAMIC DRESSING

makes ½ cup   *prep time* 5 minutes

EGG-FREE / NUT-FREE / DAIRY-FREE / PALEO-FRIENDLY / VEGAN

This dressing is hands down one of my favorites. Simple, delicious ingredients come together to make a wonderfully creamy dressing that is the perfect addition to any salad.

ingredients:

⅓ cup avocado oil or extra-virgin olive oil

¼ cup balsamic vinegar

2 teaspoons Dijon mustard

2 teaspoons pure maple syrup

Pinch of fine sea salt

directions:

1. Place all of the ingredients in a blender and blend until smooth.

2. Store the dressing in a closed container in the refrigerator for up to 1 week.

use on:

138

Winter Harvest
Salad

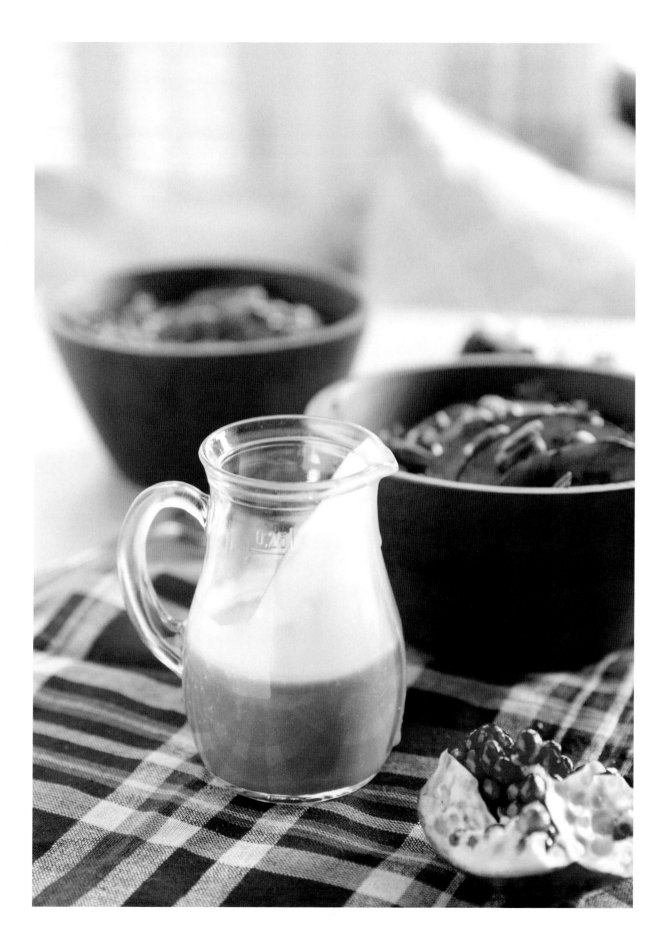

GINGER DRESSING

makes ⅓ to ½ cup *prep time* 5 minutes

EGG-FREE / NUT-FREE / DAIRY-FREE / PALEO-FRIENDLY

I simply cannot get enough of this dressing! It is creamy and flavorful and pairs perfectly with ahi tuna or salmon. It's delicious on any salad, really!

ingredients:

1½ tablespoons peeled and grated fresh ginger

1 tablespoon avocado oil or extra-virgin olive oil

1 tablespoon coconut aminos

1 tablespoon Dijon mustard

2 teaspoons lemon juice

1 teaspoon honey

1 clove garlic, crushed to a paste

Pinch of fine sea salt

Pinch of freshly ground black pepper

directions:

1. Place all of the ingredients in a small bowl and whisk together until blended.

2. If you'd like your dressing smoother, transfer it to a small jar blender and blend on high speed for 5 seconds.

3. Store the dressing in a closed container in the refrigerator for up to 4 days.

use on:

Sesame Seared Ahi Tuna Salad

Ahi Tuna Bites

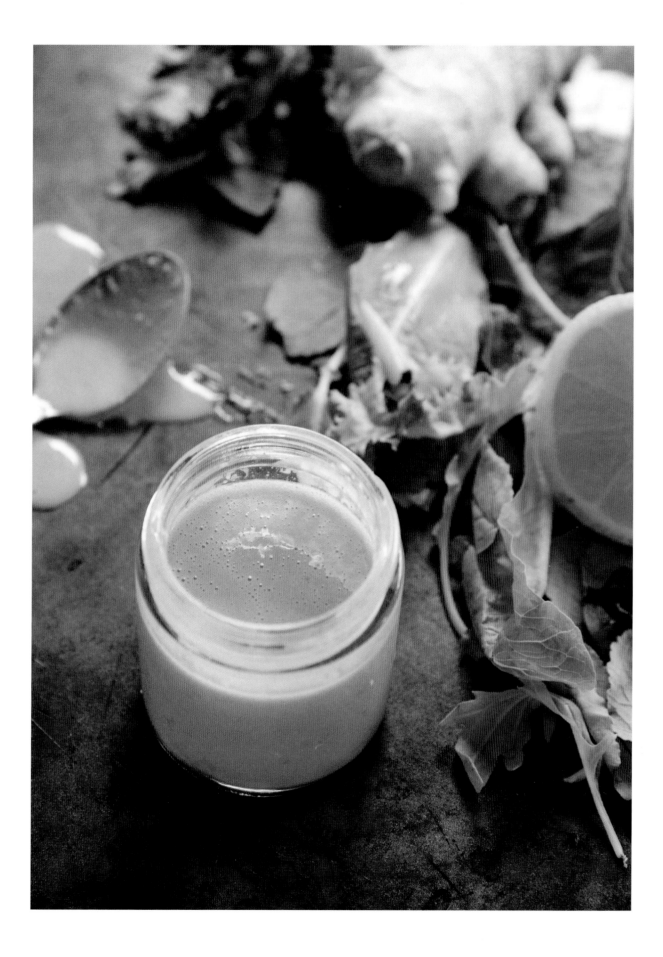

LEXI'S GREEN DRESSING

makes ½ cup   *prep time* 5 minutes

EGG-FREE / NUT-FREE / DAIRY-FREE / PALEO-FRIENDLY

A creamy salad dressing for when you want some extra greens in your life!

ingredients:

½ cup destemmed and roughly chopped kale

¼ cup extra-virgin olive oil or avocado oil

1 tablespoon apple cider vinegar

1 tablespoon water

2 teaspoons honey

1 teaspoon lemon juice

1 small bunch fresh flat-leaf parsley

1 small chunk fresh ginger (about ½ inch), peeled and chopped

1 clove garlic, chopped

note: If you use a high-speed blender to make this dressing, there's no need to chop the ginger and garlic. Simply peel the chunk of ginger and the garlic clove and drop them into the blender whole.

directions:

1. Place all of the ingredients in a blender and blend on high for 30 to 60 seconds, until smooth.

2. Store the dressing in a closed container in the refrigerator for up to 2 days.

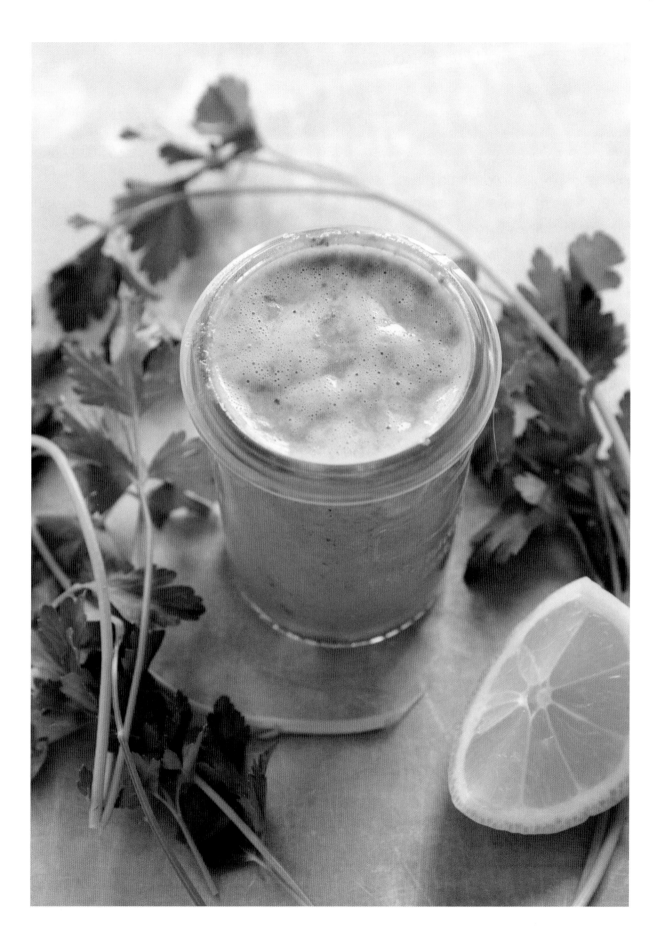

SWEET & SMOKY BBQ SAUCE

makes 2 cups   *prep time* 5 minutes   *cook time* 15 minutes

EGG-FREE / NUT-FREE / DAIRY-FREE / PALEO-FRIENDLY
VEGAN OPTION: use molasses instead of honey

Every place we travel, I pick up a unique hot sauce or BBQ sauce to try. I have an entire section in my refrigerator dedicated to these sauces. True story. By this point you know how much I care about reading labels and checking the ingredients in the products I buy. More often than not, I'm surprised to find hidden sugars, soy, wheat, and all sorts of undesirable ingredients in sauces. The solution? With a quick little stir in your pot, you can make your own clean BBQ sauce. This sauce has all kinds of uses: not only is it perfect for slathering on your favorite grilled meat (I like it on chicken), but it's also delicious on ribs (visit Lexiscleankitchen.com for my Slow Cooker Ribs recipe), on pizza (page 176), as a dip for chicken nuggets (page 158), and so much more!

ingredients:

1 (15-ounce) can tomato sauce

1 (6-ounce) can tomato paste

½ cup coconut sugar

⅓ cup apple cider vinegar

1 tablespoon molasses or honey

1½ teaspoons garlic powder

1 teaspoon dry mustard

1 teaspoon onion powder

1 teaspoon paprika

1 teaspoon smoked paprika

Up to 2 teaspoons hot sauce
   (see note)

½ teaspoon fine sea salt

½ teaspoon freshly ground black
   pepper

Optional: 1 teaspoon cayenne
   pepper

directions:

1. Place all of the ingredients in a large pot (it will splatter slightly when cooking, so avoid using a small pot) and mix well to combine. Bring to a boil, then reduce the heat and simmer for 10 minutes, until the sauce becomes fragrant.

2. Transfer the sauce to a blender and blend until smooth. Taste and adjust the balance of sweet and heat to your liking by adding more sweetener or hot sauce and/or cayenne pepper as desired.

3. Store the sauce in a jar in the refrigerator for up to 1 week.

note: Use ½ teaspoon of hot sauce if you prefer just a hint of chili heat or up to 2 teaspoons for a very hot sauce. The exact amount will depend on the heat level of the hot sauce you are using and your personal taste.

use on:

BBQ Chicken
Pizza

Chopped
BBQ Chicken
Cobb Salad

variation:

Pumpkin BBQ Sauce. Make your BBQ sauce more fall festive by adding pumpkin to it! This version pairs wonderfully with pork. To make, omit the smoked paprika and add ⅓ cup of pumpkin puree and 1 tablespoon of pumpkin pie spice.

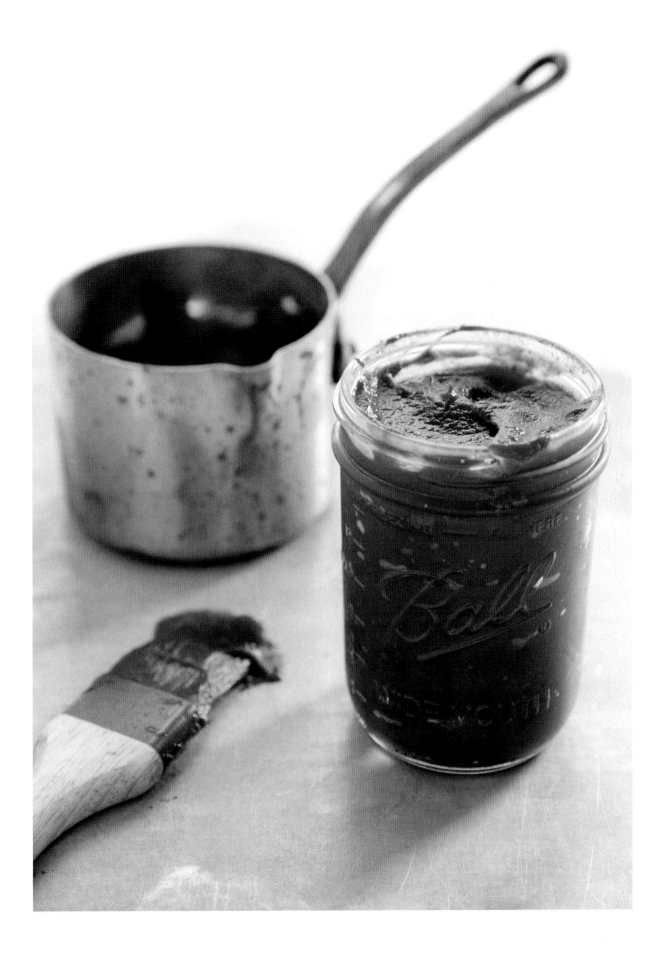

QUICK & EASY JAM

makes 1 cup   *prep time* 5 minutes   *cook time* 15 minutes

EGG-FREE / NUT-FREE / DAIRY-FREE / PALEO-FRIENDLY

While I was growing up, jam was a household staple. There were always one or two jars in the refrigerator. For breakfast we would slather it on toast, pancakes, waffles, and biscuits, sometimes with nut butter; we'd even slather it on roasted chicken at lunch or dinnertime! I love this recipe because after twenty short minutes you have delicious fresh jam without any of the added refined sugars and preservatives that store-bought jam contains. This recipe is also unique in that it uses chia seeds. I love chia seeds in jam (and in smoothies) because they create a wonderful thickness.

ingredients:

2 cups fresh fruit (see notes)

2 tablespoons honey

1 tablespoon lemon juice

2 tablespoons chia seeds (see notes)

directions:

1. In a bowl, toss the fruit with the honey and lemon juice.

2. Transfer the fruit mixture to a medium-sized saucepan and cook over medium heat until the fruit begins to break down and is soft and bubbling, about 5 minutes.

3. Reduce the heat to medium-low, add the chia seeds, and mix to combine. Bring the jam to a simmer and continue to simmer, stirring often, until it begins to thicken, about 10 minutes. Turn off the heat and let cool before transferring to a jar.

4. Store the jam in the refrigerator for up to 2 weeks.

notes: My favorite fruits for this jam are quartered or halved strawberries, whole blueberries, whole raspberries, and roughly chopped figs. If you use fruit with a lot of seeds, like raspberries or figs, reduce the amount of chia seeds to 1 tablespoon.

Because it contains chia seeds, I don't recommend canning this jam.

use in:

296
Jam Crumb Bars

serve with:

74
Buttery Drop Biscuits

94
The Ultimate Meat & Cheese Board

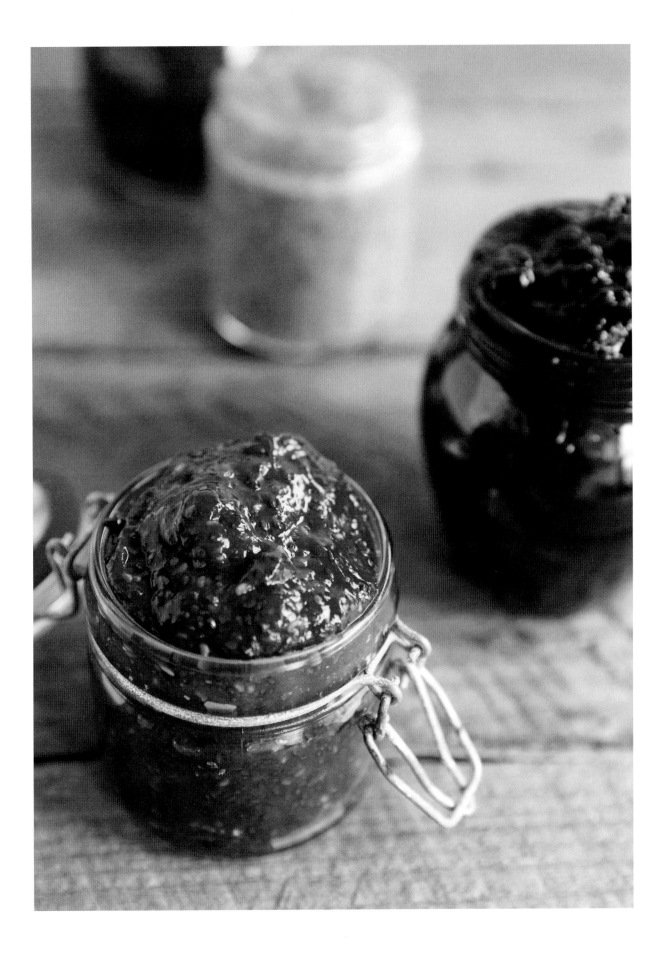

CARAMELIZED ONIONS

makes about 1 packed cup   *prep time* 5 minutes   *cook time* 30 minutes

EGG-FREE / NUT-FREE / PALEO-FRIENDLY OPTION: **use ghee instead of butter**

Caramelized onions are divine with just about everything! And they are easier to make than you might think. All you need is a little patience.

ingredients:

3 tablespoons ghee (page 350) or unsalted butter

2 large yellow onions, thinly sliced (about 5 cups)

½ teaspoon fine sea salt

note: Fond refers to the flavorful brown bits that begin to build up on the bottom of the pan.

directions:

1. Heat the ghee in a medium-sized heavy-bottomed sauté pan or skillet over medium-high heat. When the ghee is good and hot, add the onions. (The ghee is hot enough when it shimmers and bubbles after you add a drop of water to the pan.) Cook, untouched, until a fond (see note) starts to build up or the onions start to stick to the pan, about 5 minutes. Stir the onions.

2. Continue to stir once every 5 minutes for 20 to 25 minutes, adding a tablespoon of water if needed to deglaze the pan (adding water to the pan helps the onions caramelize quicker and helps redistribute the fond throughout the onions), until the onions begin to take on a deep brown color. If they begin to burn, reduce the heat to medium-low.

3. Once the onions are browned and caramelized, remove from the heat and use as desired. Store in the refrigerator for up to 1 week.

use in:

54
Kitchen Sink Frittata

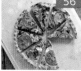
56
Quiche

164
Chicken Enchiladas

use on:

146
Chopped BBQ Chicken Cobb Salad

198
All-American Burgers

102
Prosciutto Flatbread with Grilled Peaches & Caramelized Onions

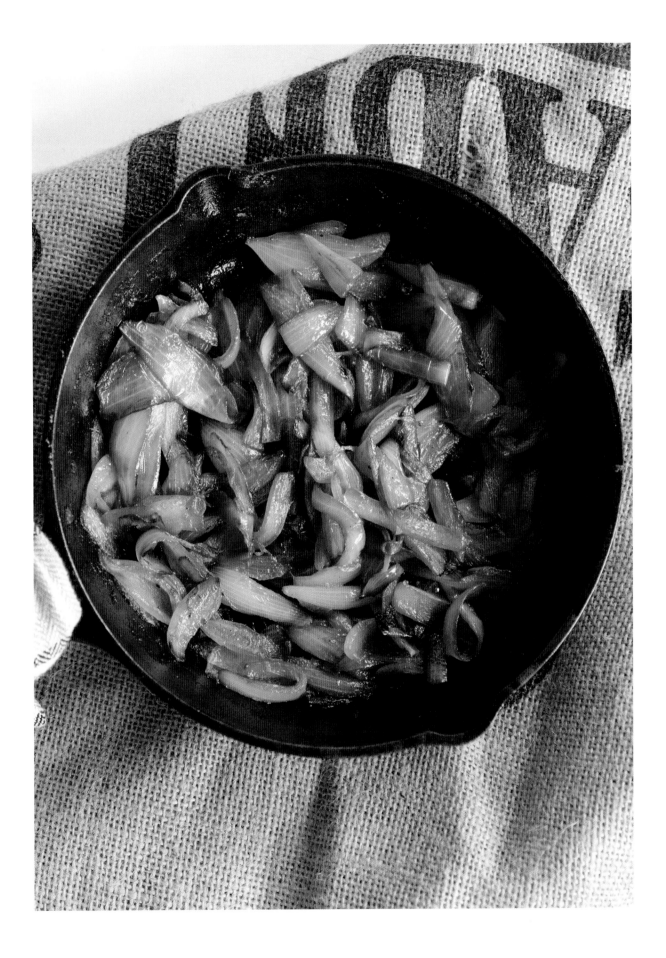

BALSAMIC GLAZE

makes ½ cup   *prep time* 2 minutes   *cook time* 20 minutes

EGG-FREE / NUT-FREE / DAIRY-FREE / PALEO-FRIENDLY / VEGAN

You can drizzle this glaze over bruschetta, bacon-wrapped scallops, grilled chicken or fish, pork tenderloin, or a caprese salad or serve it on strawberries for a snack. Try it on my Prosciutto Flatbread (page 102)!

ingredients:

1 cup good-quality balsamic vinegar (see note)

2 tablespoons granulated maple sugar or coconut sugar

¼ teaspoon fine sea salt

note: When reducing balsamic vinegar to make a glaze, I highly recommend using a good-quality vinegar. It'll affect the taste of the glaze dramatically. I try to buy local balsamic vinegar whenever possible, and I always look at expiration dates to make sure that it's fresh!

directions:

1. In a small saucepan, stir together the balsamic vinegar, sugar, and salt until combined. Bring the mixture to a boil over medium heat, stir once more, and then allow it to gently boil until it is reduced by about half and becomes thick and syrupy, 15 to 20 minutes.

2. Remove from the heat and let cool to room temperature. The glaze will thicken as it cools. If it becomes too thick, simply reheat it briefly over low heat before serving.

use in:

96
Bruschetta Bites with Balsamic Glaze

100
Bacon-Wrapped Scallops with Balsamic Glaze

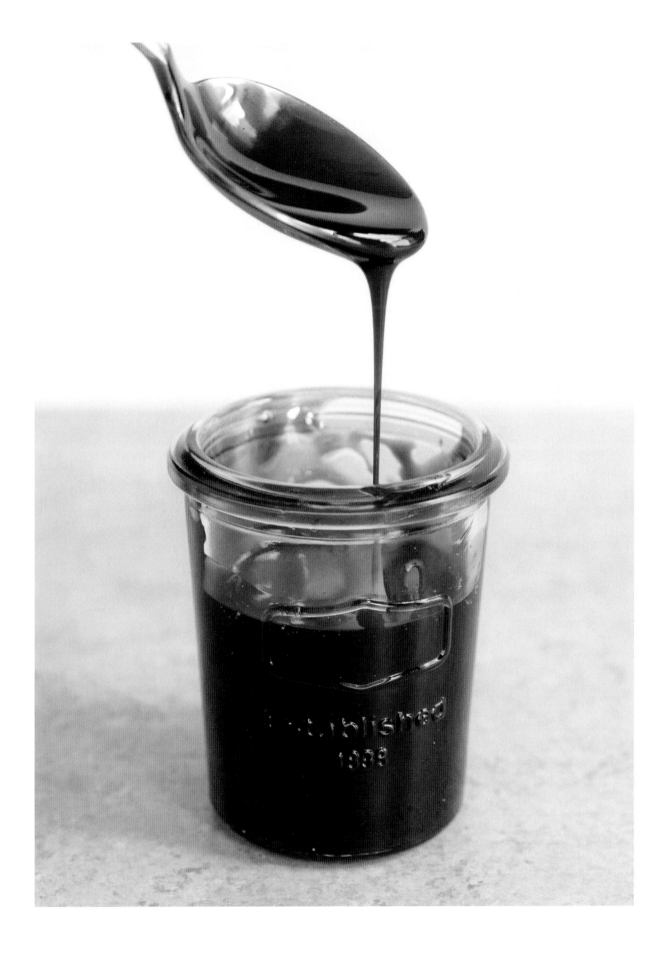

PERFECT BLENDER SALSA

makes 4 cups   *prep time* 10 minutes

EGG-FREE / NUT-FREE / DAIRY-FREE / PALEO-FRIENDLY

What makes restaurant salsa so different from store-bought salsa? Maybe it's the freshness! With this recipe, in less than fifteen minutes you'll have a fantastic salsa that is reminiscent of your favorite restaurant salsa, and you just might have the ingredients sitting in your pantry already. A high-speed blender makes this recipe come together really quickly—no chopping necessary—but it can also be made in a regular blender (see notes below).

ingredients:

1 (23-ounce) jar diced tomatoes, with juices (about 2½ cups)

1 (4-ounce) can diced green chiles

2 tablespoons tomato paste

⅓ cup fresh cilantro leaves

1 small white onion, roughly chopped

1 clove garlic

1 jalapeño pepper

Juice of 1 lime

1 teaspoon honey

1 teaspoon chili powder

1 teaspoon ground cumin

Pinch of fine sea salt

Optional: Pinch of red pepper flakes, or to taste

directions:

1. Place all of the ingredients in a high-speed blender. Pulse until the ingredients are roughly chopped and combined but the texture is still chunky. Continue to pulse until the salsa reaches your desired consistency—a quick pulse for chunky salsa or longer for smooth salsa.

2. Store the salsa in a closed container in the refrigerator for up to 2 weeks.

notes: I prefer to purchase jarred rather than canned tomato products because tomatoes packed in jars are free of additives. My go-to brand is Muir Glen. If buying canned, look for BPA-free. I also love Tuttorosso tomato products.

To make this salsa in a regular blender, roughly chop the onion, garlic, and jalapeño pepper before adding them to the blender.

use in:

134

Chicken Fajita Salads

use on:

78

Veggies, plantain chips, and/or crackers as a snack

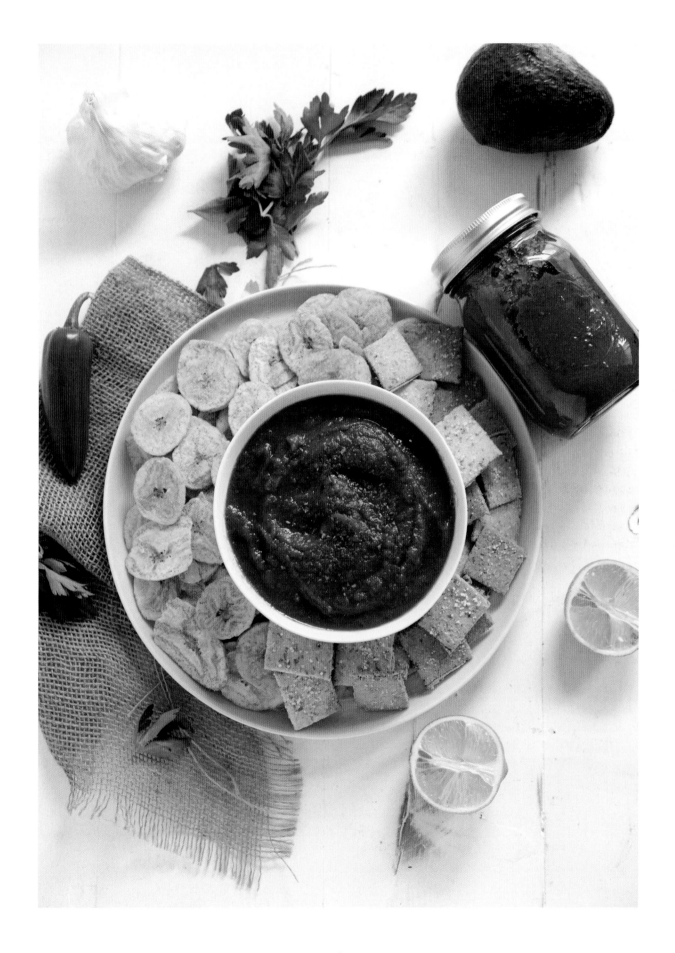

ALL-PURPOSE MARINARA SAUCE

makes 4 cups   *prep time* 5 minutes   *cook time* 20 minutes

EGG-FREE / NUT-FREE / DAIRY-FREE / PALEO-FRIENDLY /
VEGAN OPTION: use vegetable broth (page 356) instead of chicken broth

A flavorful marinara sauce is the key to a great dish! This go-to sauce is versatile enough for any type of "pasta" dish or pizza.

ingredients:

5 cloves garlic, minced

3 tablespoons extra-virgin olive oil

1 (15-ounce) can tomato sauce

1 (14½-ounce) can diced tomatoes

½ cup chicken broth, homemade (page 354) or store-bought

Leaves from 1 large sprig fresh basil or 1 teaspoon dried basil

1 teaspoon dried oregano leaves

1 teaspoon fine sea salt

½ teaspoon freshly ground black pepper

¼ teaspoon red pepper flakes

directions:

1. In a medium-sized saucepan over medium-high heat, sauté the garlic in the oil for 2 minutes, or until fragrant.

2. Add the tomato sauce, tomatoes, chicken broth, basil, oregano, salt, black pepper, and red pepper flakes to the pan. Bring to a boil, then reduce the heat and simmer for 20 minutes, until thickened. Taste and adjust the seasonings and spices as desired.

3. Once cool, store the sauce in a closed container in the refrigerator for up to 2 weeks.

note: If you wish, you can use whole canned tomatoes instead of diced. If using whole tomatoes, break them up with a wooden spoon while cooking.

use on:

Pizza Crust   Loaded Italian Meatballs

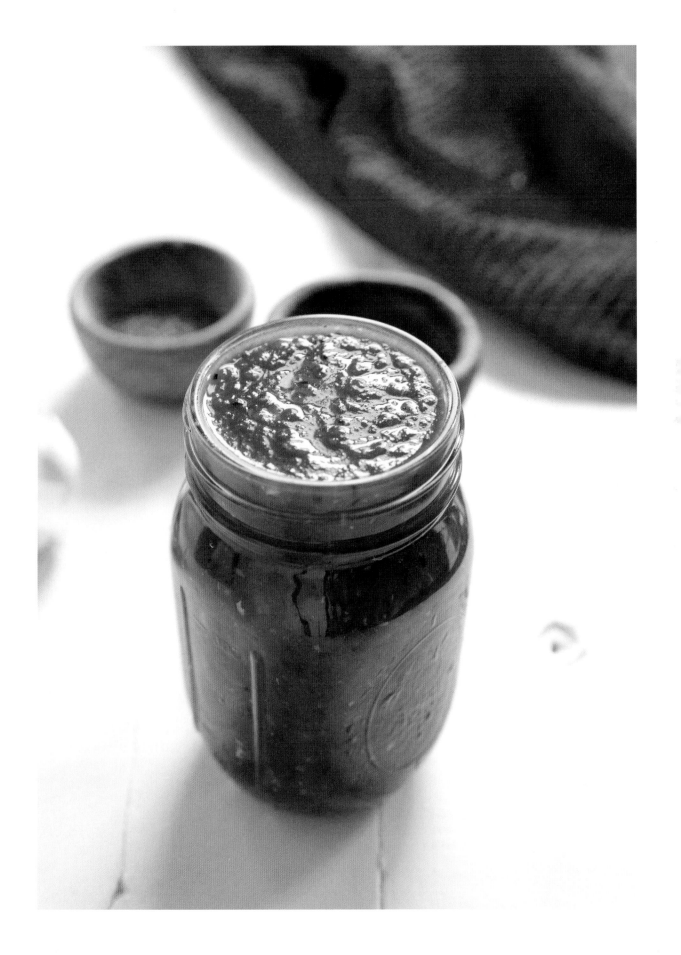

ALLA VODKA SAUCE

makes about 4½ cups   *prep time* 10 minutes   *cook time* 40 minutes

....

EGG-FREE / NUT-FREE / DAIRY-FREE OPTION: **use olive oil instead of butter**
PALEO-FRIENDLY OPTION: **use olive oil instead of butter**

....

Growing up, I just *loved* penne alla vodka. My best friend was equally into the dish, and we tried just about every rendition from the local Italian restaurants. I've developed this recipe for you so that you can make this flavorful sauce at home, store it in the refrigerator, and have it on hand for simple weeknight dinners. Set your traditional sauce aside and opt for alla vodka sauce instead! Throw in some chicken, too!

ingredients:

1 tablespoon unsalted butter or extra-virgin olive oil

3 cloves garlic, minced

1 onion, minced

1 shallot, minced

4 ounces prosciutto, chopped

1 (15-ounce) can crushed tomatoes

1 (14½-ounce) can diced tomatoes

⅓ cup gluten-free vodka (such as Tito's)

½ cup full-fat coconut milk

2 to 3 tablespoons chopped fresh basil

½ teaspoon red pepper flakes, or more to taste

Dash of fine sea salt, or more to taste

Dash of freshly ground black pepper, or more to taste

directions:

1. Melt the butter in a medium-sized skillet over medium heat. Add the garlic, onion, and shallot and cook for 5 minutes, until fragrant. Add the prosciutto and cook for about 5 minutes more, until the prosciutto is crispy and the onion is soft.

2. Add the crushed tomatoes, diced tomatoes, and vodka. Stir to combine, then reduce the heat to low and simmer for 10 minutes, until the vodka begins to evaporate and the sauce is reduced slightly.

3. Add the coconut milk, basil, red pepper flakes, salt, and black pepper. Bring to a boil over medium heat, then reduce the heat to low and simmer for 25 minutes, until the sauce has thickened slightly and is fragrant. Taste and add additional salt, pepper, and red pepper flakes, if desired.

4. Use immediately or allow to cool to room temperature before storing in a closed container. The sauce will keep in the refrigerator for up to 1 week.

use on:

248

Zucchini Noodles or Spaghetti Squash Noodles

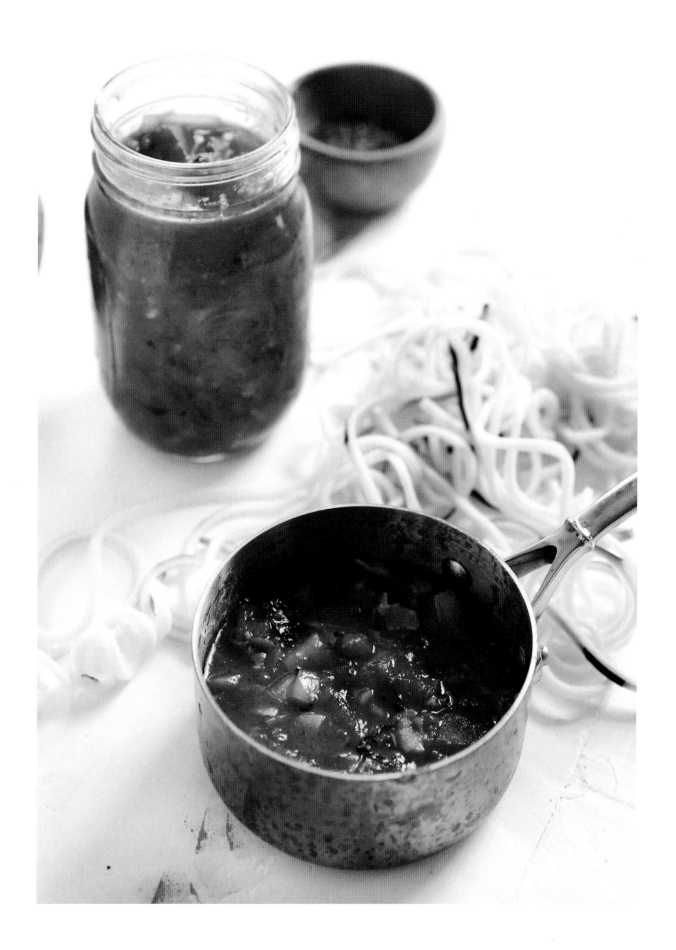

KETCHUP

makes 2 cups *prep time* 5 minutes *cook time* 10 minutes

EGG-FREE / NUT-FREE / DAIRY-FREE / PALEO-FRIENDLY

Who doesn't love ketchup? It's hard to think of a more beloved condiment. But too often, store-bought options are filled with ingredients that you don't want to eat. This one leaves out all of the added junk! If you feel like making your own ketchup, this is my go-to recipe.

ingredients:

1 cup crushed plum tomatoes

1 (6-ounce) can tomato paste

½ cup apple cider vinegar

¼ cup water, or more if you want a thinner consistency

3 tablespoons coconut sugar

2 tablespoons honey

2 teaspoons garlic powder

2 teaspoons onion powder

1½ teaspoons dry mustard

½ teaspoon fine sea salt

directions:

1. Place all of the ingredients in a blender and blend on high speed until well combined.

2. Transfer the mixture to a saucepan. Bring to a boil, then lower the heat and simmer for 5 minutes, until the color darkens slightly. Make sure to lower the heat right when the ketchup begins to boil; if left at a boil for too long, it will begin to splatter.

3. Taste and add more onion powder, garlic powder, or dry mustard, if desired.

4. Pour the ketchup back into the blender and process on high speed again, until fully smooth. Let cool completely before serving or bottling. Store in the refrigerator for up to 2 weeks.

use in:

Cocktail Sauce — 92

Thai BBQ Salmon — 188

use on:

Sweet Potato Truffle Fries — 226

All-American Burgers — 198

Classic Baked Chicken Nuggets — 158

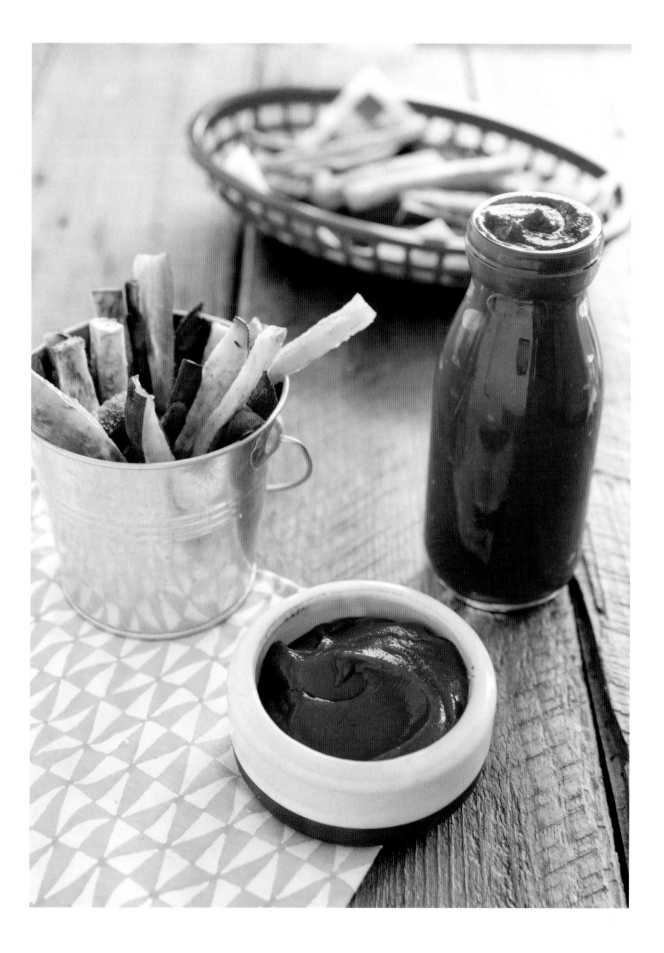

AVOCADO CREMA

makes ⅓ to ½ cup   *prep time* 5 minutes

EGG-FREE / NUT-FREE / DAIRY-FREE / PALEO-FRIENDLY / VEGAN

I'm about to transform taco night! Avocado crema takes less than five minutes to throw together, and it makes a wonderful addition to so many dishes.

ingredients:

1 avocado, peeled and pitted

1 tablespoon full-fat coconut milk

1 teaspoon lime juice

Pinch of fine sea salt

Pinch of freshly ground black pepper

directions:

Place all of the ingredients in a blender and blend on high speed for 30 seconds, or until smooth. The crema is best consumed as soon as it's made.

use on:

Fish Tacos — 190

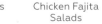
Chicken Fajita Salads — 134

Patatas Bravas — 108

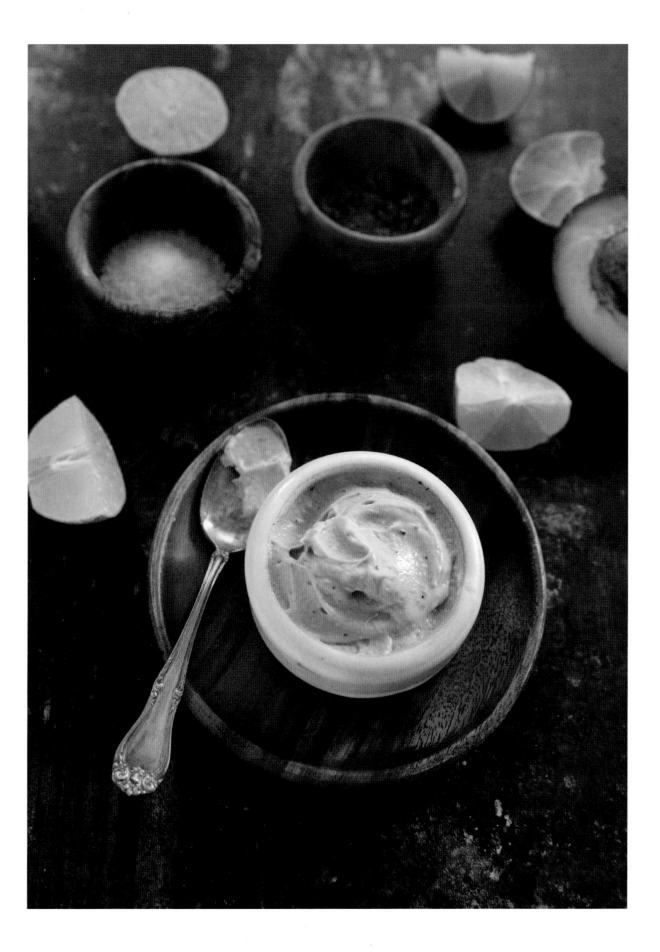

HOMEMADE PREPARED HORSERADISH

makes 1 cup   *prep time* 15 minutes

EGG-FREE / NUT-FREE / DAIRY-FREE / PALEO-FRIENDLY / VEGAN

Don't be intimidated by this recipe! Making homemade horseradish is easy peasy—you just have to follow a few precautions (see the tips below). I love making my own because it's so much more potent and flavorful than store-bought, and it's made without added ingredients. Plus, it's cheaper! It will make your next batch of cocktail sauce taste fresher and more flavorful than you can imagine, and it makes the best creamy horseradish sauce for meat. And you must try sprinkling some on top of seafood!

ingredients:

2 cups peeled and cubed fresh horseradish root (about 1 pound)

¼ cup water

3 tablespoons white vinegar

Pinch of fine sea salt

directions:

1. Place the horseradish root and water in a food processor. Pulse until the horseradish is ground into small pieces about the size of rice.

2. Transfer the horseradish to an 8-ounce jar (be careful here; ground horseradish is potent!). If you like a very hot horseradish, wait about 5 minutes, then add the vinegar and mix to combine. If you like a milder horseradish, add the vinegar right away. Stir in the salt. Secure the lid and store the horseradish in the refrigerator for up to 3 weeks.

Tips for Working with Fresh Horseradish:

After working with fresh horseradish, be mindful to wash your hands and all of the equipment you used thoroughly.

Once the root is ground, it is very potent and releases strong vapors that can sting your eyes. So don't lean in and take a whiff! Work in a well-ventilated room and keep the root at arm's length.

use in:

Cocktail Sauce

Horseradish Mayo

Beef Tenderloin with Creamy Horseradish Sauce

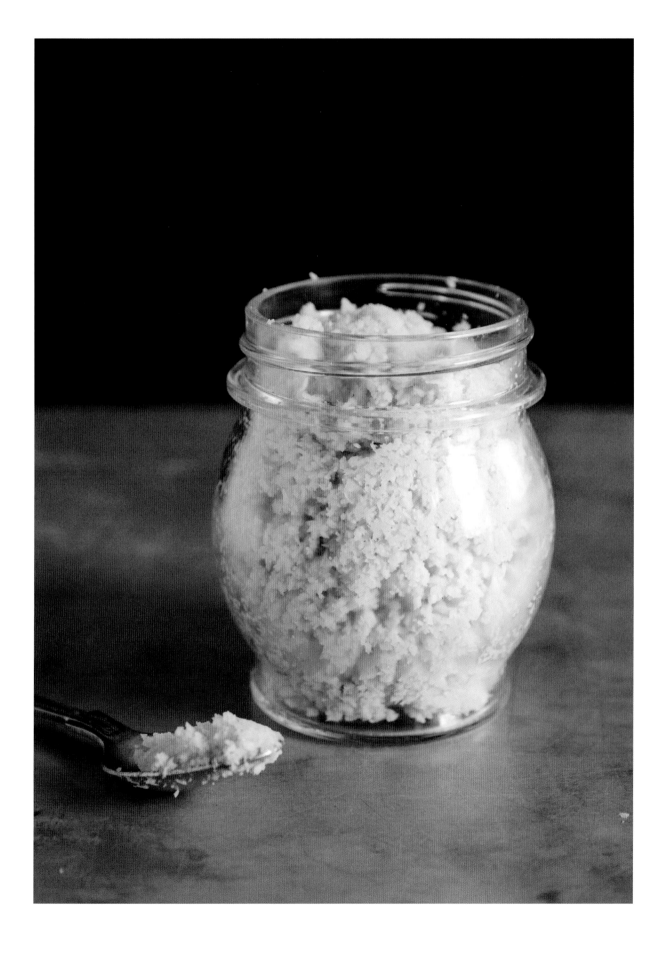

SLOW COOKER APPLESAUCE

makes about 2 cups   *prep time* 10 minutes   *cook time* 2 or 4 hours

EGG-FREE / NUT-FREE / DAIRY-FREE / PALEO-FRIENDLY / VEGAN

Ah, homemade applesauce. The flavor of store-bought simply does not compare! This applesauce is delicious on its own and even more delicious when used to top a potato pancake or in baking. You can also use this recipe to make apple butter; it just requires a bit more cooking time.

ingredients:

10 to 12 cooking apples, cored, peeled, and halved (see note)

1 cup apple juice, apple cider, or water

1 teaspoon lemon juice

½ teaspoon vanilla extract

½ teaspoon ground cinnamon

¼ teaspoon ground cloves

¼ teaspoon ground nutmeg

¼ teaspoon fine sea salt

directions:

1. Place all of the ingredients in a slow cooker, cover, and cook on high for 2 hours or low for 4 hours. Allow to cool to room temperature.

2. If you prefer chunky applesauce, gently mash with a fork or potato masher. If you prefer smooth applesauce, blend with an immersion blender or transfer to a blender and blend until smooth.

3. Transfer the applesauce to a closed container and store in the refrigerator for up to 2 weeks.

note: I use a mix of McIntosh and Cortland apples for applesauce, but any sweet and tart cooking apples will work.

variation: **Slow Cooker Apple Butter.** Complete Step 1, but cook the mixture on low for 8 hours. Once done, blend the mixture with an immersion blender or in a jar blender until it is completely smooth. Transfer the mixture to a medium-sized saucepan and simmer over medium-low heat for 20 to 30 minutes, until it is thick and spreadable. Once cool, transfer to a closed container and store in the refrigerator for up to 2 weeks.

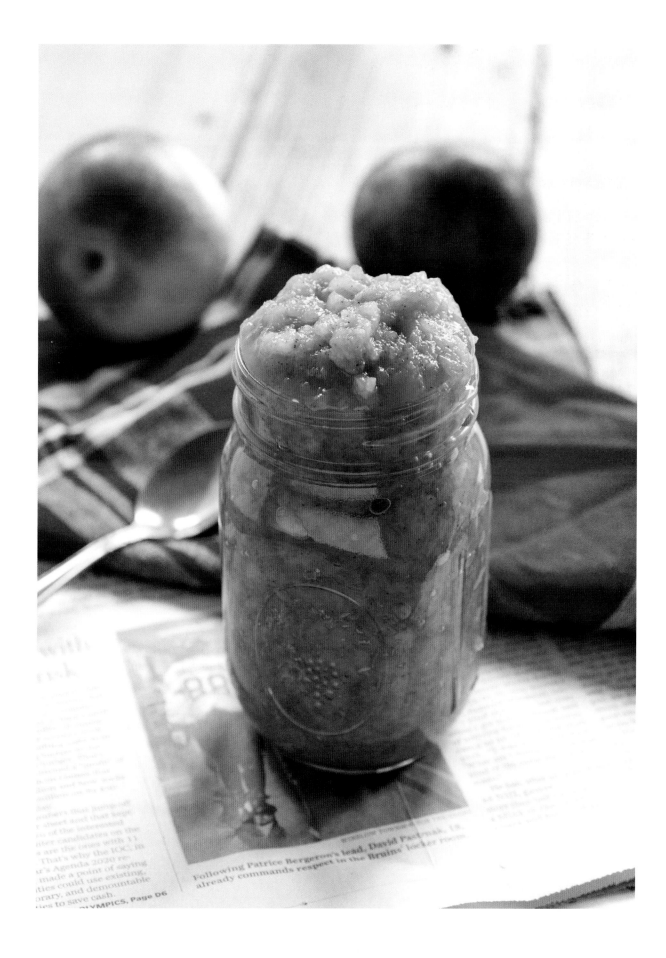

GHEE

makes about 1 cup   *prep time* less than 1 minute   *cook time* 20 minutes

EGG-FREE / NUT-FREE / PALEO-FRIENDLY

Because ghee is butter with the milk solids removed, it is a wonderful alternative for many people who want to cook with butter but can't tolerate the lactose in dairy. I love making my own ghee because it saves me money and is simple to prepare. I use it to make roasted potatoes, roasted chicken, and sautéed veggies and even in baking!

ingredients:

1 cup (2 sticks) unsalted butter, cubed

directions:

1. Melt the butter in a small saucepan over medium-low heat. Once melted, the butter will separate into three layers: a foam layer will appear on the top, and the milk solids will migrate to the bottom of the pan. The clarified butter will float between the other two layers.

2. Let the butter come to a simmer and continue to simmer until the middle layer becomes fragrant, more golden, and clear and the milk solids at the bottom begin to brown, about 5 minutes.

3. Turn off the heat and use a spoon to skim the top layer of foam into a bowl. Pour the clear, golden layer through a fine-mesh strainer into a jar, leaving the milk solids at the bottom of the pan.

4. The ghee will keep at room temperature for up to 3 months.

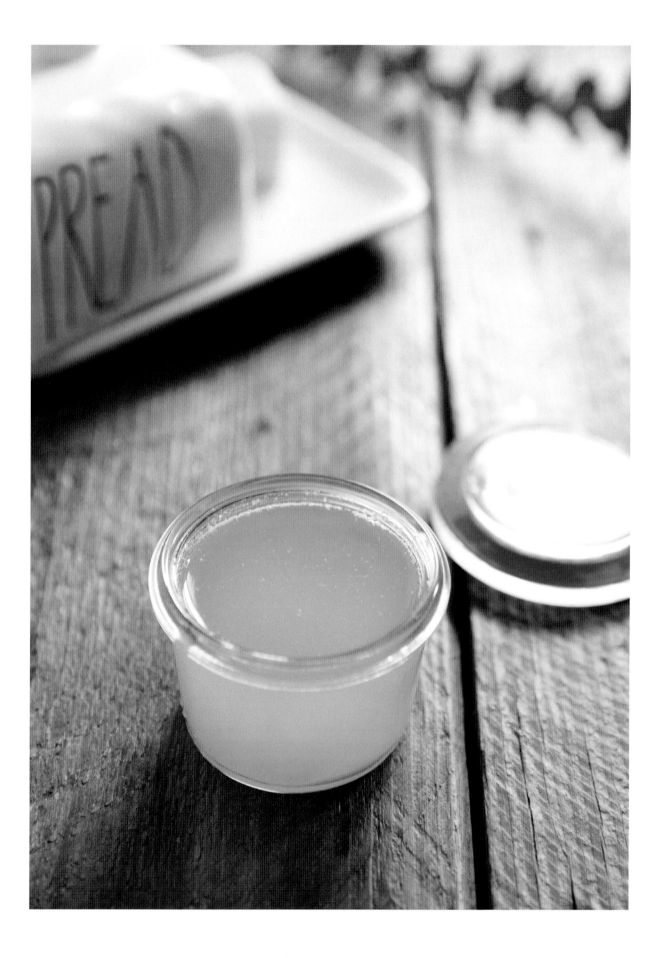

CHIMICHURRI

makes about ½ cup   *prep time* 5 minutes

EGG-FREE / NUT-FREE / DAIRY-FREE / PALEO-FRIENDLY / VEGAN

Is chimichurri the ultimate steak topper or what? (Or is it just me who thinks that?) Chimichurri is also amazing on potatoes and seafood. Basically, it's amazing on just about everything! It is simply every flavor you could want in one simple little sauce.

ingredients:

1 packed cup fresh flat-leaf parsley leaves
½ packed cup fresh cilantro leaves
⅓ cup extra-virgin olive oil
2 tablespoons apple cider vinegar
2 cloves garlic, roughly chopped
½ teaspoon ground cumin
½ teaspoon red pepper flakes
¼ teaspoon fine sea salt

directions:

1. Place all of the ingredients in a food processor or blender and puree until smooth.

2. Store the sauce in a closed container in the refrigerator for up to 1 week.

note: If you use a high-speed blender to make this sauce, there's no need to chop the garlic. Simply peel the cloves and drop them into the blender whole.

use on:

226
Sweet Potato Truffle Fries

194
Chimichurri Shrimp

212
Grilled Steak

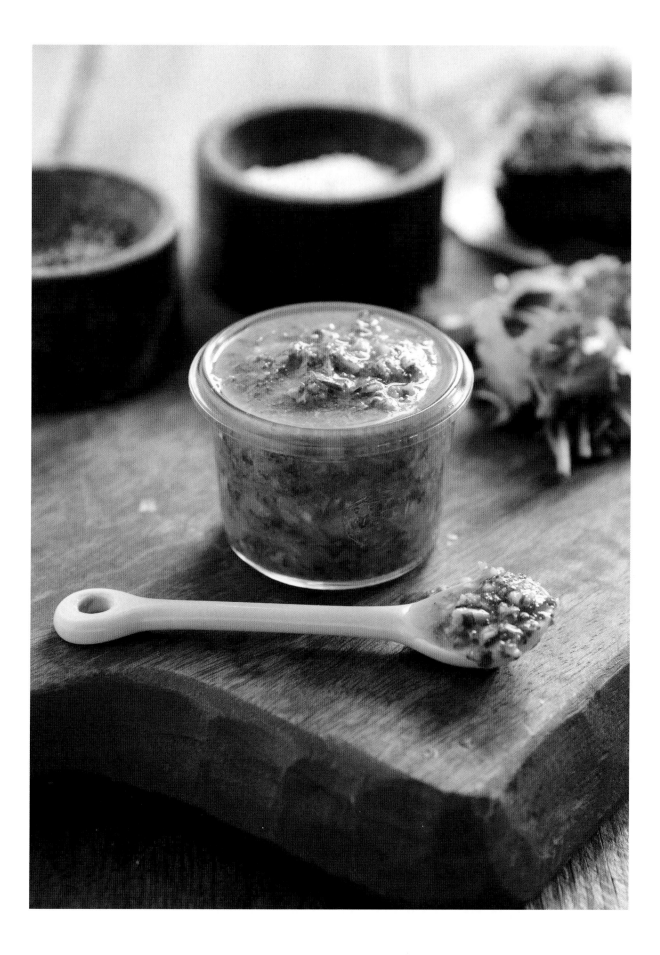

EASY CHICKEN BROTH

makes about 1 quart   *prep time* 10 minutes
cook time 45 minutes (in a pressure cooker) or 8 to 10 hours (in a slow cooker)

EGG-FREE / NUT-FREE / DAIRY-FREE / PALEO-FRIENDLY

I use chicken broth as a base in many of my dishes and on its own as a cure when I'm feeling under the weather. It's one of those classic flavors that instantly make me think of home, childhood, and family holidays. If you have the time to make your own, it's so worth it! With the pressure cooker option, you'll have rich broth in no time. If you're serving the broth on its own, you can make it more flavorful by adding some chopped fresh parsley leaves and additional salt and pepper to taste.

ingredients:

1 onion
1 large carrot
1 large leek
3 cloves garlic
3 pounds assorted chicken bones
1 tablespoon apple cider vinegar
1 teaspoon fine sea salt
1 bay leaf (for slow cooker method only)
6 to 8 cups water

tips: Try freezing the broth in ice cube trays for easy use!

When cooking white rice, use chicken broth instead of water as the cooking liquid to enhance the flavor.

variation:

Easy Beef Broth. Swap out the chicken bones for beef bones.

Pressure Cooker Directions:

1. Roughly chop the veggies and garlic and place them in a pressure cooker. Add the bones, vinegar, and salt. (Do not use a bay leaf if making the broth in a pressure cooker.)

2. Pour just enough water over the vegetables and bones to cover them (6 to 8 cups).

3. Cover and seal the pressure cooker. Using the manual timer, set the pressure cooker to high for 45 minutes. Once done, shut off the heat and let sit for 15 minutes before opening. After 15 minutes, open the pressure cooker and strain the broth through a fine-mesh sieve into jars. Taste and add more salt, if desired.

4. Store the broth in a closed container in the refrigerator for up to 5 days or in the freezer for up to a year.

Slow Cooker Directions:

1. Roughly chop the veggies and garlic and place them in a slow cooker. Add the bones, vinegar, salt, and bay leaf.

2. Pour just enough water over the vegetables and bones to cover them (6 to 8 cups).

3. Cover the slow cooker, set it to low, and cook the broth for 8 to 10 hours. Once done, strain the broth through a fine-mesh sieve into jars. Taste and add more salt, if desired.

4. Store the broth in a closed container in the refrigerator for up to 5 days or in the freezer for up to a year.

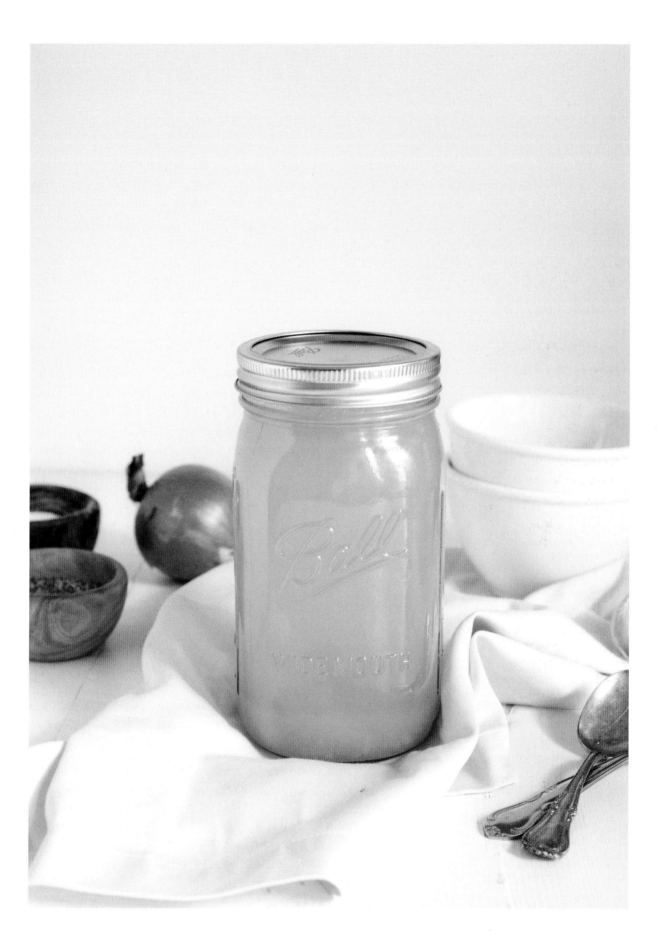

EASY VEGETABLE BROTH

makes about 5 cups   *prep time* 10 minutes   *cook time* 50 minutes

EGG-FREE / NUT-FREE / DAIRY-FREE / PALEO-FRIENDLY / VEGAN

ingredients:

1 tablespoon extra-virgin olive oil

3 carrots, peeled and chopped (see notes)

3 stalks celery, chopped

2 onions, chopped

2 cloves garlic, peeled

FOR THE BOUQUET GARNI:

3 sprigs fresh flat-leaf parsley

8 black peppercorns

2 bay leaves

Optional: 1 teaspoon grated lemon zest

8 cups water, or enough to cover the vegetables by 1 inch

1 teaspoon fine sea salt

SPECIAL EQUIPMENT (OPTIONAL):

Cheesecloth

Butcher's twine

directions:

1. Heat the oil in a large stockpot over medium heat. Add the veggies and garlic and cook, stirring often, until tender, about 5 minutes.

2. Make the bouquet garni: Set the ingredients on a piece of cheesecloth, then wrap the cloth up and around them to form a bundle. Use a piece of butcher's twine to tie it closed.

3. To the pot, add the water, bouquet garni, and salt, along with any vegetable scraps you have on hand (like onion peels and radish tops, rinsed beforehand).

4. Cover the pot and bring to a boil, then lower the heat and simmer, partially covered, for 45 minutes, until the vegetables are completely soft and the broth is fragrant.

5. Discard the bouquet garni, then strain the broth through a fine-mesh sieve into jars. Taste and add more salt, if desired.

6. Store the broth in a closed container in the refrigerator for up to 5 days or in the freezer for up to a year.

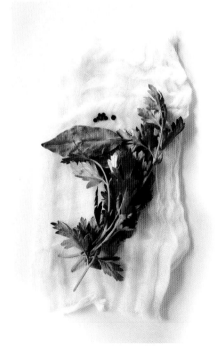

notes: If you use organic carrots, you don't need to peel them.

If you have some on hand, add halved radishes, peeled and cubed turnips, mushroom stems, and/or cored tomatoes.

A bouquet garni is handy because it makes straining easier. However, if you don't have cheesecloth, you can simply add the bouquet garni ingredients directly to the pot in Step 3 since you are straining the broth anyway.

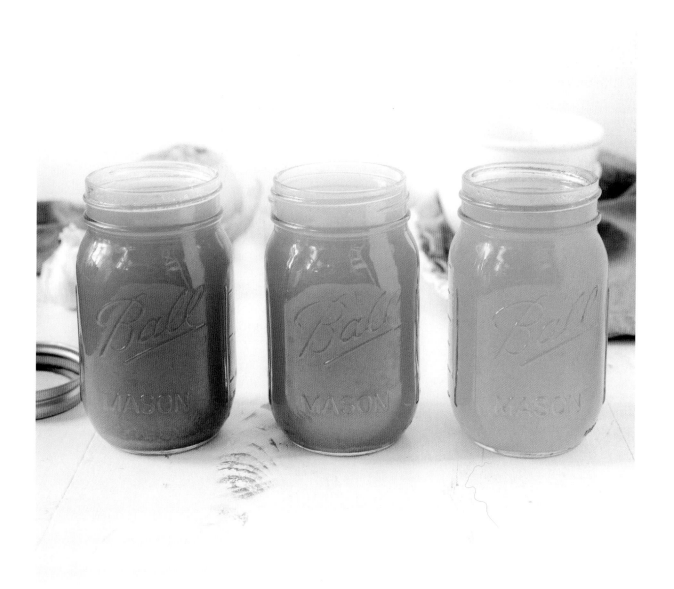

HOMEMADE CHOCOLATE HAZELNUT SPREAD

makes 1½ cups   *prep time* 10 minutes   *cook time* 20 minutes

EGG-FREE / DAIRY-FREE / PALEO-FRIENDLY

Chocolaty, creamy, indulgent, and delicious: This spread brings me back to those good old high school and college days when eating Nutella by the spoonful was acceptable. Wait, it's not now? Well, not exactly, but this version is a healthy alternative. Simply put, this spread is divine. You'll want to eat it by the spoonful, use it to top your waffles, and slather it on just about everything! Try it as a snack with a banana, some strawberries, and fresh granola (page 44 or 46). It's fabulous on pizza crust topped with fresh fruit as a dessert pizza, too!

ingredients:

2 cups raw hazelnuts

¼ cup coconut sugar

2 tablespoons cocoa powder

1 tablespoon coconut oil, melted, plus more if needed

1 teaspoon vanilla extract

Pinch of fine sea salt

1 cup dark chocolate chunks (about 70% cacao)

1 tablespoon honey

directions:

1. Preheat the oven to 400°F.

2. Spread the hazelnuts on a rimmed baking sheet and bake for 10 minutes, until the nuts have darkened and the skins have begun to flake off. Watch closely to avoid burning the hazelnuts. Remove from the oven and let cool for 5 minutes.

3. Place the hazelnuts in the center of a large kitchen towel, gather the sides of the towel together to form a pouch, and rub and shake until the brown skins of the nuts start to peel off. When most of the skins have been removed—don't worry if a few stubborn ones remain—transfer the nuts to a food processor and process for roughly 5 minutes, until a smooth butter forms, scraping down the sides as needed while processing.

4. Add the coconut sugar, cocoa powder, coconut oil, vanilla, and salt to the food processor and blend for another 3 to 5 minutes, until smooth.

use on:

Best-Ever Fluffy Waffles

Best-Ever Fluffy Pancakes

French Vanilla Muffins

Pizza Crust

5. Melt the chocolate: Fill the bottom of a double boiler with water so that the water level is ½ inch below the upper pan. (You can use a heatproof bowl set on top of a pot if you don't have a double boiler.) Place over low heat, put the chocolate and honey in the top pan, and stir constantly until the chocolate is melted. Do not allow the water to come to a boil.

6. Pour the melted chocolate mixture into the food processor and blend until smooth, about 5 minutes. Add additional coconut oil if the spread isn't as smooth as you'd like.

7. Store the spread in a closed container in the pantry for up to 2 weeks.

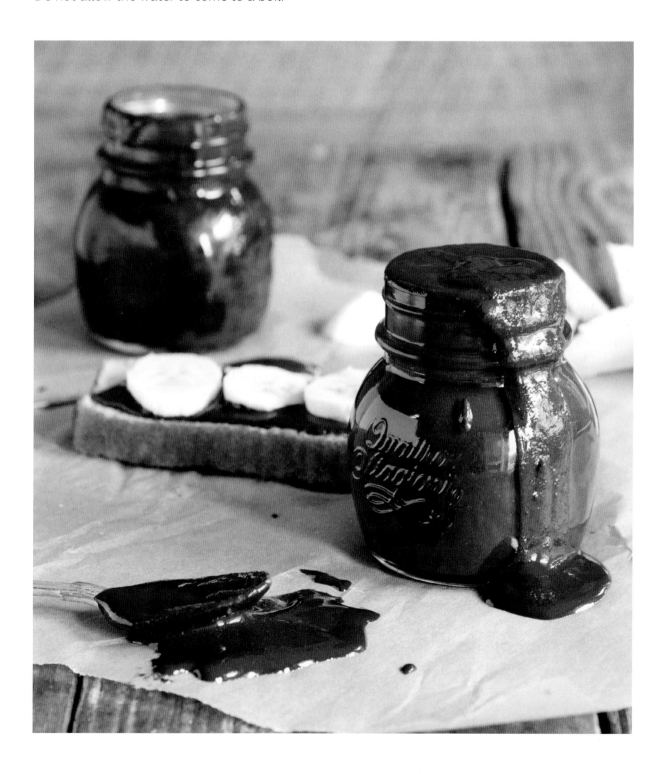

ALL-PURPOSE CARAMEL SAUCE

makes ½ cup   *prep time* 2 minutes   *cook time* 40 minutes

EGG-FREE / NUT-FREE / PALEO-FRIENDLY OPTION: use ghee instead of butter

I call this caramel sauce "all-purpose" because what *isn't* caramel sauce good on? I'll answer that for you—it's basically perfect on everything! The vanilla bean adds a little extra touch of delight to this classic caramel.

ingredients:

1 cup full-fat coconut milk

½ cup honey or pure maple syrup

1 tablespoon unsalted butter or ghee (page 350)

½ teaspoon vanilla extract

Seeds scraped from ½ vanilla bean

Pinch of fine sea salt

directions:

1. Combine all of the ingredients in a saucepan, then bring the mixture to a boil over medium heat. If it begins to boil over, quickly stir it down and/or momentarily slide the pan off the heat. Reduce the heat to low and simmer for about 30 minutes, until the caramel begins to thicken and coats the back of a spoon. For thicker caramel, simmer longer.

2. Remove from the heat, let cool for 5 minutes, and then serve immediately.

3. Store the cooled caramel sauce in a closed container in the refrigerator for up to 2 weeks. Bring to room temperature before serving.

use on:

60

Chocolate Turtle Chia Pudding

306

Caramel Brownie Cupcakes

40

Crepes

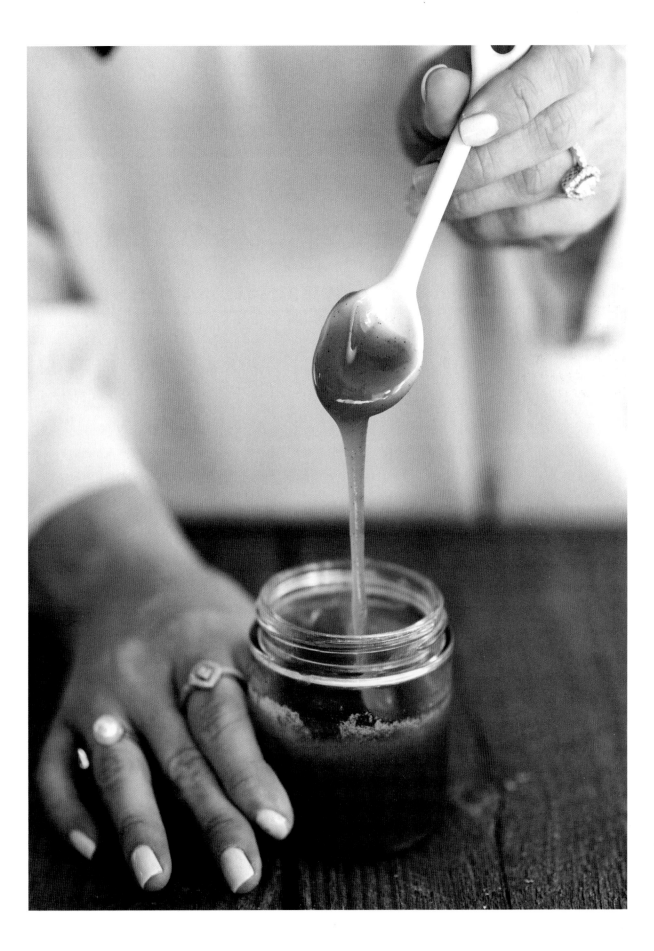

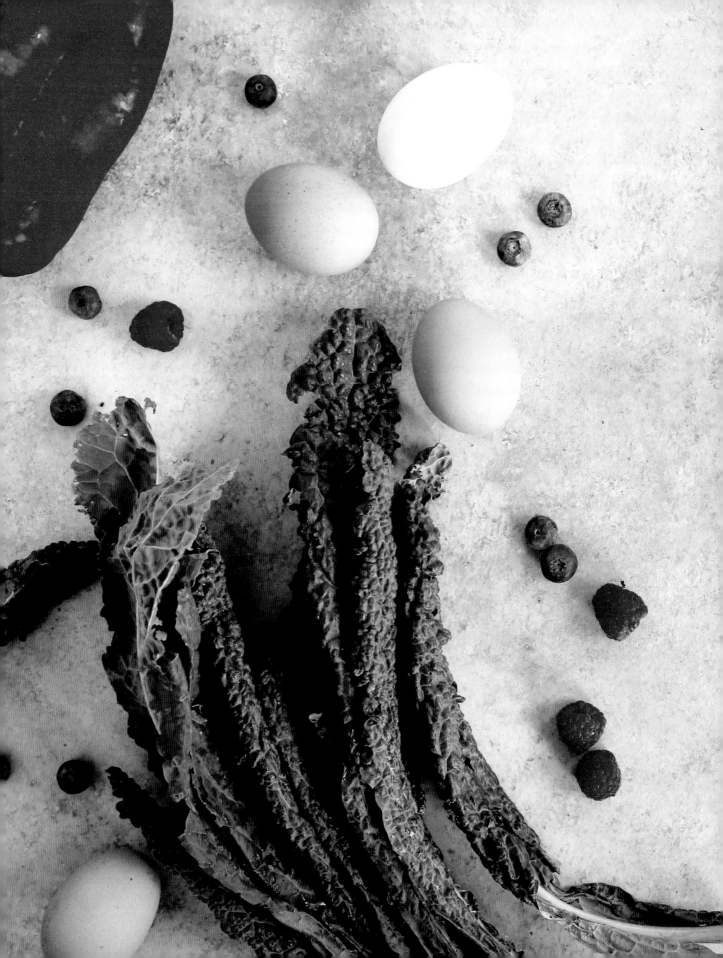

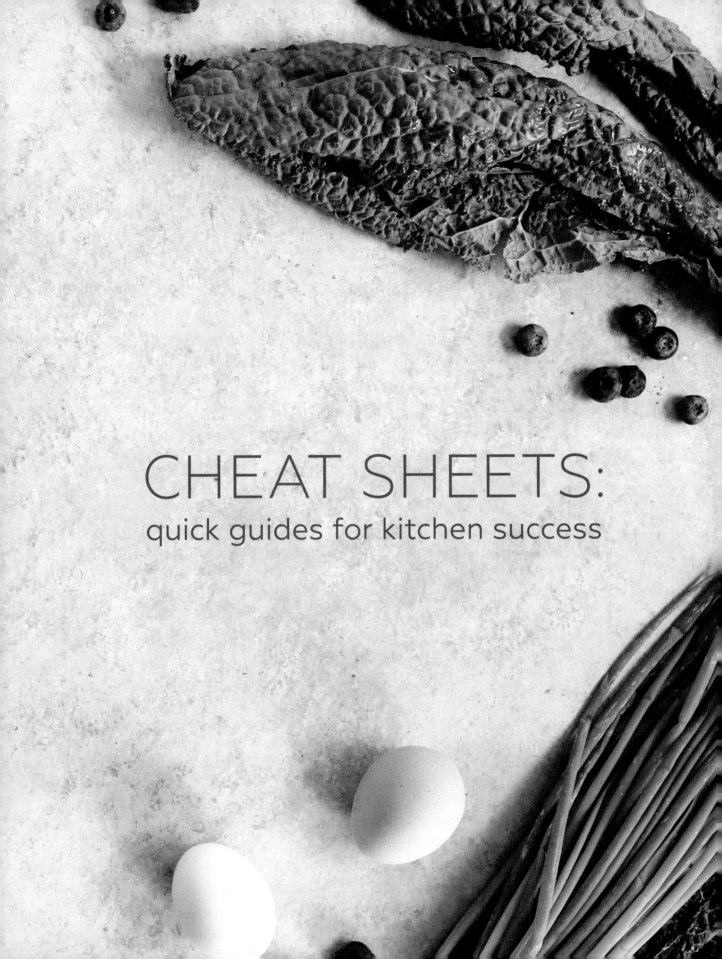

CHEAT SHEETS:
quick guides for kitchen success

BUILD A JUICE AT HOME

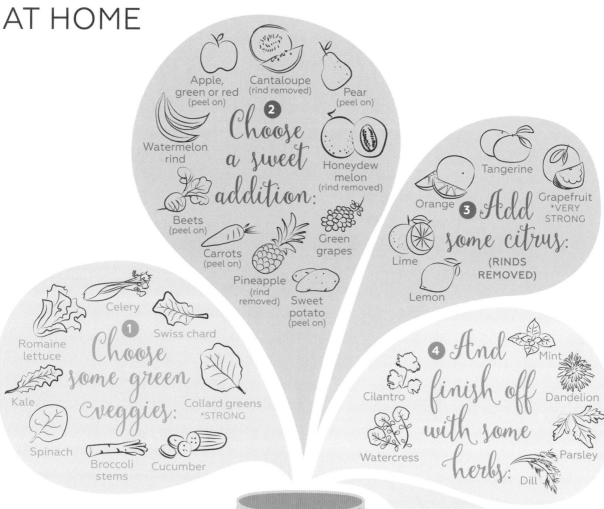

2 Choose a sweet addition:

- Apple, green or red (peel on)
- Cantaloupe (rind removed)
- Pear (peel on)
- Watermelon rind
- Honeydew melon (rind removed)
- Beets (peel on)
- Carrots (peel on)
- Green grapes
- Pineapple (rind removed)
- Sweet potato (peel on)

3 Add some citrus: (RINDS REMOVED)

- Tangerine
- Orange
- Grapefruit *VERY STRONG
- Lime
- Lemon

1 Choose some green veggies:

- Celery
- Swiss chard
- Romaine lettuce
- Kale
- Collard greens *STRONG
- Spinach
- Broccoli stems
- Cucumber

4 And finish off with some herbs:

- Cilantro
- Mint
- Dandelion
- Watercress
- Parsley
- Dill

5 And/or some healing powers:

- Fresh ginger
- Cayenne pepper
- Fresh turmeric or turmeric powder
- Fresh garlic

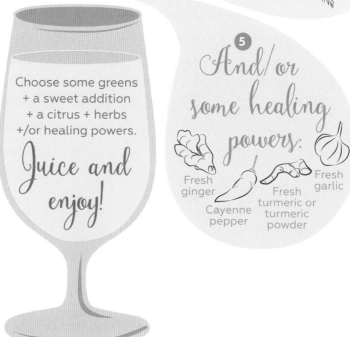

Choose some greens + a sweet addition + a citrus + herbs +/or healing powers.

Juice and enjoy!

note:

For one 8-ounce serving of juice, I like to pick one or two green veggies, one sweet addition, one citrus, and one herb and/or healing power. Depending on the juice, the green veggies and sweet additions shouldn't be used in equal amounts. I use more green veggies than I do sweet.

Best if enjoyed right away.

Will keep in the fridge for 1 day.

BUILD THE PERFECT SMOOTHIE

3 Make it green: (1 CUP)

- Avocado, diced
- Romaine lettuce
- Spinach
- Kale

EXTRAS

Make it thick and creamy: (1 TO 2 TABLESPOONS)

- Nut butter: sunflower seed or almond (no added sugars)
- Coconut meat
- Gluten-free oats
- Chia seeds
- Ice

2 Choose some fresh or frozen fruit: (1 TO 2 CUPS)*

- Mango slices
- Raspberries
- Blueberries
- Apples, cut into large pieces
- Pineapple chunks
- Strawberries
- Frozen açai
- Peach slices
- Bananas, cut into chunks

*Use less fruit if frozen, more if fresh.

EXTRAS

Give it a boost:

- Bee pollen
- Protein powder of choice
- Flaxseed
- Fresh ginger
- Coconut oil or MCT oil

1 Choose a base: (1 CUP)

- Almond milk
- Iced green tea
- Water
- Coconut milk
- Coconut water
- Fresh juice
- Iced coffee

Assemble:

Place the smoothie ingredients of choice in a blender and puree until smooth: 1 to 2 minutes in a high-speed blender or longer in a regular blender.

EXTRAS

A little something sweet:

- Figs
- Cinnamon
- Pure maple syrup
- Vanilla extract
- Dates
- Raw honey

banana tip: Always keep a bag of peeled and cut-up bananas in your freezer! They are superior to ice for creating a thick and creamy texture, not to mention a sweet flavor.

MAKE A SOUP

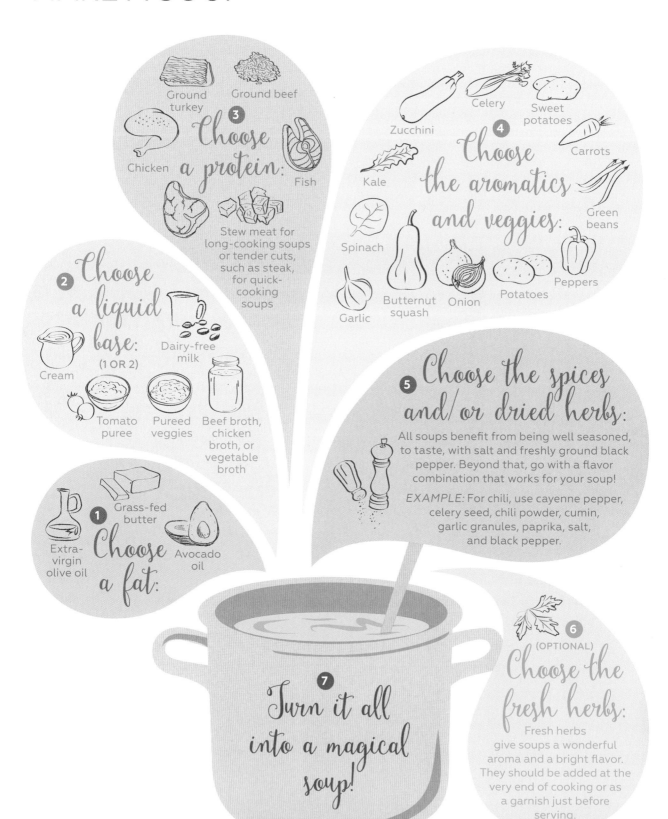

Ground turkey

Ground beef

3 Choose a protein:

Chicken

Fish

Stew meat for long-cooking soups or tender cuts, such as steak, for quick-cooking soups

Zucchini

Celery

Sweet potatoes

Carrots

4 Choose the aromatics and veggies:

Kale

Green beans

Spinach

Garlic

Butternut squash

Onion

Potatoes

Peppers

2 Choose a liquid base:
(1 OR 2)

Dairy-free milk

Cream

Tomato puree

Pureed veggies

Beef broth, chicken broth, or vegetable broth

5 Choose the spices and/or dried herbs:

All soups benefit from being well seasoned, to taste, with salt and freshly ground black pepper. Beyond that, go with a flavor combination that works for your soup!

EXAMPLE: For chili, use cayenne pepper, celery seed, chili powder, cumin, garlic granules, paprika, salt, and black pepper.

1 Grass-fed butter

Extra-virgin olive oil

Choose a fat:

Avocado oil

6 (OPTIONAL) **Choose the fresh herbs:**
Fresh herbs give soups a wonderful aroma and a bright flavor. They should be added at the very end of cooking or as a garnish just before serving.

7 Turn it all into a magical soup!

Turn it all into a magical soup!

1. Heat some fat in a stockpot or other large pot, like a Dutch oven. Add some aromatics (like onion and garlic) and sauté for 3 to 5 minutes, then add some meat to the pot and brown it.

2. Add long-cooking veggies like carrots and potatoes and cook for 5 to 10 minutes, until fork-tender. Add softer veggies, like spinach, toward the end.

3. Add the liquid base(s) and spices and mix well to combine. Add more liquid base for a thinner soup or less for a thicker soup (note that pureeing the soup will also create a thicker consistency).

4. Bring to a boil, then reduce the heat and simmer, covered, until the meat is fully cooked and tender. Remove any bones from the meat.

5. Add cream if you want a cream soup. Transfer a portion or all of the soup to a blender if you want a partially or fully pureed soup. (*Note:* Do not overfill your blender with hot soup. Puree the soup in batches, if needed.)

6. Taste for seasoning and adjust if needed. Garnish, if desired, and enjoy!

Tips:

 • Choose a meat that complements your base (for example, chicken with chicken broth).

 • Consider using two bases, such as chicken broth and diced tomatoes or pureed tomatoes and cream.

 • Use whatever veggies you have on hand, but go in with a game plan for the type of soup you want to create!

 • Taste as you go and add more salt and/or spices incrementally to avoid over-seasoned or over-spiced soup!

WHAT'S IN SEASON WHEN?

Peak Season •••	Spring	Summer	Fall	Winter
Apples			••••••••••••••••••••••••••••	
Blueberries		••••••••••		
Cherries	••••••••••••••••••••			
Grapes		••••••••••••••••		
Melons		••••••••••		
Peaches		••••••••••		
Pears			••••••••••••••••••••••••	
Raspberries		••••••••••		
Strawberries	••••••••••			
Watermelon		••••••••••		
Artichokes	••••••••••		••••••••••	
Asparagus	••••••••••			
Basil		••••••••••		
Beets		••••••••••••••••••••		
Broccoli	••••••••••		••••••••••	••••••••••
Brussels sprouts			••••••••••	••••••••••
Cabbage			••••••••••	••••••••••
Carrots	••••••••••		••••••••••	••••••••••
Cauliflower	••••••••••		••••••••••	
Cilantro		••••••••••		
Corn		••••••••••••••••		
Cucumber		••••••••••••••••		

Peak Season •••	Spring	Summer	Fall	Winter
Dill		•••••••••		
Eggplant		•••••••••		
Fennel	•••••		••••••••••••••••••••••	
Garlic	••			
Green beans		••••••••••••••		
Kale	•••••••••	••••••••••••••••••		
Leeks	••••••••		•••••••••••••••••••••	
Lettuce	•••••••••••••••••••••••••••••			
Onions	••			
Parsley		•••••••••••••••••		
Peppers		•••••••••••••••••		
Potatoes	•••			
Pumpkin			••••••••••••••••••	
Radishes	•••••••••••••••••••••••••			
Scallions	•••			
Spinach	•••••••••••••••••••••••••••••••			
Summer squash		••••••••••		
Sweet potatoes			•••••••••••••••••••••••••••	
Thyme	••••••••••••••••••••••••••••••••••			
Tomatoes		••••••••••••••••		
Turnips	••••••••		••••••••••••••••••	
Winter squash			••••••••••••••••••••••••	

KITCHEN CONVERSIONS: QUICK REFERENCE

Ounces to Grams

½ ounce	=	14 g
1 ounce	=	28 g
2 ounces	=	57 g
3 ounces	=	85 g
4 ounces	=	113 g
5 ounces	=	142 g
6 ounces	=	170 g
7 ounces	=	198 g
8 ounces	=	226 g
12 ounces	=	340 g
16 ounces	=	454 g

Tablespoons to Ounces to Cups

1	=	½ ounce	=	1/16 cup
2	=	1 ounce	=	⅛ cup
4	=	2 ounces	=	¼ cup
8	=	4 ounces	=	½ cup
12	=	6 ounces	=	¾ cup
16	=	8 ounces	=	1 cup

Teaspoons to Milliliters

¼	=	1 ml
½	=	2½ ml
¾	=	4 ml
1	=	5 ml
2	=	9 ml
3	=	15 ml

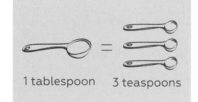

1 tablespoon = 3 teaspoons

Liquids

8 fluid ounces	=	1 cup	=	½ pint	=	¼ liter
16 fluid ounces	=	2 cups	=	1 pint	=	½ liter
32 fluid ounces	=	4 cups	=	1 quart	=	1 liter
128 fluid ounces	=	16 cups	=	1 gallon	=	3½ liters

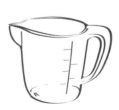

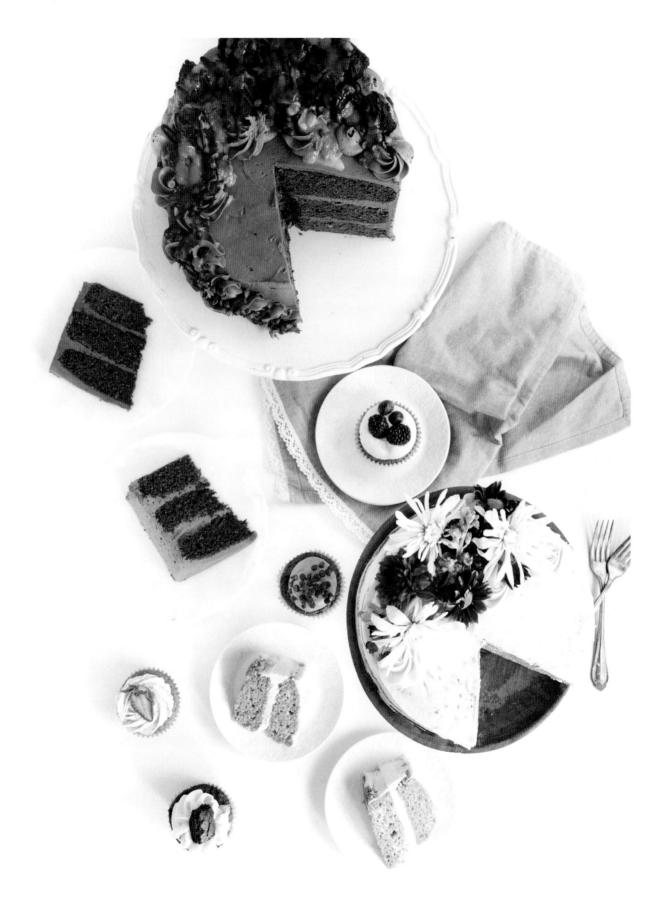

recite index

RISE & SHINE

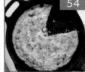

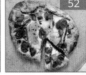

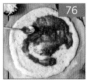

BREADS, CRUSTS & CRACKERS

LITTLE BITES

Lexi's Best Guacamole — 88

Garlic Roasted Cauliflower No-Bean Hummus — 90

Sweet Beet No-Bean Hummus — 90

The Best Shrimp Cocktail — 92

The Ultimate Meat & Cheese Board — 94

Bruschetta Bites with Balsamic Glaze — 96

Ahi Tuna Bites — 98

Bacon-Wrapped Scallops with Balsamic Glaze — 100

Prosciutto Flatbread with Grilled Peaches & Caramelized Onions — 102

Wings Three Ways — 104

Chicken Satay Skewers with Dipping Sauce — 106

Patatas Bravas Two Ways — 108

Buffalo Chicken Bites — 112

Mexican Meatballs — 114

Spinach Dip Stuffed Mushrooms — 116

DELICIOUS SOUPS & HEARTY SALADS

Classic Chili — 120

Slow Cooker Spicy Chicken Soup — 122

Cioppino Stew — 124

Greek-Inspired Lemon Chicken Soup — 126

Creamy Pumpkin Soup with Roasted Pumpkin Seeds — 128

Easy Chorizo & Kale Soup — 130

Curry Butternut Squash Soup — 132

Chicken Fajita Salads — 134

Sriracha Lime Grilled Chicken Salad — 136

Winter Harvest Salad — 138

Watermelon & Mint Salad — 140

Kale Caesar Salad — 142

Chopped Antipasto & Grilled Chicken Salad — 144

Chopped BBQ Chicken Cobb Salad — 146

Strawberry Date Salad with Poppy Seed Dressing — 148

Sesame Seared Ahi Tuna Salad with Ginger Dressing — 150

Chicken Salad Three Ways — 152

Shredded Brussels Sprouts Salad — 154

THE MAIN COURSE

 158
Classic Baked Chicken Nuggets

 160
Nanny's Potted Chicken

 162
The Best Grilled Chicken

 164
Chicken Enchiladas

 168
Jerk Chicken with Caribbean Rice & Mango Salsa

172
Chicken in Mushroom Sauce

  174
Creamy Chicken Bacon Spaghetti Squash Boats

 176
BBQ Chicken Pizza

  178
Creamy Cajun Chicken Pasta

180
Easy One-Pan Arroz con Pollo

182
Loaded Italian Meatballs

184
Thai Meatballs

  186
Maple-Crusted Salmon

 188
Thai BBQ Salmon

 190
Fish Tacos with Tropical Salsa, Spicy Slaw & Quick Pickled Cabbage

  192
Scallops Provençal

194
Chimichurri Shrimp

196
New England Lobster Rolls

  198
All-American Burgers

 200
Mediterranean Grilled Lamb Kebabs

 202
Slow Cooker Beef Barbacoa

  204
Balsamic Braised Short Ribs

206
Beef Tenderloin with Creamy Horseradish Sauce

208
Beef & Broccoli Stir-Fry

 210
Pasta with Meat Sauce

 212
Grilled Steak

 214
Pad Thai

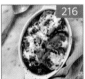 216
Baked Eggplant Parmesan

ON THE SIDE

220
Caramelized Butternut Squash

222
Kung Pao Cauliflower

224
Maple Bacon Brussels Sprouts

226
Sweet Potato Truffle Fries

228
Summer's Best Grainy Mustard Potato Salad

230
Burnt Broccoli

232
Asian Summer Slaw

234
Garlicky Blistered Green Beans

236
Pork Belly Brussels Sprouts with Lemon Dressing

238
Creamy Mashed Roots Two Ways

240
Better-Than-Takeout Chicken & Pineapple Fried Rice

242
Stir-Fried Veggies

244
Lemon Herb Spring Vegetable Risotto

246
Rice Four Ways

248
Pasta Alternatives

BEVERAGES

252
Classic Margarita

254
Classic Sangria

256
Apple Cider Sangria

258
Sunday Brunch Bloody Marys

260
Watermelon Mojito

262
Refreshing Lemonade

264
Cold-Brew Concentrate

266
Almond Milk

268
Creamy Hot Chocolate with Marshmallow Topping

270
Banana Coffee Smoothie

272
Island Blast Green Smoothie

274
Vanilla Chai Spice Smoothie

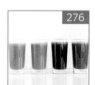
276
Juicing at Home Four Ways

SOMETHING SWEET

 280
S'mores
Pots de Crème

 282
Caribbean
Dessert Parfaits

 284
No-Bake Sea
Salt Cookie
Dough Cups

 286
Carrot Cake
Bars

 288
Vanilla
Buttercream
Frosting

 290
Pear Tartlets

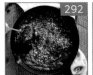 292
Flourless
Skillet Brownies

 294
Crunchy
Chocolate
Cookies

 296
Jam Crumb
Bars

 298
Chocolate Chunk
Cookie Bars

 300
Yellow
Birthday Cake

302
Chocolate
Birthday Cake

   304
Classic Vanilla
Cupcakes

306
Double
Chocolate
Cupcakes

308
Brown Butter
Apple Crisp

LEXI'S BASICS

 312
Easy Homemade
Mayo

 314
Everything Bagel
Spread

 316
Lexi's Pesto

 318
Ranch Dressing

 320
Creamy Caesar
Dressing

 322
Maple Balsamic
Dressing

 324
Ginger Dressing

 326
Lexi's Green
Dressing

 328
Sweet & Smoky
BBQ Sauce

 330
Quick & Easy
Jam

 332
Caramelized
Onions

 334
Balsamic Glaze

 336
Perfect
Blender Salsa

 338
All-Purpose
Marinara Sauce

 340
Alla Vodka
Sauce

 342
Ketchup

 344
Avocado Crema

 346
Homemade
Prepared
Horseradish

 348
Slow Cooker
Applesauce

 350
Ghee

 352
Chimichurri

354
Easy Chicken
and Vegetable
Broth

 358
Homemade
Chocolate
Hazelnut Spread

 360
All-Purpose
Caramel Sauce

general index